T0198196

Therapy in Neurology

Editor

JOSÉ BILLER

NEUROLOGIC CLINICS

www.neurologic.theclinics.com

Consulting Editor
RANDOLPH W. EVANS

February 2021 • Volume 39 • Number 1

ELSEVIER

1600 John F. Kennedy Boulevard • Suite 1800 • Philadelphia, Pennsylvania, 19103-2899

http://www.theclinics.com

NEUROLOGIC CLINICS Volume 39, Number 1
February 2021 ISSN 0733-8619, ISBN-13: 978-0-323-71281-1

Editor: Stacy Eastman
Developmental Editor: Donald Mumford

Neurologic Clinics (ISSN 0733-8619) is published quarterly by Elsevier Inc., 360 Park Avenue South, New York, NY 10010–1710. Months of issue are February, May, August, and November. Periodicals postage paid at New York, NY, and additional mailing offices. Subscription prices are $333.00 per year for US individuals, $881.00 per year for US institutions, $100.00 per year for US students, $408.00 per year for Canadian individuals, $938.00 per year for Canadian institutions, $461.00 per year for international individuals, $938.00 per year for international institutions, $210.00 for foreign students/residents, and $100.00 for Canadian students/residents. To receive student/resident rate, orders must be accompanied by name of affiliated institution, date of term, and the *signature* of program/residency coordinator on institution letterhead. Orders will be billed at individual rate until proof of status is received. Foreign air speed delivery is included in all *Clinics* subscription prices. All prices are subject to change without notice. **POSTMASTER:** Send address changes to *Neurologic Clinics*, Elsevier Health Sciences Division, Subscription Customer Service, 3251 Riverport Lane, Maryland Heights, MO 63043. **Customer Service: Telephone: 1-800-654-2452 (U.S. and Canada); 314-447-8871 (outside U.S. and Canada). Fax: 314-447-8029. E-mail: journalscustomerservice-usa@elsevier.com (for print support); journalsonlinesupport-usa@elsevier.com (for online support).**

Reprints. For copies of 100 or more of articles in this publication, please contact the Commercial Reprints Department, Elsevier Inc., 360 Park Avenue South, New York, New York, 10010-1710; Tel.: +1-212-633-3874; Fax: +1-212-633-3820, and E-mail: reprints@elsevier.com.

Neurologic Clinics is also published in Spanish by Nueva Editorial Interamericana S.A., Mexico City, Mexico.

Neurologic Clinics is covered in *Current Contents/Clinical Medicine, MEDLINE/PubMed (Index Medicus), EMBASE/Excerpta Medica, and PsycINFO, and ISI/BIOMED.*

Printed in the United States of America.

Contributors

CONSULTING EDITOR

RANDOLPH W. EVANS, MD
Clinical Professor, Department of Neurology, Baylor College of Medicine, Houston, Texas, USA

EDITOR

JOSÉ BILLER, MD, FACP, FAAN, FAHA, FANA
Professor and Chair, Department of Neurology, Loyola University Chicago, Stritch School of Medicine, Maywood, Illinois, USA

AUTHORS

ALLEN J. AKSAMIT Jr, MD
Professor, Department of Neurology, Mayo Clinic College of Medicine, Mayo Clinic, Rochester, Minnesota, USA

CYNTHIA BODKIN, MD
Associate Professor, Clinical Neurology, Associate Professor, Physical Medical Rehabilitation, Indiana University School of Medicine, Indiana University Health, Indianapolis, Indiana, USA

BENJAMIN H. BRINKMANN, PhD
Mayo Clinic, Rochester, Minnesota, USA

MATTHEW R. BURNS, MD, PhD
Clinical Fellow, The Fixel Institute for Neurological Diseases, Department of Neurology, The University of Florida, Gainesville, Florida, USA

EDOARDO CARONNA, MD
Department of Medicine, Headache and Neurological Pain Research Group, Vall d'Hebron Research Institute, Universitat Autònoma de Barcelona, Barcelona, Spain

GREGORY D. CASCINO, MD, FAAN, FANA, FACNS, FAES
Mayo Clinic, Rochester, Minnesota, USA

SHANNON Y. CHIU, MD
Assistant Professor, The Fixel Institute for Neurological Diseases, Department of Neurology, The University of Florida, Gainesville, Florida, USA

CAROLYN GOLDSCHMIDT, DO
Mellen Center U-10, Cleveland Clinic, Cleveland, Ohio, USA

JOAQUIN B. GONZALEZ, MD
Interventional Cardiology, Department of Cardiology, Advocate Illinois Masonic Medical Center, Chicago, Illinois, USA

ROBERT C. GRIGGS, MD
Professor of Neurology, Medicine, Pediatrics, Pathology & Laboratory Medicine, Center for Health + Technology, University of Rochester Medical Center, Rochester, New York, USA

AKI KAWASAKI, MD, PhD
Associate Professor of Biology and Medicine, University of Lausanne, Hôpital Ophtalmique Jules Gonin, Fondation Asile des Aveugles, Lausanne, Switzerland

ILYA KISTER, MD
Associate Professor, Department of Neurology, Comprehensive MS Center, NYU Grossman School of Medicine, New York, New York, USA

RIMAS V. LUKAS, MD
Department of Neurology, Northwestern University; Lou & Jean Malnati Brain Tumor Institute of the Robert H. Lurie Comprehensive Cancer Center, Chicago, Illinois, USA

IRENE A. MALATY, MD
Associate Professor, The Fixel Institute for Neurological Diseases, Department of Neurology, The University of Florida, Gainesville, Florida, USA

MARISA P. McGINLEY, DO, MSc
Mellen Center U-10, Cleveland Clinic, Cleveland, Ohio, USA

SOTIRIS G. MITROPANOPOULOS, MD
Assistant Professor, Department of Neurology and Epilepsy, The University of Florida, Gainesville, Florida, USA

ROBERT M. PASCUZZI, MD
Professor, Chair, Neurology Department, Indiana University School of Medicine, Indiana University Health, Indianapolis, Indiana, USA

ANUP D. PATEL, MD
Section Chief, Neurology, Nationwide Children's Hospital, Associate Professor of Clinical Pediatrics and Neurology, The Ohio State University College of Medicine, Columbus, Ohio, USA

BHAVANA PATEL, DO
Assistant Professor, The Fixel Institute for Neurological Diseases, Department of Neurology, The University of Florida, Gainesville, Florida, USA

KATHERINE B. PETERS, MD, PhD
Department of Neurology, Duke University School of Medicine, Durham, North Carolina, USA

VIKRAM C. PRABHU, MD
Department of Neurological Surgery, Loyola University Stritch School of Medicine, Maywood, Illinois, USA

ADOLFO RAMIREZ-ZAMORA, MD
Associate Professor, The Fixel Institute for Neurological Diseases, Department of Neurology, The University of Florida, Gainesville, Florida, USA

BHASKAR ROY, MBBS, MMST
Department of Neurology, Yale School of Medicine, New Haven, Connecticut, USA

MICHAEL J. SCHNECK, MD
Professor, Departments of Neurology and Neurosurgery, Vice Chairman, Department of Neurology, Loyola University Chicago, Stritch School of Medicine, Maywood, Illinois, USA

EUGENE R. SCHNITZLER, MD
Professor, Departments of Neurology and Pediatrics, Loyola University Chicago, Stritch School of Medicine, Director Division of Pediatric Neurology, Loyola University Medical Center, Maywood, Illinois, USA

AMAAL J. STARLING, MD, FAHS, FAAN
Associate Professor, Department of Neurology, Mayo Clinic, Scottsdale, Arizona, USA

FERNANDO D. TESTAI, MD, PhD, FAHA
Stroke Section, Department of Neurology and Rehabilitation, University of Illinois College of Medicine at Chicago, Chicago, Illinois, USA

JIGISHA P. THAKKAR, MD
Department of Neurology, Division of Neuro-oncology, Loyola University Chicago, Stritch School of Medicine, Maywood, Illinois, USA

MATTHEW J. THURTELL, MD
Associate Professor of Ophthalmology and Neurology, Departments of Ophthalmology and Visual Sciences, and Neurology, University of Iowa, Iowa City, Iowa, USA

MATTHEW TREMBLAY, MD, PhD
Neurologist, MS Comprehensive Care Center, RWJ Barnabas Health, Livingston, New Jersey, USA

ASYA IZRAELIT WALLACH, MD
Neurologist, Alfiero and Lucia Palestroni MS Comprehensive Care Center, Holy Name Medical Center, Teaneck, New Jersey, USA

JOSHUA K. WONG, MD
Clinical Fellow, The Fixel Institute for Neurological Diseases, Department of Neurology, The University of Florida, Gainesville, Florida, USA

LAWRENCE A. ZEIDMAN, MD, FAAN
Associate Professor of Neurology and Bioethics, Director, Neuromuscular-EMG Division, Department of Neurology, Loyola University Chicago, Loyola University Medical Center, Stritch School of Medicine, Maywood, Illinois, USA

Contents

The discovery of calcitonin gene-related peptide (CGRP) and its role in migraine has promoted a new era in migraine treatment: CGRP antagonism. Two classes of medications are currently available: small molecules targeting the CGRP receptor and monoclonal antibodies targeting the CGRP receptor or CGRP ligand. The revolution of these medications is represented by blurring the borders between acute and preventive treatments, episodic and chronic migraine, naïve and refractory patients and even between migraine and other headache disorders.

Multiple sclerosis is a relatively common, immune-mediated neurologic disease of the central nervous system that can cause significant disability and lead to reduced quality of life. There are several currently approved disease-modifying therapies, and more in the pipeline being developed and tested. As the field learns more about the pathophysiology and natural course of the disease, the treatment approaches are also being investigated. This article reviews data on available treatments along with a discussion of future treatment targets under investigation.

Neuromyelitis optica spectrum disorder (NMOSD) is a rare, relapsing-remitting neuroinflammatory disorder of the central nervous system. Advances in the understanding of NMOSD pathogenesis and identification of the NMO-specific pathogenic anti-AQP4 autoantibody have led to the development of highly effective disease-modifying strategies. Five placebo-controlled, randomized trials for NMOSD have been successfully completed as of 2020. These trials support the efficacy of rituximab and tocilizumab and led to the FDA approval of eculizumab, satralizumab and inebilizumab for NMOSD. Our review provides an update on these evidence-based disease-modifying therapies and discussed the treatment of acute relapses in NMOSD.

Up to a third of strokes are cryptogenic. The prevalence of patent foramen ovale (PFO) in patients with cryptogenic stroke is higher than in individuals with stroke of known origin. It has been proposed that some cryptogenic strokes can be caused by paradoxic embolism across a PFO. The treatment of PFO includes medical treatment with antithrombotic agents and percutaneous PFO closure. There is limited evidence to support PFO closure in unselected cases of cryptogenic stroke. However, large randomized clinical trials confirmed the superiority of transcatheter PFO closure compared with medical treatment in young patients with cryptogenic stroke.

Deep brain stimulation is a safe and effective therapy for the management of a variety of neurologic conditions with Food and Drug Administration or humanitarian exception approval for Parkinson disease, dystonia, tremor, and obsessive-compulsive disorder. Advances in neurophysiology, neuroimaging, and technology have driven increasing interest in the potential benefits of neurostimulation in other neuropsychiatric conditions including dementia, depression, pain, Tourette syndrome, and epilepsy, among others. New anatomic or combined targets are being investigated in these conditions to improve symptoms refractory to medications or standard stimulation.

Increased understanding of disease pathophysiology and advances in gene therapies and drug technologies are revolutionizing treatment of muscular dystrophies and motor neuron disorders (MNDs). New drugs have been approved for Duchenne muscular dystrophy, spinal muscular atrophy, and amyotrophic lateral sclerosis. For other diseases, new targets have been identified, and new therapies are in clinical trials. The impact of such therapies will be fully understood only in the next decades. Cost burden and accessibility are major challenges in the wide application of new drugs. This article reviews advances in gene therapies, newly approved drugs, and therapeutic promises in muscular dystrophies and MNDs.

Small fiber neuropathy (SFN) is a prevalent neurologic syndrome. Testing methods have emerged in recent years to better diagnose it, including autonomic tests and skin punch biopsy. SFN can present in a non–length-dependent fashion and can be mistaken for syndromes such as fibromyalgia and complex regional pain syndrome. SFN is caused by a variety of metabolic, infectious, genetic, and inflammatory diseases. Recently treatments have emerged for TTR amyloid neuropathy and Fabry disease, and novel biomarkers have been found both in genetic and inflammatory SFN syndromes. Ongoing trials attempt to establish the efficacy of intravenous immunoglobulin in inflammatory SFN syndromes.

NEUROLOGIC CLINICS

FORTHCOMING ISSUES

May 2021
Neurologic Emergencies
Joseph D. Burns and Anna M. Cervantes-Arslanian, *Editors*

August 2021
Pediatric Neurology
Gary D. Clark and James J. Riviello, *Editors*

November 2021
Electromyography
Devon I. Rubin, *Editor*

RECENT ISSUES

November 2020
Applied Neurotoxicology
Michael R. Dobbs and Mam I. Ibraheem, *Editors*

August 2020
Case Studies in Neuromuscular Disorders
Aziz Shaibani, *Editor*

May 2020
Treatment of Movement Disorders
Joseph Jankovic, *Editor*

RELATED SERIES

Neurosurgery Clinics
https://www.neurosurgery.theclinics.com/
Neuroimaging Clinics
www.neuroimaging.theclinics.com
Psychiatric Clinics
https://www.psych.theclinics.com/
Child and Adolescent Psychiatric Clinics
https://www.childpsych.theclinics.com/

Preface

Therapy in Neurology

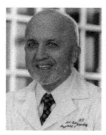

José Biller, MD, FACP, FAAN, FAHA, FANA
Editor

A decade ago, I had the privilege of serving as guest editor for an issue of the *Neurologic Clinics* dedicated to Advances in Neurologic Therapy. Who would have anticipated the proliferation of the newer, ongoing, and more selective therapeutic interventions that the current neurology practitioner has at his or her disposition? I humbly accepted serving once again as a guest editor with the specific intent of highlighting some of these state-of-the-art contemporary therapeutic advances, accepting the realization that therapeutic suggestions, although up-to-date as of this writing, most likely were going to be superseded by newer advances in research.

This issue begins with an in-depth update of calcitonin gene–related peptide antagonists in the abortive or preventive treatment of migraines. This is followed by comprehensive reviews of the ever-expanding advances in the treatment of multiple sclerosis, and neuromyelitis optica spectrum disorder, a distinct central nervous system inflammatory demyelinating disorder characterized by bilateral or recurrent optic neuritis with or without longitudinally extensive spinal cord lesions. The next article addresses current advances and remaining controversies in patent foramen ovale closure among patients who had a cryptogenic stroke, including a scholarly and balanced discussion of recent randomized clinical trials in patients younger than 60 years. Current and emergent management aspects in neuromodulation and neurostimulation in Parkinson disease, essential tremor, dystonia, Tourette syndrome, tardive dyskinesia, chorea, epilepsy, and pain are elegantly and concisely covered in the next article. The 3 subsequent articles deal with selective neuromuscular disorders and scholarly advances in the treatment of muscular dystrophies and motor neuron disorders, progress in the management of small-fiber neuropathy, and a meticulous update in the management of myasthenia gravis and the Lambert-Eaton myasthenic syndrome. Separate consideration is given to the current management of idiopathic intracranial hypertension (pseudotumor cerebri). A rigorous review of what is new in neurooncology is extensively analyzed by a multidisciplinary group of colleagues. As part of the

Neurol Clin 39 (2021) xiii–xiv
https://doi.org/10.1016/j.ncl.2020.09.016
0733-8619/21/© 2020 Published by Elsevier Inc.

neurologic.theclinics.com

therapeutic advances in epilepsy, surgical management of drug-resistant focal epilepsy in the adult patient is painstakingly discussed in another scholarly overview article. A subsequent article provides a comprehensive approach to the treatment of herpetic and nonherpetic viral encephalitides, including progressive multifocal leukoencephalopathy. An update on the expanding indications for botulinum toxin use in neurology, and the use of cannabinoids in neurologic illnesses, including certain forms of epilepsy, such as Lennox-Gastaut and Dravet syndrome, multiple sclerosis, movement disorders, Tourette syndrome, headaches, and migraine, are presented in the ensuing 2 articles. The section concludes with a provocative discussion about the transition of neurologic patients from pediatric to adult health care providers.

I am greatly indebted to the many contributors for their scholarly material who made this issue possible. I greatly acknowledge the editorial assistance provided by Donald Mumford, Senior Developmental Editor at Elsevier. A special thanks to Linda Turner, for her support during this project.

José Biller, MD, FACP, FAAN, FAHA, FANA
Department of Neurology
Loyola University Chicago
Stritch School of Medicine
2160 S. First Avenue
Building 105, Room 2700
Maywood, IL 60153, USA

E-mail address:
jbiller@lumc.edu

Update on Calcitonin Gene-Related Peptide Antagonism in the Treatment of Migraine

Edoardo Caronna, MD[a], Amaal J. Starling, MD[b],*

KEYWORDS

- Migraine • Treatment • CGRP • Gepants • Monoclonal antibodies • Efficacy
- Safety

KEY POINTS

- Medications that antagonize calcitonin gene-related peptide (CGRP) activity represent the first treatment specifically designed for migraine as both therapy acute and preventive therapy.
- Gepants are small molecules that antagonize the CGRP receptor, are approved for migraine acute treatment (ubrogepant and rimegepant), and currently are being studied for migraine prevention (rimegepant and atogepant).
- Monoclonal antibodies targeting the CGRP receptor (erenumab) or CGRP ligand (galcanezumab, fremanezumab, and eptinezumab) all have been approved for migraine prevention in the United States.
- Clinical trials have demonstrated similar efficacy of anti-CGRP therapy as well as good safety profile; however, real-world data from clinical practice still are needed to better evaluate this new class of medication with respect to efficacy and safety.

INTRODUCTION

Migraine is a prevalent condition, affecting 10% of the overall population,[1] causing severe disability, and is ranked as second among the most disabling diseases according to the Global Burden of Disease study.[2] Since the discovery of the calcitonin gene-related peptide (CGRP) and its prominent role in migraine,[3] several medications that antagonize the CGRP activity have been approved, representing the first preventive treatment to be designed specifically for migraine. This explains the enthusiasm

a Department of Medicine, Headache and Neurological Pain Research Group, Vall d'Hebron Research Institute, Universitat Autònoma de Barcelona, Ps. Vall d'Hebron 119-129, Barcelona 08035, Spain; b Department of Neurology, Mayo Clinic, 13400 East Shea Boulevard, Scottsdale, AZ 85259, USA
* Corresponding author.
E-mail address: starling.amaal@mayo.edu
Twitter: @CaronnaEdoardo (E.C.); @AmaalStarlingMD (A.J.S.)

Neurol Clin 39 (2021) 1–19
https://doi.org/10.1016/j.ncl.2020.09.001
0733-8619/21/© 2020 Elsevier Inc. All rights reserved.

with which this new class has been welcomed and it represents not only a progress in migraine treatment but also an opportunity to better understand aspects of migraine pathophysiology.

This review aims to give an update on CGRP antagonism in migraine treatment, underlying how classic dichotomies that used to be relevant in choosing the right treatment no longer may be relevant. With this new class of medications, borders between migraine and other headache types, acute and preventive treatments, EM and CM, and naïve and refractory patients are becoming less defined.

CALCITONIN GENE-RELATED PEPTIDE MECHANISM

CGRP is a 37 amino acid peptide expressed in several tissues in the human body, although it has been specifically defined as a neuropeptide with a complex role in brain functioning.[4] Concerning migraine, the role of CGRP has been demonstrated by the finding of elevated levels during migraine attacks[3] as well as interictal phases with higher levels in CM.[5]

This role of CGRP in migraine pathophysiology is believed to be exerted mainly peripherally in the trigeminovascular system, although the presence of CGRP in central nervous system areas involved in migraine pathophysiology[6,7] highlights that a central modulation mediated by CGRP in migraine is possible too.

ANTI–CALCITONIN GENE-RELATED PEPTIDE MECHANISMS

Two classes of medications have been developed for CGRP antagonism in migraine: the gepants and the anti-CGRP monoclonal antibodies (mAbs). **Table 1** compares the main characteristics for both gepants and mAbs. These drugs have been designed as acute or preventive treatments.

Gepants

Gepants are small molecules that specifically inhibit the CGRP receptor. Olcegepant[8] was the first anti-CGRP molecule to be designed that showed efficacy in reducing headache frequency; however, its low bioavailability and intravenous administration prevented from its full development. Telcagepant was the first oral compound to be investigated in phase 2 and phase 3 studies[9,10] and showed efficacy compared with placebo; however, due to hepatotoxicity, its development ended. MK-3207 also was discontinued due to possible hepatotoxicity.[11] After the failure of these compounds, a second generation of gepants has been developed. Ubrogepant

Table 1
Comparison between small molecules and monoclonal antibodies

Characteristics	Small Molecules	Monoclonal Antibodies
Target specificity	Low	High
Clearance	Liver, kidney	Reticuloendothelial system
Half-life	Minutes to hours	3–7 wk
Size	0.5–0.6 kDa	143–146 kDa
Ability to cross blood-brain barrier	Possible (controversial)	No
Administration	Oral	Parenteral
Immunogenicity	No	Yes

successfully underwent phase 2[12] and phase 3 studies (ACHIEVE II[13] and ACHIEVE I[14]), leading to approval by the US Food and Drug administration (FDA) on December 2019 for the acute treatment of migraine. After positive results in phase 2 and phase 3 studies,[15–17] another small molecule, rimegepant, was approved by the FDA on February 2020. At the time of this article, it still is under investigation as a preventive treatment.[18] For atogepant, first results of clinical trials in migraine prevention have been published.[19] A new intranasal gepant, vazegepant, is being studied as an acute treatment of migraine with results available.[20] **Table 2** reviews the different characteristics of each gepant, and **Table 3** presents phase 2 and phase 3 studies for the currently investigated gepants.

Monoclonal Antibodies

The risk for hepatotoxicity observed for the first generation of gepants motivated the design of mAbs. mAbs are large synthetized IgG molecules with high stability, resulting in long half-lives, specificity, and affinity for their target.

The first mAb to be developed, erenumab,[21] targets the CGRP receptor, whereas the other 3, galcanezumab,[22] fremanezumab,[23] and eptinezumab,[24] target the CGRP ligand. All 4 mAbs have been studied for prevention in both episodic migraine (EM) and chronic migraine (CM). Erenumab, fremanezumab, and galcanezumab have been approved for EM and EM by both FDA and the European Medicines Agency (EMA), whereas eptinezumab only by the FDA.

Table 2 reviews the different characteristics of each mAb, and **Table 4** presents phase 2 and phase 3 studies for each mAb.

EFFICACY AND SAFETY

In clinical studies, all the current anti-CGRP treatments have demonstrated efficacy by achieving their primary endpoints with limited adverse events.

Gepants

Efficacy for acute treatment

Reflecting the real-world setting, where patients experience not only pain as a bothersome symptom but also photophobia, phonophobia, and nausea/vomiting, clinical trials have started using not only freedom from pain at 2 hours but also freedom from most bothersome symptoms after 2 hours as coprimary endpoints.[25] Ubrogepant and rimegepant have achieved these coprimary endpoints in phase 2 and 3 trials, as shown in **Table 3**.

Efficacy for prevention

Results for atogepant as a preventive for EM have been partially published.[19] The primary endpoint, change in mean monthly migraine days in the 12-week study period, has been achieved by all studies (see **Table 3**). Results from the rimegepant trial[18] in migraine prevention are not yet available.

Adverse events and special medical concerns

Clinical trials have observed a low frequency of AEs. Nausea was the most common adverse events for both rimegepant[17] and ubrogepant[13] in approximately 2% of the cases. Urinary tract infections were observed in the rimegepant phase 3 trial (1.5% in the rimegepant group and 1.1% in the placebo group). Somnolence and dry mouth were AEs observed for ubrogepant in ACHIEVE I.[14]

No serious adverse events were reported in clinical trials.

Table 2
Main characteristics for currently investigated gepants and monoclonal antibodies

	Erenumab	Galcanezumab	Fremanezumab	Eptinezumab	Ubrogepant	Rimegepant	Atogepant	Vazegepant
Design	Prevention (EM, CM)	Prevention (EM, CM, eCH, cCH)	Prevention (EM, CM, eCH, cCH)	Prevention (EM, CM)	Acute (migraine)	Acute and prevention (migraine)	Prevention (EM)	Acute (migraine)
Target	CGRP receptor	CGRP ligand	CGRP ligand	CGRP ligand	CGRP receptor	CGRP receptor	CGRP receptor	CGRP receptor
Administration	Monthly SC	Monthly SC	Monthly or quarterly SC	Quarterly IV	Oral	Oral	Oral	Intranasal
IgG type	IgG2, human	IgG4, humanized	IgG2a, humanized	IgG1, humanized	N/A	N/A	N/A	N/A
Approval	FDA/EMA	FDA/EMA for EM, CM; FDA for eCH	FDA/EMA for EM and CM	FDA	FDA	FDA (acute)	N/A	N/A
Doses approved	70 mg or 140 mg	Migraine: 120 mg (240 mg loading dose) eCH: 300 mg	225 mg monthly or 675 mg quarterly	100 mg or 300 mg	50 mg or 100 mg	75 mg	N/A	N/A

Abbreviations: cCH, chronic cluster headache; eCH, episodic cluster headache; IV, intravenous; SC, subcutaneous injection.

Table 3
Phase 2 and phase 3 studies for currently investigated gepants in migraine treatment

Drug	Study	Doses	Primary Endpoints	Statistically Significant Results	Reference
Ubrogepant	Phase 2b (dose-ranging) Acute	1 mg 10 mg 25 mg 50 mg 100 mg Placebo	Pain freedom and headache response at 2 h	Pain freedom (100 mg: 25.5% vs placebo: 8.9%) Headache response[a]	Voss et al,[12] 2016
	Phase 3 Acute ACHIEVE I	100 mg 50 mg Placebo	Coprimary: pain freedom and absence of MBS at 2 h	Pain freedom: 100 mg (21.2%), 50 mg (19.2%), Placebo (11.8%) MBS: 100 mg (37.7%), 50 mg (38.6%), placebo (27.8%)	Dodick et al,[14] 2019
	Phase 3 Acute ACHIEVE II	50 mg 25 mg Placebo	Coprimary: pain freedom and absence of MBS at 2 h	Pain freedom (absolute difference vs placebo): 50 mg (7.5%); 25 mg (6.4%) MBS (absolute difference vs placebo): 50 mg (11.5%); 25 mg (6.7%)[a]	Lipton et al,[13] 2019
	Phase 3 Acute UBR-MD-04 (OLE of ACHIEVE I–II)	50 mg 100 mg Usual care arm (to treat up to 8 migraine attacks a month)	Safety and tolerability (over 56 wk)	No severe AEs No hepatotoxicity	Ailani et al,[63] 2020
	Phase 2 Acute 31,110-105-002	Intermittent 100 mg alternating with placebo (for 2 d each) over an 8-wk period in healthy volunteers	Safety	No hepatotoxicity. Most common AEs included headache, oropharyngeal pain, and nasopharyngitis (>5%)	[71]

(continued on next page)

Table 3
(continued)

Drug	Study	Doses	Primary Endpoints	Statistically Significant Results	Reference
Rimegepant	Phase 2 (dose-ranging) Acute	10 mg 25 mg 75 mg 150 mg 300 mg 600 mg 100 mg of sumatriptan Placebo	Pain freedom at 2 h	10 mg[a] 25 mg[a] 75 mg (31.4%) 150 mg (32.9%) 300 mg (29.7%) 600 mg (24.4%) Sumatriptan (35.0%) Placebo (15.3%)	Marcus et al,[15] 2014
	Phase 3 Acute	75 mg Placebo	Coprimary: pain freedom and absence of MBS at 2 h	Pain freedom: 19.6% vs 12.0%; MBS: 37.6% vs 25.2%	Lipton et al,[17] 2019
	Phase 3 Acute	75 mg (orally disintegrating tablet) Placebo	Coprimary: pain freedom and absence of MBS at 2 h	Pain freedom: 21% vs 11%; MBS: 35% vs 27%	Croop et al,[16] 2019
	Phase 2/3 Preventive (EM-CM until 18 headache d/mo)	75 mg Placebo	Mean change in MMD (wk 9–12)	N/A	[18]
Atogepant	Phase 2 b/3 Prevention (EM)	10 mg QD 30 mg QD 30 mg BID 60 mg QD 60 mg BID Placebo	Mean change in MMD (wk 1–12)	10 mg QD (−4.0 d) 30 mg QD (−3.8 d) 30 mg BID (−4.2 d) 60 mg QD (−3.5 d) 60 mg BID (−4.1 d) Placebo (−2.8 d)	Goadsby et al,[19] 2019
Vazegepant	Phase 2/3 Acute	5mg 10 mg 20 mg Placebo (intranasal)	Pain freedom at 2 h	Pain freedom: 5 mg (19.6%)[a], 10 mg (22.5%), 20 mg (23.1%), placebo (15.5%) MBS: 5 mg (39.0%)[a], 10 mg (41.9%), 20 mg (42.5%), placebo (33.7%)	[20]

Abbreviations: AE, adverse event; BID, twice per day; MBS, most bothersome symptom reported by participants; MMD, monthly migraine days; OLE, open-label extension; QD, daily.

[a] Not statistically significant.

Table 4
Phase 2 and phase 3 studies for monoclonal antibodies for migraine prevention

Drug	Study	Doses	Primary Endpoint(s)	Statistically Significant Results	Reference
Erenumab	Phase 2, EM (dose-ranging)	7 mg 21 mg 70 mg Placebo (monthly SC)	Change in MMD (wk 9–12)	7 mg (−2.2 d)[a] 21 mg (−2.4 d)[a] 70 mg (−3.4 d) Placebo (−2.3 d)	Sun et al,[21] 2016
	Phase 3, EM ARISE	70 mg Placebo (monthly SC)	Change in MMD (wk 9–12)	70 mg (−2.9 d) Placebo (−1.8 d)	Dodick et al,[31] 2018
	Phase 3, EM STRIVE	70 mg 140 mg Placebo (monthly SC)	Change in MMD (wk 13–24)	70 mg (−3.2 d) 140 mg (−3.7 d) Placebo (−1.8 d)	Goadsby et al,[32] 2017
	Phase 2, CM	70 mg 140 mg Placebo (monthly SC)	Change in MMD (wk 9–12)	70 mg (−6.6 d) 140 mg (−6.6 d) PBO (−4.2 d)	Tepper et al,[36] 2017
	Phase 2 EM (OLE)	Initially received 70 mg A protocol amendment increased the dosage to 140 mg (monthly SC)	Safety and tolerability (interim analysis of 3-plus year results from a 5-y OLE)	No severe AEs No increase in cardiovascular risk	Ashina et al,[53] 2019
	Phase 2 CM (OLE)	Initially received 70 mg A protocol amendment increased the dosage to 140 mg (monthly SC)	Safety and tolerability (over 52 wk)	No severe AEs. (not fully published)	Tepper et al,[55] 2020
	Phase 3b, EM with 2–4 unsuccessful preventive treatments LIBERTY	140 mg Placebo (monthly SC)	50% or greater reduction in the mean MMD (wk 9–12)	Erenumab was superior to placebo (odds ratio 2.7)	Reuter et al,[45] 2018

(continued on next page)

Table 4
(continued)

Drug	Study	Doses	Primary Endpoint(s)	Statistically Significant Results	Reference
Galcanezumab	Phase 2, EM	150 mg Placebo (every 2 wk SC)	Change in MMD (wk 9–12)	150 mg (−4.2 d) Placebo (−3.0 d)	Dodick et al,[22] 2014
	Phase 2, EM (dose-ranging)	5mg 50 mg 120 mg 300 mg Placebo (monthly SC)	Change in MMD (wk 9–12)	120 mg was superior than placebo (99.6% posterior probability −4.8 vs 95% superiority threshold [bayesian analysis] −3.7 d)	Skljarevski et al,[72] 2018
	Phase 3, EM EVOLVE-1	120 mg 240 mg Placebo (monthly SC)	Mean change in MMD (mo 1–6)	120 mg (−4.7 d) 240 mg (−4.5 d) Placebo (−2.8 d)	Stauffer et al,[73] 2018
	Phase 3, EM EVOLVE-2	120 mg 240 mg Placebo (monthly SC)	Mean change in MMD (mo 1–6)	120 mg (−4.3 d) 240 mg (−4.2 d) Placebo (−2.3 d)	Skljarevski et al,[34] 2018
	Phase 3, CM REGAIN	120 mg (with a 240-mg loading dose) 240 mg Placebo (monthly SC)	Mean change in MMD (mo 1–3)	120 mg (−4.8 d) 240 mg (−4.6 d) Placebo (−2.7 d)	Detke et al,[38] 2018
	Phase 3, EM and CM (open label)	120 mg (with a 240-mg loading dose) 240 mg (monthly SC)	Safety and tolerability (over 1 y)	Safety was consistent with phase 2 and phase 3 studies	Camporeale et al,[54] 2018
	Phase 3, EM and CM with unsuccessful preventive treatments CONQUER	Galcanezumab Placebo (monthly SC)	Mean change in MMD (mo 1–3)	Not available	[74]

Drug	Phase	Dosing	Outcome	Results	Reference
Fremanezumab	Phase 2b, HFEM	225 mg 675 mg (monthly SC)	Change in MMD (wk 9–12)	225 mg (−6.27 d) 675 (−6.09 d) Placebo (−3.46 d)	Bigal et al,[23] 2015
	Phase 2b, CM	675/225/225 900/900/900 PBO/PBO/PBO (3 cycles: monthly SC)	Change in number of headache hours of any severity (wk 9–12)	675/225/225 (−59.8 h) 900/900/900 (−67.5 h) PBO/PBO/PBO (−37.1 h)	Bigal et al,[75] 2015
	Phase 3, EM HALO	225 mg/225/225 675 mg/ PBO/PBO PBO/PBO/PBO (3 cycles: monthly SC)	Mean change in MMD (wk 1–12)	225/225/225 (−4.2 d) 675/PBO/PBO (−4.0 d) PBO/PBO/PBO (−2.7 d)	Dodick et al,[33] 2018
	Phase 3, CM HALO-2	675 mg/PBO/PBO 675 mg/ 225/225 PBO/PBO (3 cycles: monthly SC)	Mean change in number of moderate-severe headache days (wk 1–12)	675/225/225 (−4.6 d) 675/PBO/PBO (−4.3 d) PBO/PBO/PBO (−2.5 d)	Silberstein et al,[37] 2017
	Phase 3b, EM and CM with 2–4 unsuccessful preventive treatments FOCUS	675 mg/PBO/PBO 675 mg/ 225/225 (CM) or 225 mg/ 225/225 (EM) PBO/PBO/PBO (3 cycles: monthly SC)	Mean change in MMD (wk 1–12)	675 mg/PBO/PBO (LSM difference vs placebo −3.1); 675 mg/225/225 or 225/225/ 225 (LSM difference vs placebo −3.5)	Ferrari et al,[46] 2019
Eptinezumab	Phase 2, EM	1000 mg Placebo (single IV)	Change in MMD (wk 5–8)	1000 mg (−5.6 d) Placebo (−4.6 d)	Dodick et al,[24] 2014
	Phase 3, EM PROMISE-1	30 mg 100 mg 300 mg Placebo (up to 4 IV administration)	Mean change in MMD (wk 1–12)	30 mg (−4.0 d)	Ashina et al,[35] 2020
	Phase 2b, CM	10 mg 30 mg 100 mg 300 mg Placebo (single IV)	≥75% reduction in MMD (wk 1–12)	10 mg, 26.8%[a] 30 mg, 28.2%[a] 100 mg, 31.4%[a] 300 mg, 33.3% Placebo, 20.7%	Dodick et al,[76] 2019
	Phase 3, CM PROMISE-2	100 mg 300 mg Placebo (IV administration on d 0 and wk 12)	Mean change in MMD (wk 1–12)	100 mg (−7.7 d) 300 mg (−8.2 d) Placebo (−5.6 d)	Lipton et al,[39] 2020

Abbreviations: AE, adverse event; HFEM, high-frequency episodic migraine; IV, intravenous; LSM, least-squares mean; MMD, monthly migraine days; OLE, open-label extension; PBO, placebo; SC, subcutaneous injection.
[a] Not statistically significant.

Although long-term safety in a real-world setting is still lacking, 3 considerations could be made about gepants according to clinical trials

Hepatotoxicity Considering the fact that telcagepant[26] showed liver toxicity, liver function has been monitored in clinical trials. Trials for the acute use of rimegepant[17] and ubrogepant[13,14] have not observed significant increase in liver enzymes more than 3 times the upper limit of the normal range, whereas in atogepant preventive trial,[19] 10 patients reported this AE, although they were balanced across study groups.

Risk of addiction, rebound, and medication overuse headache Medication overuse headache (MOH), as defined by the International Headache Society,[27,28] currently has been described with other acute medications. Considering that CGRP antagonism is being investigated for migraine prevention, it is logical to hypothesize that it is unlikely to cause MOH.

Risk of vasoconstriction Considering the vasodilating function of CGRP, the risk of vasoconstriction and its possible implication in people with cardiovascular disease have been studied. Telcagepant has been tested, however, in patients with coronary artery disease and stable angina,[28,29] not detecting increased risk of vasoconstriction. More recently, the effect of ubrogepant and atogepant has been investigated on human isolated coronary, cerebral, and middle meningeal arteries.[30] In intracranial arteries, both blockers antagonized the CGRP-induced relaxations more potently compared with the inhibition observed in distal human coronary arteries; however, in the distal human coronary arteries, both gepants are devoid of relevant vasoconstrictive properties.

These findings seem to support the use of anti-CGRP small molecules as a therapeutic option for migraine attacks in patients with cardiovascular contraindications for the use of triptans.

Monoclonal Antibodies

Efficacy
Reduction in migraine days Changes in mean migraine days have been assessed as a primary endpoint by the majority of studies at 9 weeks to 12 weeks (3-month studies). All the reported phase 3 studies in EM observed a statistically significant change in mean migraine days for the doses tested compared with placebo.[31–35] Results observed for EM also were confirmed by phase 2 and 3 studies in CM.[36–39] **Table 4** shows the reduction in migraine days in each trial.

Disability, impact, and quality of life Migraine has a high burden of disease. Most studies have focused on changes in Migraine Disability Assessment (MIDAS) and Headache Impact Test (HIT-6) scores as well as the Migraine-Specific Quality of Life Questionnaire to evaluate disability. Statistically significant improvement has been reported for all 4 medications compared with placebo.[40–43]

Efficacy in different clinical conditions
Efficacy in patients with concomitant preventive treatment Most studies allowed the stable concomitant use of preventive treatment. A post hoc analysis of phase 2 studies on fremanezumab[44] to analyze the subgroup of patients with concomitant preventive treatment demonstrated efficacy of the active drug compared with placebo. No drug-drug interactions were observed that possibly could reduce efficacy or increase incidence of adverse events.

These data report efficacy and safety for anti-CGRP antibodies as an add-on therapy to other preventive treatments and are extremely important, considering that in clinical practice a majority of patients may be on other preventive therapies.

Efficacy in patients with more than one preventive failure Most of the studies have excluded patients with more than 2 or 3 preventive treatment failures due to lack of efficacy and/or unacceptable tolerability, resulting in difficult interpretation of clinical efficacy in refractory patients. The active drug showed greater reduction in the mean number of monthly migraine days for EM patients with unsuccessful response to between 2 and 4 preventive drugs were for erenumab[45] and for both EM and CM for fremanezumab.[46]

It is important to remark the benefits of the anti-CGRP antibodies in refractory patients, especially considering that in those countries with greater restriction in treatment prescription, this population probably will be the first one to receive it.

Efficacy in patients with medication overuse Acute medication intake is an important aspect to consider while evaluating treatment efficacy and anti-CGRP antibodies have achieved statistically greater reduction than placebo, especially for CM patients.[36–39] A subgroup analysis in CM patients with MOH has been conducted with erenumab, showing in the treated population greater reduction in migraine frequency and in migraine-specific medication treatment days.[47] These data suggest that anti-CGRP antibodies are effective in reducing acute medication intake even in those patients who overuse medication, representing a useful tool to achieve acute drug discontinuation.

Considerations on efficacy: super-responders and nonresponders
High response rates A 50% or greater reduction in the number of migraine days in at least 50% of patients is considered clinically significant in EM trials. Smaller proportions but still significantly higher than placebo are observed for greater than or equal to 75% response in both EM and CM patients. The most interesting results, however, come from the analysis of the 100% responders. Specifically, a post hoc analysis from the EVOLVE-1 and EVOLVE-2 trials[48] observed 13.5% of patients with galcanezumab, 120 mg, and 14.3% of patients with galcanezumab, 240 mg, with 100% response rate on an average month in the 6-month period (placebo, 5.9%).

These data raise the question whether for some patients the CGRP pathway is the unique pathogenic mechanism.

Nonresponders Patients not reaching a certain cutoff, usually fixed on 50% response in reduction in migraine days, are considered nonresponders. Whether or not these patients may experience later improvement and convert into responders is an important question. A post hoc analysis of phase 3 studies for galcanezumab,[49] which classified nonresponders according to the level of reduction in migraine days at first month observed a greater likelihood to achieve response over time in those with initial response closer to the threshold. These data support, in clinical practice, the administration of more than 1 cycle of active drug in order to define the patients' response to treatment as it may be achieved at later time points.

Considerations on efficacy: short term and long term
Rapid onset of response For galcanezumab and erenumab, the onset of efficacy has been described within 1 week.[50,51] For eptinezumab,[35] the probability of migraine 1 day after infusion was used, showing a statistically significant reduction with eptinezumab compared with placebo. These results have encouraged the design of a new trial (RELIEF) to evaluate efficacy of eptinezumab administered intravenously in subjects experiencing acute migraine attacks, currently ongoing.[52]

The fact that all 4 anti-CGRP antibodies show rapid response, both for EM and CM, is a desirable characteristic for preventive treatments because it may improve adherence.

Long-term response and duration of effect Results from a 3-year interim analysis of the open-label phase 2 study on erenumab in EM[53] show sustained efficacy. For galcanezumab, sustained efficacy was confirmed by 1-year interim analysis of an open-label phase 3 study in both EM and CM.[54]

The duration of effect in patients who discontinued anti-CGRP antibodies raises disease-modifying possibilities. A recent retrospective pooled analysis, including completers of the open-label extension study phase for the preventive treatment of CM with galcanezumab[38] and erenumab[55] with 9-month and 12-month follow-ups, respectively, showed therapeutic effect of mAbs after termination up to 12 weeks.[56] The persistence of therapeutic effects after discontinuation raises the question whether anti-CGRP may act as disease-modifying drugs.

Adverse events and special medical concerns
Safety profile of anti-CGRP antibodies was analyzed in phase 2 and phase 3 studies, showing similar results for the 4 drugs. Patients receiving the active drug compared with placebo reported more treatment-emergent adverse events, including injection-site reactions, erythema, pruritus, and pain.[38,54,57,58] Constipation has been reported in approximately 3% in clinical trials for erenumab.[59] Open-label extension trials provided data on similar safety profile over time.[54,57,60]

Special concerns were raised on the basis of the potent vasodilator role of CGRP and the consequential potential cardiovascular effect with CGRP inhibition. Although all the studies have excluded patients with significant cardiovascular disease or vascular ischemia, patients with cardiovascular risk factors were included. The population with high cardiovascular risk was addressed specifically in just 1 study.[61] Erenumab showed no significant changes in exercise treadmill test. Another study analyzed[62] the coadministration of erenumab with a vasoconstrictive drug, such as sumatriptan, with no additional cardiovascular effects.

Hepatotoxicity also was evaluated in anti-CGRP antibodies studies due to the findings observed in first trials of gepants without significant cases reported.

Concerning immunogenicity, for all 4 anti-CGRP antibodies, treatment-emergent antidrug antibodies have tested positive in active drug groups at low variable proportions (3%–14%)[22,31,34,37] but still significantly higher than placebo. Among treatment-emergent antidrug antibodies, neutralizing antibodies were detected in some of them at low titers, without effect on efficacy, safety, and tolerability. Long-term efficacy of mAbs support the idea that antidrug antibodies do not seem to exert major effects.

Short clinical trials do not represent the ideal setting to observe dropouts due to lack of efficacy but can give information on discontinuation secondary to treatment-emergent adverse events. Anti-CGRP antibodies have shown a good tolerability profile, with less than 5% of discontinuation rate,[54] due to the low rate of adverse events. Treatment-emergent adverse events related to site injection usually are transient within few days and do not predict dropouts.

UNANSWERED QUESTIONS

The rich and complex scenario of CGRP antagonism represents a revolution in the headache medicine, although several questions need to be addressed.

Long-Term Efficacy and Safety

Despite the promising open-label extension studies for mAb[53,54] and ubrogepant,[63] data from real-world experience are needed to evaluate these treatments fully. Possible treatment wearing off must be investigated. Another central issue is the decision on when to discontinue treatment. Discontinuation occurs in patients with good response that are willing to stop the medication or in patients who lack of improvement. On this matter, guidelines from the European Headache Federation[64] recommend considering discontinuation after 6 months to 12 months of treatment, whereas the American Headache Society[65] recommends evaluating response after 3 months and continuing treatment if reduction in monthly migraine days is greater than or equal to 50% compared with baseline or a clinically meaningful improvement is achieved in the MIDAS or HIT-6 scores. In this context, future research should aim to investigate the presence of biomarkers that could predict anti-CGRP treatment response and, therefore, guide clinicians' decision on prescribing or discontinuing such treatments.

Gender Differences and Ethnicity

Considering that clinical trials included mainly women, in whom migraine is more prevalent, questions on the efficacy in the male population still have to be clarified.

Studies on anti-CGRP antibodies were conducted mainly on white subjects. EVOLVE-2 study and PROMISE-2[66] recruited patients worldwide in order to have a broader ethnicity sample; however, specific data on different ethnicities are lacking.

Pediatric Migraine

Clinical trials have excluded patients under 18 year old. Considering the need for preventive treatments with a low AE profile, it is logical to consider that anti-CGRP antibodies may represent a good treatment option. In this context, galcanezumab currently is being tested among patients with 6 years to 17 years of age, suffering from EM.[67] Another trial has been started to investigate erenumab in pediatric patients with CM.[68]

Pregnancy and Breastfeeding

No data are available for the pregnancy and breastfeeding populations because they were excluded from clinical trials. Anti-CGRP drugs must be avoided in these situations, especially considering the preclinical data that showed increased fetal mortality in rats[69] and considering the role of CGRP in the control of human fetoplacental vascular tone.[70]

SUMMARY

CGRP currently is revolutionizing headache medicine. CGRP antagonism is providing insights into migraine pathophysiology and shared therapeutic pathways that can provide both acute and preventive treatments strategies with good responses in terms of efficacy and safety.

Clinical trials' results are encouraging but real-world data are awaited to further validate findings.

DISCLOSURE

E. Caronna has nothing to disclose. A.J. Starling has received consulting fees from Alder, Allergan, Amgen, Axsome Therapeutics, eNeura, Eli Lilly & Company, Impel,

Lundbeck, Med-IQ, Medscape, Novartis, Teva, and Theranica; research funding from Migraine Research Foundation and Mayo Clinic; and honoraria from Migraine World Summit.

REFERENCES

1. Burch R, Rizzoli P, Loder E. The prevalence and impact of migraine and severe headache in the United States: figures and trends from government health studies. Headache 2018. https://doi.org/10.1111/head.13281.
2. James SL, Abate D, Abate KH, et al. Global, regional, and national incidence, prevalence, and years lived with disability for 354 Diseases and Injuries for 195 countries and territories, 1990-2017: A systematic analysis for the Global Burden of Disease Study 2017. Lancet 2018. https://doi.org/10.1016/S0140-6736(18)32279-7.
3. Goadsby PJ, Edvinsson L, Ekman R. Vasoactive peptide release in the extracerebral circulation of humans during migraine headache. Ann Neurol 1990. https://doi.org/10.1002/ana.410280213.
4. Warfvinge K, Edvinsson L. Distribution of CGRP and CGRP receptor components in the rat brain. Cephalalgia 2019. https://doi.org/10.1177/0333102417728873.
5. Cernuda-Morollón E, Larrosa D, Ramón C, et al. Interictal increase of CGRP levels in peripheral blood as a biomarker for chronic migraine. Neurology 2013. https://doi.org/10.1212/WNL.0b013e3182a6cb72.
6. Eftekhari S, Gaspar RC, Roberts R, et al. Localization of CGRP receptor components and receptor binding sites in rhesus monkey brainstem: A detailed study using in situ hybridization, immunofluorescence, and autoradiography. J Comp Neurol 2016. https://doi.org/10.1002/cne.23828.
7. Eftekhari S, Salvatore CA, Calamari A, et al. Differential distribution of calcitonin gene-related peptide and its receptor components in the human trigeminal ganglion. Neuroscience 2010. https://doi.org/10.1016/j.neuroscience.2010.05.016.
8. Olesen J, Diener HC, Husstedt IW, et al. Calcitonin gene-related peptide receptor antagonist BIBN 4096 BS for the acute treatment of migraine. N Engl J Med 2004. https://doi.org/10.1056/NEJMoa030505.
9. Ho TW, Ferrari MD, Dodick DW, et al. Efficacy and tolerability of MK-0974 (telcagepant), a new oral antagonist of calcitonin gene-related peptide receptor, compared with zolmitriptan for acute migraine: a randomised, placebo-controlled, parallel-treatment trial. Lancet 2008. https://doi.org/10.1016/S0140-6736(08)61626-8.
10. Connor KM, Shapiro RE, Diener HC, et al. Randomized, controlled trial of telcagepant for the acute treatment of migraine. Neurology 2009. https://doi.org/10.1212/WNL.0b013e3181b87942.
11. Hewitt DJ, Aurora SK, Dodick DW, et al. Randomized controlled trial of the CGRP receptor antagonist MK-3207 in the acute treatment of migraine. Cephalalgia 2011. https://doi.org/10.1177/0333102411398399.
12. Voss T, Lipton RB, Dodick DW, et al. A phase IIb randomized, double-blind, placebo-controlled trial of ubrogepant for the acute treatment of migraine. Cephalalgia 2016. https://doi.org/10.1177/0333102416653233.
13. Lipton RB, Dodick DW, Ailani J, et al. Effect of ubrogepant vs placebo on pain and the most bothersome associated symptom in the acute treatment of migraine: The achieve ii randomized clinical trial. JAMA 2019. https://doi.org/10.1001/jama.2019.16711.

14. Dodick DW, Lipton RB, Ailani J, et al. Ubrogepant for the treatment of migraine. N Engl J Med 2019;381(23):2230–41.
15. Marcus R, Goadsby PJ, Dodick D, et al. BMS-927711 for the acute treatment of migraine: A double-blind, randomized, placebo controlled, dose-ranging trial. Cephalalgia 2014. https://doi.org/10.1177/0333102413500727.
16. Croop R, Goadsby PJ, Stock DA, et al. Efficacy, safety, and tolerability of rimege-pant orally disintegrating tablet for the acute treatment of migraine: a rando-mised, phase 3, double-blind, placebo-controlled trial. Lancet 2019. https://doi.org/10.1016/S0140-6736(19)31606-X.
17. Lipton RB, Croop R, Stock EG, et al. Rimegepant, an oral calcitonin gene-related peptide receptor antagonist, for migraine. N Engl J Med 2019. https://doi.org/10.1056/NEJMoa1811090.
18. Biohaven Pharmaceuticals I. Efficacy and Safety Trial of Rimegepant for Migraine Prevention in Adults. Available at: https://clinicaltrials.gov/ct2/show/NCT03732638.
19. Goadsby PJ, Dodick DW, Trugman JM, et al. Orally administered atogepant was efficacious, safe, and tolerable for the prevention of migraine: results from a phase 2b/3 Study (S17.001). Neurology 2019;92(15 Sup).
20. New Haven CBP. Biohaven achieves positive topline results in pivotal phase 2/3 study of & vazegepant, the first and only intranasal CGRP receptor antagonist in clinical development for the acute treatment of migraine.
21. Sun H, Dodick DW, Silberstein S, et al. Safety and efficacy of AMG 334 for pre-vention of episodic migraine: A randomised, double-blind, placebo-controlled, phase 2 trial. Lancet Neurol 2016. https://doi.org/10.1016/S1474-4422(16)00019-3.
22. Dodick DW, Goadsby PJ, Spierings ELH, et al. Safety and efficacy of LY2951742, a monoclonal antibody to calcitonin gene-related peptide, for the prevention of migraine: A phase 2, randomised, double-blind, placebo-controlled study. Lan-cet Neurol 2014. https://doi.org/10.1016/S1474-4422(14)70128-0.
23. Bigal ME, Dodick DW, Rapoport AM, et al. Safety, tolerability, and efficacy of TEV-48125 for preventive treatment of high-frequency episodic migraine: A multi-centre, randomised, double-blind, placebo-controlled, phase 2b study. Lancet Neurol 2015. https://doi.org/10.1016/S1474-4422(15)00249-5.
24. Dodick DW, Goadsby PJ, Silberstein SD, et al. Safety and efficacy of ALD403, an antibody to calcitonin gene-related peptide, for the prevention of frequent episodic migraine: A randomised, double-blind, placebo-controlled, exploratory phase 2 trial. Lancet Neurol 2014. https://doi.org/10.1016/S1474-4422(14)70209-1.
25. Dodick DW, Tepper SJ, Friedman DI, et al. Use of most bothersome symptom as a coprimary endpoint in migraine clinical trials: a post-hoc analysis of the pivotal ZOTRIP randomized, controlled trial. Headache 2018. https://doi.org/10.1111/head.13327.
26. Ho TW, Connor KM, Zhang Y, et al. Randomized controlled trial of the CGRP re-ceptor antagonist telcagepant for migraine prevention. Neurology 2014. https://doi.org/10.1212/WNL.0000000000000771.
27. Headache Classification Committee of the International Headache Society (IHS) The International Classification of Headache Disorders, 3rd edition. Cephalalgia 2018. https://doi.org/10.1177/0333102417738202.
28. Ho TW, Ho AP, Chaitman BR, et al. Randomized, controlled study of telcagepant in patients with migraine and coronary artery disease. Headache 2012. https://doi.org/10.1111/j.1526-4610.2011.02052.x.

29. Chaitman BR, Ho AP, Behm MO, et al. A randomized, placebo-controlled study of the effects of telcagepant on exercise time in patients with stable angina. Clin Pharmacol Ther 2012. https://doi.org/10.1038/clpt.2011.246.

30. Rubio-Beltran E, Chan KY, Danser AJ, et al. Characterisation of the calcitonin gene-related peptide receptor antagonists ubrogepant and atogepant in human isolated coronary, cerebral and middle meningeal arteries. Cephalalgia 2019. https://doi.org/10.1177/0333102419884943.

31. Dodick DW, Ashina M, Brandes JL, et al. ARISE: A Phase 3 randomized trial of erenumab for episodic migraine. Cephalalgia 2018. https://doi.org/10.1177/0333102418759786.

32. Goadsby PJ, Uwe R, Hallstrom Y, et al. A controlled trial of erenumab for episodic migraine. N Engl J Med 2017. https://doi.org/10.1056/NEJMoa1705848.

33. Dodick DW, Silberstein SD, Bigal ME, et al. Effect of Fremanezumab compared with placebo for prevention of episodic migraine a randomized clinical trial. JAMA 2018. https://doi.org/10.1001/jama.2018.4853.

34. Skljarevski V, Matharu M, Millen BA, et al. Efficacy and safety of galcanezumab for the prevention of episodic migraine: Results of the EVOLVE-2 Phase 3 randomized controlled clinical trial. Cephalalgia 2018. https://doi.org/10.1177/0333102418779543.

35. Ashina M, Saper J, Cady R, et al. Eptinezumab in episodic migraine: A randomized, double-blind, placebo-controlled study (PROMISE-1). Cephalalgia 2020; 40(3):241–54. https://doi.org/10.1177/0333102420905132.

36. Tepper S, Ashina M, Reuter U, et al. Safety and efficacy of erenumab for preventive treatment of chronic migraine: a randomised, double-blind, placebo-controlled phase 2 trial. Lancet Neurol 2017. https://doi.org/10.1016/S1474-4422(17)30083-2.

37. Silberstein SD, Dodick DW, Bigal ME, et al. Fremanezumab for the preventive treatment of chronic migraine. N Engl J Med 2017. https://doi.org/10.1056/NEJMoa1709038.

38. Detke HC, Goadsby PJ, Wang S, et al. Galcanezumab in chronic migraine: The randomized, double-blind, placebo-controlled REGAIN study. Neurology 2018. https://doi.org/10.1212/WNL.0000000000006640.

39. Lipton RB, Goadsby PJ, Smith J, et al. Efficacy and safety of eptinezumab in patients with chronic migraine. Neurology 2020;94(13):e1365–77.

40. Ford JH, Ayer DW, Zhang Q, et al. Two randomized migraine studies of galcanezumab: Effects on patient functioning and disability. Neurology 2019. https://doi.org/10.1212/WNL.0000000000007856.

41. VanderPluym J, Dodick DW, Lipton RB, et al. Fremanezumab for preventive treatment of migraine: Functional status on headache-free days. Neurology 2018. https://doi.org/10.1212/01.wnl.0000544321.19316.40.

42. Buse DC, Lipton RB, Hallström Y, et al. Migraine-related disability, impact, and health-related quality of life among patients with episodic migraine receiving preventive treatment with erenumab. Cephalalgia 2018. https://doi.org/10.1177/0333102418789072.

43. Dodick D, Goadsby P, Silberstein S, et al. 75% responder rates provide improvement in HIT-6 scores from week 4 through 12 following a single infusion of ALD403, or placebo. Neurology 2017;88:165.

44. Cohen JM, Dodick DW, Yang R, et al. Fremanezumab as add-on treatment for patients treated with other migraine preventive medicines. Headache 2017. https://doi.org/10.1111/head.13156.

45. Reuter U, Goadsby PJ, Lanteri-Minet M, et al. Efficacy and tolerability of erenumab in patients with episodic migraine in whom two-to-four previous preventive treatments were unsuccessful: a randomised, double-blind, placebo-controlled, phase 3b study. Lancet 2018. https://doi.org/10.1016/S0140-6736(18)32534-0.
46. Ferrari MD, Diener HC, Ning X, et al. Fremanezumab versus placebo for migraine prevention in patients with documented failure to up to four migraine preventive medication classes (FOCUS): a randomised, double-blind, placebo-controlled, phase 3b trial. Lancet 2019. https://doi.org/10.1016/S0140-6736(19)31946-4.
47. Tepper SJ, Diener HC, Ashina M, et al. Erenumab in chronic migraine with medication overuse: Subgroup analysis of a randomized trial. Neurology 2019. https://doi.org/10.1212/WNL.0000000000007497.
48. Rosen N, Pearlman E, Ruff D, et al. 100% response rate to galcanezumab in patients with episodic migraine: a post hoc analysis of the results from phase 3, randomized, double-blind, placebo-controlled EVOLVE-1 and EVOLVE-2 Studies. Headache 2018. https://doi.org/10.1111/head.13427.
49. Nichols R, Doty E, Sacco S, et al. Analysis of initial nonresponders to galcanezumab in patients with episodic or chronic migraine: results from the EVOLVE-1, EVOLVE-2, and REGAIN randomized, double-blind, placebo-controlled studies. Headache 2019. https://doi.org/10.1111/head.13443.
50. Goadsby PJ, Dodick DW, Martinez JM, et al. Onset of efficacy and duration of response of galcanezumab for the prevention of episodic migraine: A post-hoc analysis. J Neurol Neurosurg Psychiatry 2019. https://doi.org/10.1136/jnnp-2018-320242.
51. Schwedt T, Reuter U, Tepper S, et al. Early onset of efficacy with erenumab in patients with episodic and chronic migraine. J Headache Pain 2018. https://doi.org/10.1186/s10194-018-0923-6.
52. H. Lundbeck A/S. Evaluate Efficacy & Safety of Eptinezumab Administered Intravenously in Subjects Experiencing Acute Attack of Migraine (RELIEF). Available at: https://clinicaltrials.gov/ct2/show/NCT04152083.
53. Ashina M, Goadsby PJ, Reuter U, et al. Long-term safety and tolerability of erenumab: Three-plus year results from a five-year open-label extension study in episodic migraine. Cephalalgia 2019. https://doi.org/10.1177/0333102419854082.
54. Camporeale A, Kudrow D, Sides R, et al. A phase 3, long-term, open-label safety study of Galcanezumab in patients with migraine. BMC Neurol 2018. https://doi.org/10.1186/s12883-018-1193-2.
55. Tepper SJ, Ashina M, Reuter U, et al. Long-term safety and efficacy of erenumab in patients with chronic migraine: Results from a 52-week, open-label extension study. Cephalalgia 2020;40(6):543–53.
56. Raffaelli B, Mussetto V, Israel H, et al. Erenumab and galcanezumab in chronic migraine prevention: Effects after treatment termination. J Headache Pain 2019. https://doi.org/10.1186/s10194-019-1018-8.
57. Detke H, Pozo-Rosich P, Reuter U, et al. Aurora Neurology Apr 2019;92(15 Supplement):10-010.
58. Hong P, Wu X, Liu Y. Calcitonin gene-related peptide monoclonal antibody for preventive treatment of episodic migraine: A meta analysis. Clin Neurol Neurosurg 2017. https://doi.org/10.1016/j.clineuro.2017.01.009.
59. Ashina M, Kudrow D, Reuter U, et al. Long-term tolerability and nonvascular safety of erenumab, a novel calcitonin gene-related peptide receptor antagonist for prevention of migraine: A pooled analysis of four placebo-controlled trials with

long-term extensions. Cephalalgia 2019. https://doi.org/10.1177/0333102419888222.

60. Ashina M, Dodick D, Goadsby PJ, et al. Erenumab (AMG 334) in episodic migraine: Interim analysis of an ongoing open-label study. Neurology 2017. https://doi.org/10.1212/WNL.0000000000004391.

61. Depre C, Antalik L, Starling A, et al. A randomized, double-blind, placebo-controlled study to evaluate the effect of erenumab on exercise time during a treadmill test in patients with stable angina. Headache 2018. https://doi.org/10.1111/head.13316.

62. de Hoon J, Van Hecken A, Vandermeulen C, et al. Phase 1, randomized, parallel-group, double-blind, placebo-controlled trial to evaluate the effects of erenumab (AMG 334) and concomitant sumatriptan on blood pressure in healthy volunteers. Cephalalgia 2019. https://doi.org/10.1177/0333102418776017.

63. Ailani J, Lipton RB, Hutchinson S, et al. Long-term safety evaluation of ubrogepant for the acute treatment of migraine: phase 3, randomized, 52-week extension trial. Headache 2020;60(1):141–52.

64. Sacco S, Bendtsen L, Ashina M, et al. European headache federation guideline on the use of monoclonal antibodies acting on the calcitonin gene related peptide or its receptor for migraine prevention. J Headache Pain 2019. https://doi.org/10.1186/s10194-018-0955-y.

65. American Headache Society. The American Headache Society position statement on integrating new migraine treatments into clinical practice. Headache 2019. https://doi.org/10.1111/head.13456.

66. Lipton RB, Goadsby PJ, Smith J, et al. Efficacy and safety of eptinezumab in patients with chronic migraine: PROMISE-2. Neurology 2020 Mar 31;94(13):e1365–77. https://doi.org/10.1212/WNL.0000000000009169. Epub 2020 Mar 24. PMID: 32209650; PMCID: PMC7274916.

67. Eli Lilly and Company. A Study of Galcanezumab (LY2951742) in Participants 6 to 17 Years of Age With Episodic Migraine (REBUILD).

68. Amgen. Efficacy and Safety of Erenumab in Pediatric Subjects With Chronic Migraine (OASIS (CM)).

69. Gangula PRR, Dong YL, Wimalawansa SJ, et al. Infusion of pregnant rats with calcitonin gene-related peptide (CGRP)8-37, a CGRP receptor antagonist, increases blood pressure and fetal mortality and decreases fetal growth1. Biol Reprod 2002. https://doi.org/10.1095/biolreprod67.2.624.

70. Dong YL, Vegiraju S, Chauhan M, et al. Involvement of calcitonin gene-related peptide in control of human fetoplacental vascular tone. Am J Physiol Heart Circ Physiol 2004. https://doi.org/10.1152/ajpheart.00140.2003.

71. Allergan announces completion of two positive safety studies for ubrogepant – An oral CGRP receptor antagonist for the acute treatment of migraine.

72. Skljarevski V, Oakes TM, Zhang Q, et al. Effect of different doses of Galcanezumab vs Placebo for episodic migraine prevention a randomized clinical trial. JAMA Neurol 2018. https://doi.org/10.1001/jamaneurol.2017.3859.

73. Stauffer VL, Dodick DW, Zhang Q, et al. Evaluation of galcanezumab for the prevention of episodic migraine: The EVOLVE-1 randomized clinical trial. JAMA Neurol 2018. https://doi.org/10.1001/jamaneurol.2018.1212.

74. Eli Lilly and Company. A Study of Galcanezumab (LY2951742) in Adults With Treatment-Resistant Migraine (CONQUER). Available at: https://clinicaltrials.gov/ct2/show/results/NCT03559257.

75. Bigal ME, Edvinsson L, Rapoport AM, et al. Safety, tolerability, and efficacy of TEV-48125 for preventive treatment of chronic migraine: A multicentre, randomised, double-blind, placebo-controlled, phase 2b study. Lancet Neurol 2015. https://doi.org/10.1016/S1474-4422(15)00245-8.
76. Dodick DW, Lipton RB, Silberstein S, et al. Eptinezumab for prevention of chronic migraine: A randomized phase 2b clinical trial. Cephalalgia 2019. https://doi.org/10.1177/0333102419858355.

Advances in the Treatment of Multiple Sclerosis

Carolyn Goldschmidt, DO, Marisa P. McGinley, DO, MSc*

KEYWORDS

• Multiple sclerosis • Disease-modifying treatment • Remyelination therapies
• Neuroprotection therapies • Treatment approaches

KEY POINTS

• Multiple sclerosis (MS) is a chronic, immune-mediated neurologic disease that affects nearly 1 million people in the United States, is a major cause of disability, and can lead to a reduced quality of life.

• There are currently more than a dozen approved disease-modifying therapies for MS, with varying mechanisms of action, routes of administration, dosing schedule, efficacy, and side-effect profiles.

• Most disease-modifying therapies target active, inflammatory disease that defines relapsing remitting MS, with less treatments available to target neurodegenerative disease.

• The treatment targets, goals, and algorithms are changing as the field learns more about the pathophysiology of the disease.

• New therapies that target remyelination and neurodegeneration are being developed, but more robust data are needed before they are integrated into routine clinical care.

INTRODUCTION

Multiple sclerosis (MS) is an immune-mediated, inflammatory demyelinating disease of the central nervous system (CNS) that leads to irreversible disability and currently is estimated to affect 1 million people in the United States and more than 2 million people globally.[1,2] The most common disease type is relapsing remitting (85%–90%), and most treatments target this disease subtype. Some of these relapsing remitting MS (RRMS) patients will transition to a secondary progressive course. A small proportion of patients (10%) has primary progressive MS (PPMS), which is characterized by progression from onset. Treatment options for progressive disease are currently limited.

As the understanding of the disease has evolved, treatment options and treatment approaches have also advanced. The definitions of clinical courses were revised to better reflect underlying MS pathologic condition.[3] Importantly, disease activity was added as a temporal qualifier to the MS phenotypes because clinical and radiographic

Mellen Center U-10, Cleveland Clinic, 9500 Euclid Avenue, Cleveland, OH 44195, USA
* Corresponding author.
E-mail address: mcginlm@ccf.org

Neurol Clin 39 (2021) 21–33
https://doi.org/10.1016/j.ncl.2020.09.002
0733-8619/21/© 2020 Elsevier Inc. All rights reserved.

disease activity along with disability progression can occur in both relapsing and progressive disease. This balance of disease activity reflects a combination of inflammatory and neurodegenerative processes that is important to understand in treatment decision making. This review discusses the evolution of the treatment landscape of MS, treatment approaches, and future directions.

DISEASE-MODIFYING THERAPIES

The first disease-modifying therapy (DMT) was an injectable medication approved by the Food and Drug Administration (FDA) in 1993. Subsequently, there have been a variety of injectable, oral, and infusion DMTs developed that have unique risks and benefits.

Injectables

Interferon β-1b was the first FDA-approved treatment for RRMS.[4] There are currently 5 formulations of interferon injections available for RRMS. The initial phase 3 IFN-β trials showed a reduction in relapse rates by 18% to 34% in patients with relapsing MS.[5] Shortly after the interferons were approved, glatiramer acetate was approved with similar efficacy.[6] Injectable therapies were the mainstay of MS treatment for more than 15 years, until the first oral medications were approved. The injectable DMTs have the most long-term safety data, and there are patients who have remained stable on them for many years with few side effects. However, in the current landscape, use of injectable therapies has diminished because of the development of alternative DMTs with improved tolerability and higher efficacy.

Orals

Fingolimod, a sphingosine 1-phosphate (S1P) receptor modulator, was the first FDA-approved oral DMT in 2010 which was a major advancement because of the improved efficacy and new route of administration. Since this development, there have been a variety of oral options approved, changing the landscape of treatment (**Table 1**). Siponimod and ozanimod are both selective S1P receptor modulators that were recently approved. These medications, although similar to fingolimod, have unique side effects and monitoring requirements. All patients started on fingolimod require first-dose observation (FDO) because of the possibility of first-dose bradycardia from interaction with receptors on cardiac myocytes. Conversely, only patients with a cardiac history are suggested to undergo an FDO with siponimod, and there is no FDO recommendation with ozanimod. These varying recommendations are due to the more selective S1P receptor subtypes of the newer medications. Teriflunomide, like the S1P receptor modulators, has convenient once-daily dosing, but with a different mechanism of action (pyrimidine synthesis inhibition). The fumarates are another class of oral medications. The most recently approved fumarate, diroximel fumarate, has the same dosing frequency and mechanism of action as dimethyl fumarate, but was shown to have improved tolerability, specifically reduction of gastrointestinal (GI) side effects.[7,8] Finally, cladribine is unique in the oral medication group because it has an induction-type dosing schedule of two 5-day cycles 12 months apart.[9] Overall, the oral medications are more efficacious than the injectable therapies, except for teriflunomide, which is similar in efficacy to injectables, and cladribine has the highest efficacy. They are well tolerated, although their side-effect profile varies. The risk of infections is increased compared with the injectable therapies, and some may be limited because of other risks, such lymphopenia, in fingolimod or dimethyl fumarate and transaminitis with teriflunomide.

Table 1
An overview of currently approved oral disease modifying therapies (as of April 2020)

DMT	Year Approved	Dosing	Medication Class	Phase 3 Trial	Trial Design	Main Outcome	Main Side Effects
Fingolimod[10]	2010	0.5 mg daily	Sphingosine 1-phosphate receptor modulator	• FREEDOMS • TRANSFORMS	• RRMS, placebo-controlled • RRMS, active control with interferon β-1a	• 54% decrease in annualized relapse rate • 48% decrease in annualized relapse rate	Bradycardia/heart block with first dose, macular edema, elevated liver enzymes, hypertension, headache, varicella-zoster virus (VZV) reactivation
Siponimod[11]	2019	Initial titration with a final dose of 2 mg daily for CYP2C9 genotypes 1/1, 1/2, 2/2 or 1 mg daily for genotypes 1/3 or 2/3	Selective sphingosine 1-phosphate receptor modulator	EXPAND	SPMS, placebo-controlled	21% decrease in risk of 3 mo confirmed disability progression	Bradycardia with first dose, lymphopenia, elevated liver enzymes, macular edema, hypertension, VZV reactivation
Ozanimod[12,13]	2020	1 mg daily	Selective sphingosine 1-phosphate receptor modulator	• RADIANCE • SUNBEAM	• RRMS, active-controlled with interferon β-1a • RRMS, active-controlled with interferon β-1a	• 38% reduction in ARR • 48% reductions in ARR	Elevated liver enzymes, nasopharyngitis, hypertension

(continued on next page)

Table 1
(continued)

DMT	Year Approved	Dosing	Medication Class	Phase 3 Trial	Trial Design	Main Outcome	Main Side Effects
Dimethyl fumarate[14,15]	2013	240 mg bid	Anti-inflammatory/cytoprotective	• DEFINE • CONFIRM	• RRMS, placebo-controlled • RRMS, placebo-controlled	• 53% reduction in ARR • 44% reduction in ARR	Flushing, GI upset, elevated liver enzymes, lymphopenia
Diroximel fumarate[7]	2019	462 mg bid	Converted to same active metabolite as DMF	EVOLVE-MS-2	RRMS, head-to-head comparison to DMF	46% reduction in days with Individual Gastrointestinal Symptom and Impact Scale score of ≥ 2	Flushing, GI upset, elevated liver enzymes, lymphopenia
Teriflunomide[16]	2012	7 mg or 14 mg daily	Interferes with de novo pyrimidine synthesis	• TOWER • TEMSO	• RRMS, placebo-controlled • RRMS, placebo-controlled	• 36% reduction in ARR • 31.5% reduction in ARR	Elevated liver enzymes, hair thinning, headache
Cladribine[9]	2019	1.75 mg/kg in two 5-d courses 23–27 d apart in year 1 and again 43 wk later	Inhibits DNA synthesis and promote apoptosis in lymphocytes	CLARITY	RRMS, placebo-controlled	57.6% reduction in ARR	Lymphopenia, VZV reactivation, infections

Infusions

Natalizumab was the first approved infusion DMT for RRMS in 2004. It is a monoclonal antibody against α-4 integrin and is a selective adhesion molecule inhibitor, given by a monthly infusion.[17] This therapy dramatically changed the landscape of treatment not only because of its route and frequency of administration but also because of its high efficacy on relapses and MRI activity. Its use has been limited because of the serious risk of developing progressive multifocal leukoencephalopathy (PML). Risk can be stratified by JC virus (JCV) status and index level, but for patients who are seropositive and on the medication for greater than 2 years, the risk climbs to 3 cases per 1000. For this reason, this medication is primarily used in JCV-seronegative patients, and seropositive patients are not typically recommended to continue this medication beyond 2 years. There is evidence that dosing intervals can be extended, which can mitigate PML risks.[18,19]

Rituximab is a CD20 monoclonal antibody that historically has been used off label for treatment of MS supported by phase 2 placebo-controlled trial evidence demonstrating efficacy in RRMS.[20] This DMT was often used in patients with highly active disease that were JCV seropositive, thus limiting the use of natalizumab. In 2017, ocrelizumab, also a CD20 monoclonal antibody, was FDA-approved for the treatment of RRMS and PPMS based on the results of the OPERA I/II and ORATORIO studies, respectively.[21,22] Ocrelizumab is different from rituximab because it is humanized, which has the potential to decrease infusion reactions. These medications are becoming more commonly prescribed because of their high efficacy, ease of dosing, and side-effect profile.

Alemtuzumab is a humanized monoclonal antibody that targets the CD52 antigen expressed on T cells, B cells, monocytes, and eosinophils that produces rapid, profound, and prolonged lymphocyte depletion with gradual reconstitution. It is administered for 5 consecutive days during the first cycle followed by a 3-day course 1 year later, with the potential for re-treatment.[23] Even after reconstitution, the cell profile and function are altered, leading to continued efficacy that may not require further treatment. Monitoring is burdensome and includes malignancy screening with annual gynecologic and skin examinations, pretreatment laboratory workup, and monthly blood and urine testing for 4 years after treatment. The monthly monitoring is part of an Risk Evaluation Mitigation Strategy (REMS) program to monitor for autoimmune conditions, such as thyroid disease, glomerular basement membrane disease, and thrombocytopenia.[23] In addition, acyclovir 200 mg to 400 mg twice a day is given prophylactically during the course of treatment and continues until CD4$^+$ lymphocytes recover to at least 200 cells/μL, with a minimum duration of 2 months because of the risk of herpes virus infections and reactivations.[24]

STEM CELL TRANSPLANT

Stem cell therapy is of increasing interest in several neurologic conditions, including MS. Particularly, the role of immunoablation and autologous hematopoietic stem cell transplantation (AHSCT) in treatment-resistant relapsing disease is currently under investigation. Despite the variety of DMTs listed above, there is a subset of patients who have continued inflammatory disease activity or are limited by adverse events who may be candidates for AHSCT.[25] Recently, the American Society for Blood and Bone Marrow Transplantation created a task force to review the evidence and provide recommendations regarding treatment-refractory MS as an indication for AHSCT.[25] Their review of retrospective studies found an overall incidence of relapse-free survival at 5 years after transplant of 80% to 87%, with many studies showing Expanded

Disability Status Scale (EDSS) stability or improvement.[25] They also reviewed several single-arm clinical trials (NCT00278655, NCT01099930, NCT00288626, ACTRN 12613000339752) and 2 randomized controlled trials (NCT00273364, EUDRACT 2007-000064-24) that differed in inclusion criteria, conditioning regimens, primary outcomes, and comparators in the randomized trials. These trials also showed high rates of relapse-free survival, disability stability or improvement, and improved MRI measures.[25] Mortalities across these studies range from 0% to -4.2% and have significantly improved over time. Overall, it appears that AHSCT is most effective and of most benefit in patients with active, relapsing disease despite DMT, and in patients who are younger with a relatively short disease duration, but still ambulatory although accruing disability.[25] There is an ongoing randomized trial evaluating the safety, efficacy, and cost-effectiveness of AHSCT compared with best available therapy (natalizumab, CD20 monoclonal antibodies, and alemtuzumab) in treatment-refractory relapsing patients with the goal of determining the optimal use of this treatment in the current landscape (BEAT-MS, NCT04047628).

TREATMENT STRATEGIES FOR RELAPSING REMITTING MULTIPLE SCLEROSIS

There are currently 9 classes of DMTs that were discussed above. These medications vary in mechanism of action, efficacy, route of administration, and side-effect profiles. With the increasing number of approved therapies, there are a variety of treatment approaches that can be used. Treatment decisions should be tailored to each individual patient with regards to disease phenotype, risk profile, and patient preference, but there are 2 general approaches: escalation and early highly effective treatment.

For an escalation approach, the patient is started on a low- to moderate-efficacy DMT (eg, injectable or oral DMT), and if there is breakthrough disease, the patient's therapy is escalated to a highly effective choice (eg, monoclonal antibody). This approach has been commonly used because the older medications have a well-established safety profile. Although some patients will remain stable on the first DMT, some will require a change in therapy because of disease activity. Evidence of disease activity is most commonly defined as clinical relapses and/or new lesions on MRI. A stricter target that has been suggested is no evidence of disease activity (NEDA). NEDA-3 includes measures such as clinical relapses, disability progression, and MRI activity, whereas NEDA-4 adds brain volume loss to account for the neurodegenerative process.[26] NEDA has been suggested as a target outcome, but not currently used in clinical practice. With the advent of the newer DMTs, the threshold for escalation has lowered, but is still dependent on comfort of the practitioner and patients using the medications, access to the support needed for the therapies (ie, infusion centers), and cost. The benefit of escalation therapy is minimizing the risk, but the concern is for the potential for undertreatment of disease activity that may lead to accumulation of disability and disease progression.[27]

The alternative approach is to start a highly effective therapy as the first treatment option. Subgroup analysis and observational studies demonstrate starting DMT earlier in the disease course, preferably after the first clinical attack, leads to better long-term clinical outcomes.[27] A goal of the most recent 2017 McDonald criteria revisions was to facilitate earlier diagnosis, allowing for earlier treatment.[28] The DMTs that are considered highly effective include natalizumab, rituximab, ocrelizumab, and alemtuzumab.[27] The tradeoffs to higher efficacy are increased risks, such as infection, autoimmunity, and malignancy, with less long-term safety data for many of these medications. Currently in clinical practice, the decision between treatment strategies is made based on a variety of prognostic indicators and shared decision making between the patient and provider. Several demographic and disease characteristics that may suggest a more severe course include male gender, older age at presentation, increased severity and frequency of relapses, higher burden of spinal cord and infratentorial lesions, increased T2 lesions burden, increased contrast-enhancing lesion burden, and increased brain atrophy.[27] Although observational studies suggest that early high-efficacy treatment may have long-term benefits, there is currently no randomized trials that have evaluated the 2 treatment strategies. There are 2 ongoing large, randomized multicenter trials in treatment-naïve RRMS patients who will rigorously evaluate the 2 treatment approaches: Determining the Effectiveness of Early Intensive versus Escalation approaches for the Treatment of Relapsing-Remitting Multiple Sclerosis (DELIVER-MS, NCT03535298) and Traditional versus Early Aggressive Therapy for Multiple Sclerosis Trial (TREAT-MS, NCT03500328).

PROGRESSIVE DISEASE

There has been a multitude of advances in the treatment of RRMS, but developments in progressive MS treatment have been slow. All the currently available DMTs primarily target inflammatory disease activity, which is typically present to a lesser degree in progressive disease. Progressive patients can have evidence of disease activity, such as superimposed relapses on a progressive decline or MRI activity (eg, new or enhancing lesions). In progressive patients with evidence of disease activity, all the currently available DMTs are now approved for secondary progressive MS with evidence of disease activity. In 2019, the EXPAND phase 3 trial of siponimod demonstrated efficacy in a secondary progressive disease with activity, which led to its approval in both RRMS and Secondary progressive multiple sclerosis (SPMS) with activity. Around this time, the FDA also changed the approval of all DMTs to include both RRMS and active SPMS. This prescribing information change reflected the understanding that progressive disease can have inflammatory disease activity in which current DMTs may be of use. Ocrelizumab is the only approved DMT for PPMS; however, anti-CD20 treatments are likely more effective in younger individuals with evidence of disease activity.

Although the siponimod and ocrelizumab trials demonstrated efficacy in progressive populations, there are still forms of progressive MS that have little inflammatory disease and more neurodegeneration. There have been several negative trials in progressive disease with currently available DMTs.[29–34] Although these studies did not demonstrate an effect on the primary outcome of disability progression, they helped confirm there is another underlying progress beyond inflammatory activity. There is still a great amount of work needed in the field to discover and develop treatments that target the noninflammatory portion of progressive disease. Remyelination and neuroprotective therapies are 2 potential treatment targets that are now being explored.

Remyelination Therapies

Demyelination of both white and gray matter is a key pathologic feature of MS. Although remyelination does occur, the amount is variable and it decreases with age.[35] Mitochondrial dysfunction and demyelination lead to virtual hypoxia, making axons prone to degeneration and irreversible disability. Oligodendrocytes are the cells that produce myelin and appear crucial for axonal health independent of myelination.[36] It is currently thought that impaired oligodendrocyte precursor cell (OPC) differentiation is involved in remyelination failure, and subsequently that increased OPC differentiation may promote remyelination and have an impact on disability.[37] OPC recruitment into demyelinated lesions and their differentiation is decreased with age, which parallels decreased remyelination.[38] In addition, the microenvironment around the demyelinated lesion appears to also impair OPC differentiation, adding another challenge to therapy development.

Remyelination is an important target for progressive therapies, as this could theoretically halt disability accrual and potentially reverse some already accumulated disability. One compound that demonstrated potential to promote remyelination was high-dose biotin. Biotin is a cofactor for carboxylases that are expressed in oligodendrocytes in addition to supporting myelin repair by enhancing fatty acid synthesis and protecting against hypoxia-driven axonal degeneration. In 1 phase 3 placebo-controlled trial of high-dose biotin, 12.6% of treated participants compared with no placebo participants met the endpoint of a decreased in EDSS or decrease in timed 25-foot walk; however, the biotin-treated group had more new or enlarging MRI lesions.[39] Unfortunately, the definitive phase 3 trial had no effect on disability improvement.[40]

Another potential remyelination target that has gained interest is opicinumab, which is a humanized monoclonal antibody against the leucine-rich repeat neuronal protein 1 (LINGO-1). LINGO-1 is a cell-surface glycoprotein expressed on CNS neurons and oligodendrocytes and inhibits oligodendrocyte differentiation, myelination, neuronal survival, and axonal regeneration.[41] In vitro and in vivo studies showed that LINGO-1 blockade facilitates axonal remyelination; however, the phase 2 study RENEW that included individuals with a first time episode of optic neuritis failed to show an improvement in the primary outcome of visual-evoked potentials.[42] SYNERGY, another phase 2 trial, failed to show improvement in the primary outcome of disability.[41]

A high-throughput screening approach identified several already available compounds, including antihistamine, that have the potential to stimulate OPC differentiation in vivo. Clemastine is a first-generation antihistamine that has been available over the counter since 1992. It readily crosses the blood-brain barrier and has been shown to promote remyelination through an effect on human OPCs.[43,44] ReBUILD is a phase 2, randomized, placebo-controlled, cross-over study that showed reduced latency in visual-evoked potentials in MS patients with chronic optic neuropathy.[43] Although this study demonstrated a significant reduction in the primary outcome, it is unclear if the reduction in latency translates to a clinically meaningful improvement in individuals. The overall success of the trial demonstrates the utility of a high-throughput screening approach for identifying potential therapies and introduced a new trial design for evaluating efficacy.

Mesenchymal stem cells (MSCs) are an area of interest in progressive disease for potential remyelination because of their ability to differentiate into various types of cells. These cells can be isolated from bone marrow, adipose tissue, umbilical cord, and other sources.[45] Neural progenitor cells less frequently differentiate into mesodermal cells, which makes them more attractive for transplantation in MS. Although MSCs do not appear to stay in the CNS for long after intrathecal injection (IT), they may have other effects, such as secretion of neurotrophic factors inducing axonal outgrowth and increasing cell survival.[45] One study of neural progenitor MSCs transplanted IT in 3 injections in MS patients showed improved median EDSS, strength, and bladder function.[46] There are currently several studies investigating the use of MSCs in progressive MS given intravenously (IV), IT, and in combination from both autologous and umbilical sources (IV studies: NCT01377870, NCT03778333, NCT02034188, NCT00395200, NCT01745783, NCT01056471, NCT02495766; IT studies: NCT01895439, NCT01933802, NCT03355365, NCT03822858, NCT03799718,

NCT03696485; comparing IV and IT: NCT02166021, NCT03069170). Although there is potential with MSC, there are several concerns, including the risk of infection, infusion-related toxicity, and theoretic risk of malignancy or ectopic tissue formation.[45] In addition, there remain several questions regarding appropriate dosing, route of administration, cell culture protocol, and storage procedures before these therapies should be considered in clinical practice.[47]

Neuroprotective Treatments

The goal of therapies aimed at neuroprotection is to prevent irreversible disability and slow progression. Studies to date have been limited and encompass medications with a variety of mechanisms of action, including simvastatin, phenytoin, ibudilast, α-lipoic acid (ALA), and metformin.

Simvastatin has been proposed as a potential neuroprotective agent because of evidence from animal models demonstrating its impact on multiple immunomodulatory effects. MS-STAT was a phase 2, randomized study of 80 mg simvastatin versus placebo in an SPMS population with a primary outcome of whole brain atrophy. The simvastatin group had a decreased rate of whole brain atrophy compared with placebo.[48]

Ibudilast inhibits cyclic nucleotide phosphodiesterases, toll-like receptor 4, and macrophage inhibitory factor and is able to cross the blood-brain barrier. SPRINT-MS was a phase 2 randomized trial of ibudilast compared with placebo with a primary outcome of rate of brain atrophy in a progressive MS population. Ibudilast had a significantly slower rate of brain atrophy compared with placebo.[49] This study also used 5 advanced imaging metrics as secondary outcomes that may help inform future clinical trials in progressive MS. Further studies of ibudilast would be needed to better understand the impact on clinical measures of disability progression.

There have been smaller studies investigating the potential neuroprotective effects of phenytoin, ALA, and metformin. Phenytoin is a voltage-gated sodium channel inhibitor, which is a mechanism that has been shown to have neuroprotective properties in preclinical trials.[50] One randomized, placebo-controlled phase 2 trial showed that patients with acute optic neuritis who were given phenytoin within 2 weeks of onset had 30% less retinal nerve fiber layer thinning compared with placebo.[50] The clinical relevance of this is not entirely clear, and there are potential serious adverse events with phenytoin administration, such as rash and interactions with other medications, thus limiting its use. ALA has potential neuroprotective effects, as it is a cofactor for the oxidation-reduction portion of mitochondrial reactions and with anti-inflammatory properties. A small phase 2 trial showed benefit in reducing the rate of brain atrophy with a trend toward improvement of the timed 25-foot walk compared with placebo.[51] Animal studies have suggested that metformin may exhibit neuroprotective effects by protecting against oxidative stress, inducing an anti-inflammatory profile by decreasing T helper 1 (Th1) and Th17 cells, while increasing regulatory T cells, and also may induce remyelination by improving OPC responsiveness.[38]

Finally, the Multiple Sclerosis Secondary Progressive Multi-Arm Randomisation Trial was a phase 2 trial that used a unique multiarm, parallel group randomized trial design to investigate the neuroprotective effects of 3 medications: amiloride, fluoxetine, and riluzole. These 3 compounds were chosen via a systematic review of available evidence of oral neuroprotective drugs that were tested in clinical trials in various neurologic diseases as well as in Experimental autoimmune encephalomyelitis (EAE) models that all have different mechanisms of action targeting axonal pathobiology. None of the medications were superior to placebo for the primary outcome of percentage brain volume change.[52]

All the studies to date evaluating the efficacy of a neuroprotective therapy in MS have demonstrated modest or negative results. The main advances that have emerged are new techniques to identify potential components, such as high-throughput screening, and novel trial designs and outcomes to better evaluate the potential neuro-protective effects.

DISCUSSION

MS treatments have greatly advanced since the first DMT approval in 1993. Most treatments continue to target inflammatory disease activity, but there remains a dearth of options for progressive disease with predominantly neurodegenerative pathologic condition. The multitude of treatment options has changed the landscape of MS man-agement, but ongoing research will help optimize the treatment approaches to maxi-mize the benefit and minimize the risks for individuals with MS. Finally, the field is developing new methods of identifying and assessing a medication's potential for remyelination and neuroprotection, which will lead to continued advancements.

DISCLOSURE

M.P. McGinley has served on scientific advisory boards for Genzyme and Genentech, receives research support from Novartis, and receives funding from a KL2 (KL2TR002547) grant from Clinical and Translational Science Collaborative of Cleve-land, from the National Center for Advancing Translational Sciences (NCATS) compo-nent of the NIH.

REFERENCES

1. Browne P, Chandraratna D, Angood C, et al. Atlas of multiple sclerosis 2013: a growing global problem with widespread inequity. Neurology 2014;83(11): 1022–4.
2. Wallin MT, Culpepper WJ, Campbell JD, et al. The prevalence of MS in the United States: a population-based estimate using health claims data. Neurology 2019; 92(10):e1029–40.
3. Lublin FD, Reingold SC, Cohen JA, et al. Defining the clinical course of multiple sclerosis: the 2013 revisions. Neurology 2014;83(3):278–86.
4. Interferon beta-1b is effective in relapsing-remitting multiple sclerosis. I. Clinical results of a multicenter, randomized, double-blind, placebo-controlled trial. The IFNB Multiple Sclerosis Study Group. Neurology 1993;43(4):655–61.
5. Placebo-controlled multicentre randomised trial of interferon beta-1b in treatment of secondary progressive multiple sclerosis. European Study Group on interferon beta-1b in secondary progressive MS. Lancet 1998;352(9139):1491–7.
6. La Mantia L, Di Pietranton C, Rovaris M, et al. Interferons-beta versus glatiramer acetate for relapsing-remitting multiple sclerosis. Cochrane Database Syst Rev 2016;(11):CD009333.
7. Naismith RT, Wundes A, Ziemssen T, et al. Diroximel fumarate demonstrates an improved gastrointestinal tolerability profile compared with dimethyl fumarate in patients with relapsing-remitting multiple sclerosis: results from the randomized, double-blind, phase III EVOLVE-MS-2 Study. CNS Drugs 2020;34(2):185–96.
8. Naismith RT, Wolinsky JS, Wundes A, et al. Diroximel fumarate (DRF) in patients with relapsing-remitting multiple sclerosis: interim safety and efficacy results from the phase 3 EVOLVE-MS-1 study. Mult Scler 2019. https://doi.org/10.1177/1352458519881761. 1352458519881761.

9. Giovannoni G, Comi G, Cook S, et al. A placebo-controlled trial of oral cladribine for relapsing multiple sclerosis. N Engl J Med 2010;362(5):416–26.
10. Kappos L, Radue EW, O'Connor P, et al. A placebo-controlled trial of oral fingolimod in relapsing multiple sclerosis. N Engl J Med 2010;362(5):387–401.
11. Kappos L, Bar-Or A, Cree BAC, et al. Siponimod versus placebo in secondary progressive multiple sclerosis (EXPAND): a double-blind, randomised, phase 3 study. Lancet 2018;391(10127):1263–73.
12. Cohen JA, Comi G, Selmaj KW, et al. Safety and efficacy of ozanimod versus interferon beta-1a in relapsing multiple sclerosis (RADIANCE): a multicentre, randomised, 24-month, phase 3 trial. Lancet Neurol 2019;18(11):1021–33.
13. Comi G, Kappos L, Selmaj KW, et al. Safety and efficacy of ozanimod versus interferon beta-1a in relapsing multiple sclerosis (SUNBEAM): a multicentre, randomised, minimum 12-month, phase 3 trial. Lancet Neurol 2019;18(11): 1009–20.
14. Gold R, Kappos L, Arnold DL, et al. Placebo-controlled phase 3 study of oral BG-12 for relapsing multiple sclerosis. N Engl J Med 2012;367(12):1098–107.
15. Fox RJ, Miller DH, Phillips JT, et al. Placebo-controlled phase 3 study of oral BG-12 or glatiramer in multiple sclerosis. N Engl J Med 2012;367(12):1087–97.
16. Confavreux C, O'Connor P, Comi G, et al. Oral teriflunomide for patients with relapsing multiple sclerosis (TOWER): a randomised, double-blind, placebo-controlled, phase 3 trial. Lancet Neurol 2014;13(3):247–56.
17. Miller DH, Khan OA, Sheremata WA, et al. A controlled trial of natalizumab for relapsing multiple sclerosis. N Engl J Med 2003;348(1):15–23.
18. Ryerson LZ, Foley J, Chang I, et al. Risk of natalizumab-associated PML in patients with MS is reduced with extended interval dosing. Neurology 2019; 93(15):e1452–62.
19. Yamout BI, Sahraian MA, Ayoubi NE, et al. Efficacy and safety of natalizumab extended interval dosing. Mult Scler Relat Disord 2018;24:113–6.
20. Hauser SL, Waubant E, Arnold DL, et al. B-cell depletion with rituximab in relapsing-remitting multiple sclerosis. N Engl J Med 2008;358(7):676–88.
21. Hauser SL, Bar-Or A, Comi G, et al. Ocrelizumab versus interferon beta-1a in relapsing multiple sclerosis. N Engl J Med 2017;376(3):221–34.
22. Montalban X, Hauser SL, Kappos L, et al. Ocrelizumab versus placebo in primary progressive multiple sclerosis. N Engl J Med 2017;376(3):209–20.
23. Cohen JA, Coles AJ, Arnold DL, et al. Alemtuzumab versus interferon beta 1a as first-line treatment for patients with relapsing-remitting multiple sclerosis: a randomised controlled phase 3 trial. Lancet 2012;380(9856):1819–28.
24. Epstein DJ, Dunn J, Deresinski S. Infectious complications of multiple sclerosis therapies: implications for screening, prophylaxis, and management. Open Forum Infect 2018;5(8):ofy174.
25. Cohen JA, Baldassari LE, Atkins HL, et al. Autologous hematopoietic cell transplantation for treatment-refractory relapsing multiple sclerosis: position statement from the American Society for Blood and Marrow Transplantation. Biol Blood Marrow Transplant 2019;25(5):845–54.
26. Parks NE, Flanagan EP, Lucchinetti CF, et al. NEDA treatment target? No evident disease activity as an actionable outcome in practice. J Neurol Sci 2017; 383:31–4.
27. Ontaneda D, Tallantyre E, Kalincik T, et al. Early highly effective versus escalation treatment approaches in relapsing multiple sclerosis. Lancet Neurol 2019;18(10): 973–80.

28. Thompson AJ, Banwell BL, Barkhof F, et al. Diagnosis of multiple sclerosis: 2017 revisions of the McDonald criteria. Lancet Neurol 2018;17(2):162–73.
29. Andersen O, Elovaara I, Farkkila M, et al. Multicentre, randomised, double blind, placebo controlled, phase III study of weekly, low dose, subcutaneous interferon beta-1a in secondary progressive multiple sclerosis. J Neurol Neurosurg Psychiatry 2004;75(5):706–10.
30. Secondary progressive efficacy clinical trial of recombinant interferon-beta-1a in MSSG. Randomized controlled trial of interferon- beta-1a in secondary progressive MS: clinical results. Neurology 2001;56(11):1496–504.
31. Leary SM, Miller DH, Stevenson VL, et al. Interferon beta-1a in primary progressive MS: an exploratory, randomized, controlled trial. Neurology 2003;60(1):44–51.
32. Wolinsky JS, Narayana PA, O'Connor P, et al. Glatiramer acetate in primary progressive multiple sclerosis: results of a multinational, multicenter, double-blind, placebo-controlled trial. Ann Neurol 2007;61(1):14–24.
33. Lublin F, Miller DH, Freedman MS, et al. Oral fingolimod in primary progressive multiple sclerosis (INFORMS): a phase 3, randomised, double-blind, placebo-controlled trial. Lancet 2016;387(10023):1075–84.
34. Kapoor R, Ho PR, Campbell N, et al. Effect of natalizumab on disease progression in secondary progressive multiple sclerosis (ASCEND): a phase 3, randomised, double-blind, placebo-controlled trial with an open-label extension. Lancet Neurol 2018;17(5):405–15.
35. Faissner S, Gold R. Progressive multiple sclerosis: latest therapeutic developments and future directions. Ther Adv Neurol Disord 2019;12. 1756286419878323.
36. Faissner S, Plemel JR, Gold R, et al. Progressive multiple sclerosis: from pathophysiology to therapeutic strategies. Nat Rev Drug Discov 2019;18(12):905–22.
37. Schwartzbach CJ, Grove RA, Brown R, et al. Lesion remyelinating activity of GSK239512 versus placebo in patients with relapsing-remitting multiple sclerosis: a randomised, single-blind, phase II study. J Neurol 2017;264(2):304–15.
38. Neumann B, Baror R, Zhao C, et al. Metformin restores CNS remyelination capacity by rejuvenating aged stem cells. Cell Stem Cell 2019;25(4):473–85.e8.
39. Tourbah A, Lebrun-Frenay C, Edan G, et al. MD1003 (high-dose biotin) for the treatment of progressive multiple sclerosis: a randomised, double-blind, placebo-controlled study. Mult Scler 2016;22(13):1719–31.
40. MedDay reports top-line data from phase III trial "SPI2" for treatment of progressive forms of multiple sclerosis. 2020. Available at: https://www.medday-pharma.com/2020/03/10/medday-reports-top-line-data-from-phase-iii-trial-spi2-for-treatment-of-progressive-forms-of-multiple-sclerosis/. Accessed March 10, 2020.
41. Cadavid D, Mellion M, Hupperts R, et al. Safety and efficacy of opicinumab in patients with relapsing multiple sclerosis (SYNERGY): a randomised, placebo-controlled, phase 2 trial. Lancet Neurol 2019;18(9):845–56.
42. Petrillo J, Balcer L, Galetta S, et al. Initial impairment and recovery of vision-related functioning in participants with acute optic neuritis from the RENEW trial of opicinumab. J Neuroophthalmol 2019;39(2):153–60.
43. Green AJ, Gelfand JM, Cree BA, et al. Clemastine fumarate as a remyelinating therapy for multiple sclerosis (ReBUILD): a randomised, controlled, double-blind, crossover trial. Lancet 2017;390(10111):2481–9.
44. Cohen JA, Tesar PJ. Clemastine fumarate for promotion of optic nerve remyelination. Lancet 2017;390(10111):2421–2.

45. Mansoor SR, Zabihi E, Ghasemi-Kasman M. The potential use of mesenchymal stem cells for the treatment of multiple sclerosis. Life Sci 2019;235:116830.

46. Harris VK, Stark J, Vyshkina T, et al. Phase I trial of intrathecal mesenchymal stem cell-derived neural progenitors in progressive multiple sclerosis. EBioMedicine 2018;29:23–30.

47. Baldassari LE, Cohen JA. Mesenchymal stem cell-derived neural progenitor cells in progressive multiple sclerosis: great expectations. EBioMedicine 2018;29:5–6.

48. Chataway J, Schuerer N, Alsanousi A, et al. Effect of high-dose simvastatin on brain atrophy and disability in secondary progressive multiple sclerosis (MS-STAT): a randomised, placebo-controlled, phase 2 trial. Lancet 2014;383(9936): 2213–21.

49. Fox RJ, Coffey CS, Conwit R, et al. Phase 2 trial of ibudilast in progressive multiple sclerosis. N Engl J Med 2018;379(9):846–55.

50. Raftopoulos R, Hickman SJ, Toosy A, et al. Phenytoin for neuroprotection in patients with acute optic neuritis: a randomised, placebo-controlled, phase 2 trial. Lancet Neurol 2016;15(3):259–69.

51. Spain R, Powers K, Murchison C, et al. Lipoic acid in secondary progressive MS: a randomized controlled pilot trial. Neurol Neuroimmunol Neuroinflamm 2017; 4(5):e374.

52. Chataway J, De Angelis F, Connick P, et al. Efficacy of three neuroprotective drugs in secondary progressive multiple sclerosis (MS-SMART): a phase 2b, multiarm, double-blind, randomised placebo-controlled trial. Lancet Neurol 2020; 19(3):214–25.

Advances in the Treatment of Neuromyelitis Optica Spectrum Disorder

Asya Izraelit Wallach, MD[a],*, Matthew Tremblay, MD, PhD[b],
Ilya Kister, MD[c]

KEYWORDS

- Neuromyelitis optica spectrum disorder • Treatment • Immunosuppression
- Complement inhibition • Anti-IL-6 therapy • Anti-CD20 therapy • Relapses

KEY POINTS

- Acute relapses in neuromyelitis optica spectrum disorder (NMOSD) require immediate treatment. Early deployment of high-dose steroids and plasmapheresis/immunoadsorption is associated with better long-term outcomes.
- Advances in the understanding of NMOSD pathogenesis and identification of the NMO-specific pathogenic autoantibody have led to the development of highly effective disease-modifying strategies.
- Randomized clinical trials support the use of B-cell depletion (rituximab, inebilizumab), interleukin-6 signaling blockade (tocilizumab, satralizumab), and complement inhibition (eculizumab) to decrease relapse rates in NMOSD.
- Mortality in the treated contemporary NMOSD cohorts has been considerably lower (3%–7%) than in the natural history studies (22%–30%).

INTRODUCTION

Neuromyelitis optica spectrum disorder (NMOSD) is a rare, relapsing-remitting neuro-inflammatory disorder of the central nervous system (CNS) usually associated with aquaporin-4 antibody (AQP4 Ab). The International Panel for Neuromyelitis Optica Diagnosis criteria recognizes 5 core syndromes of NMOSD, of which optic neuritis and longitudinally extensive myelitis are the most common.[1] Despite being an "orphan disease," NMOSD affects about 17,000 people in the United States,[2] and 5

[a] Alfiero and Lucia Palestroni MS Comprehensive Care Center, Holy Name Medical Center, 718 Teaneck Road, Teaneck, NJ 07666, USA; [b] MS Comprehensive Care Center, RWJ Barnabas Health, 200 South Orange Avenue, Suite 124-A, Livingston, NJ 07039, USA; [c] Department of Neurology, Comprehensive MS Center, NYU Grossman School of Medicine, 240 East 38th Street, New York, NY 10016, USA
* Corresponding author.
E-mail address: ASYAWALLACH@GMAIL.COM
Twitter: ASENKAMD (A.I.W.)

Neurol Clin 39 (2021) 35–49
https://doi.org/10.1016/j.ncl.2020.09.003
0733-8619/21/© 2020 Elsevier Inc. All rights reserved.

neurologic.theclinics.com

randomized, placebo-controlled phase 2 and phase 3 clinical trials for 5 different therapies have been successfully completed for NMOSD as of 2020.[3–7] These trials confirmed the efficacy of rituximab[3] and tocilizumab[4] and led to the Food and Drug Administration (FDA) approval of eculizumab,[5] inebilizumab,[6] and satralizumab[7] for NMOSD. These landmark trials cap 2 decades of remarkable progress in the understanding of the pathogenesis of NMOSD. During this short period, NMOSD has been transformed from an obscure, ill-defined, untreatable disorder with a dismal prognosis into a distinct nosologic entity with a highly specific serologic marker and a wide range of immunomodulatory and immunosuppressive treatment options.[8]

MANAGEMENT OF RELAPSES

Relapses in NMOSD tend to be more disabling than in multiple sclerosis (MS) and may lead to vision loss and paralysis, which are often only partially reversible. Traditionally, the inexpensive, widely available intravenous (IV) steroids are used first-line. In observational studies of NMOSD/MOG Ab seropositive optic neuritis, shorter time to treatment correlated with less retiral nerve fiber layer loss[9] and better visual outcomes.[10] However, there is no high-level evidence that steroids affect long-term outcomes.[11] For plasma exchange (PLEX), on the other hand, there is class I evidence for a long-term benefit on disability outcomes based on a pivotal randomized trial of PLEX versus sham PLEX in acute CNS inflammatory relapses recalcitrant to steroids.[12] Immunoadsorption (IA), an alternative to PLEX that does not require blood exchange, seems to have similar efficacy to PLEX.[13] Recent observational studies have shown that earlier use of PLEX/IA as an add-on to steroids in NMOSD is associated with lower long-term disability and a higher proportion of patients with complete recovery.[13–18] These data support prompt initiation of PLEX/IA in any NMOSD relapse that causes moderate-to-severe disability. The typical regimen is 5 to 7 cycles. Side effects of PLEX include complications of central venous catheter placement, which can be mitigated by using peripheral access instead; line infections; hypotension; bleeding due to depletion of coagulation factors; and electrolyte abnormalities. For the subset of patients with NMOSD who are positive for MOG Ab, a course of IV immunoglobulins (IVIg) has been successfully deployed during an acute relapse.[19,20] However, in randomized clinical trials of IVIg for optic neuritis,[21,22] treatment did not improve short- or long-term outcomes.[21,22] "Catastrophic relapses" that are refractory to steroids and PLEX may benefit from high-dose IV methotrexate.[23] Any patient with motor and gait deficits due to a relapse will benefit from a multidisciplinary rehabilitation program,[24] which should be started as soon as the feasible, preferably during the acute hospitalization.

DISEASE-MODIFYING THERAPIES: B-CELL DEPLETION THERAPIES

B-lymphocytes play a prominent role in the immunopathogenesis of NMOSD via AQP4 autoantibody production, enhanced proinflammatory B cell and plasmablast activity, and other mechanisms.[25] Therefore, B-cell depletion is a rational therapeutic strategy for NMOSD.

Rituximab

Rituximab is a chimeric murine/human monoclonal antibody against the CD20 surface molecule, which is found on pre-B cells, mature B cells, and memory B cells, but not on plasma cells. Rituximab was given to 8 patients with NMOSD in an open-label study in 2005 and was found to be safe and effective.[26] Subsequently, dozens of retrospective and prospective observational studies provided evidence for the effectiveness of rituximab in both pediatric[27] and adult NMOSD, both as a first-line therapy[28] and in refractory cases.[29-32] A meta-analysis of 26 studies of rituximab in NMOSD found that the annualized relapse rate was decreased by 1.56, with 63% of patients being free of relapses during the period of observation.[32] A larger metanalyses with 46 studies showed that treatment with rituximab decreased the annualized relapse rate ratio by 0.79 and Expanded Disability Status Scale (EDSS) by an average 0.64 to 1.2 points.[31] Possibly, even more impressive results could be achieved if all patients are treated to complete suppression of CD19+ (<0.1% of total lymphocytes) and CD27+ (<0.05% of total lymphocytes) cell counts. In a Korean study of 100 patients with NMOSD treated with rituximab with the goal of complete CD27+ (memory B cell) depletion, 70% of patients were relapse-free over a median period of more than 5 years, and the annualized relapse rate was just 0.1.[33] A recently published multicenter, blinded, randomized study of rituximab versus placebo, which enrolled 38 AQP4 Ab seropositive patients in Japan, documented relapses in 7 (37%) patients in the placebo arm and none (0%) in the rituximab arm during the 72-week study period (group difference 36·8%). There were no differences in the final EDSS scores in the 2 groups, but the more sensitive quantification of nerve and spinal cord impairment scores in patients assigned to the rituximab group was significantly better than in the placebo group.[3]

In clinical practice, variable dosing strategies are deployed. Induction is typically with 1000 mg doses 2 weeks apart, or 375 mg/m^2 weekly for 4 weeks, followed by a maintenance treatment of 500 mg to 1000 mg once (or twice) every 6 months. Treatment to CD19/CD27 suppression targets is recommended and may allow for lower doses or longer interdose intervals in some patients, especially those with lower body mass index. However, smaller doses are associated with a more rapid B-cell reconstitution, and more frequent B-cell monitoring may be required.[34-38] Caution is advised when initiating rituximab within weeks of an acute relapse, as disease exacerbation in the immediate postinfusion period has been reported, presumably due to a rituximab-induced proinflammatory cytokine surge.[39] The most common adverse reactions are nonsevere infusion reactions, which can be mitigated with pretreatment and slow titration, and infections. In a recent meta-analysis, the rate of serious infections and adverse reactions in adult patients with NMOSD was 2%, and the crude mortality rate was 1.6%.[31] In rituximab-treated children with neurologic diseases, serious infections were observed in 7.6% and mortality in 2%.[40] In a large case series of patients with MS and NMO treated with rituximab, the main risk factor for serious infection was nonambulatory status, which increased the risk of serious infections nearly 9-fold in comparison to fully ambulatory patients.[41] Rare complications such as serum sickness[42] and pyoderma gangrenosum[43] have been reported in patients treated with rituximab for neurologic indications.

Inebilizumab

CD19 and CD20 surface antigens are both found on immature B cells and memory B cells, but CD19 is also found on pro-B cells, plasmablasts, and most of the plasma cells.[44] As such, targeting CD19-positive cells could be a more potent strategy for controlling B-cell–mediated diseases than anti-CD20 therapy. Inebilizumab, a humanized, affinity-optimized, afucosylated IgG1 kappa monoclonal antibody against CD19 has undergone extensive clinical development for NMOSD culminating in a double-blind, placebo-controlled phase 2/3 trial (N-Momentum).[6] The trial enrolled 230 adults with active NMOSD (at least one attack requiring treatment the year before enrollment or 2 attacks in 2 years) and EDSS of 8 or less (restricted to bed/chair or better). The cohort was predominantly women (91%), with a mean age of 43 and 92% seropositive for AQP4 Ab. Approximately 2 out of 3 patients had prior exposure to disease-modifying therapies. The patients were randomized 2:1 into the active group (N = 174) or placebo (N = 56). In the active group, patients were treated with an induction dose of inebilizumab, 300 mg, IV 2 weeks apart, and then a maintenance dose of 300 mg every 26 weeks. Only 12% of participants receiving inebilizumab had an attack, compared with 39% of participants receiving placebo, with a relative risk reduction of 73%. Because of an unequal allocation of seronegative patients across groups (only 4 seronegative patients in the placebo group, none of whom had relapses), efficacy could not be interpreted in the seronegative subset. Serious adverse events were infrequent and similarly distributed during the treatment phase. No deaths occurred during the trial, but during the open-label period, 2 patients who were started on inebilizumab had died after developing new or worsening neurologic symptoms. Based on this trial, inebilizumab (Uplizna) has been FDA approved for NMOSD. Inebilizumab is contraindicated for patients with active hepatitis B and active or untreated latent tuberculosis. Immunoglobulin levels should be measured before and during treatment, as inebilizumab may cause hypogammaglobulinemia, which is a risk factor for recurrent infections or serious opportunistic infections, and may warrant consideration to stop treatment,[45] or, possibly, supplementation with IVIg to replete immunoglobulins.

DISEASE-MODIFYING THERAPIES: INTERLEUKIN-6 ANTAGONISTS

Several lines of evidence implicate interleukin-6 (IL-6) in the pathophysiology of NMOSD. IL-6 levels are increased in cerebrospinal fluid during NMOSD relapses, but not in MS relapses, nor in other neurologic disorders.[46] Only IL-6, among multiple cytokines, demonstrated significantly higher levels in the serum of patients with NMOSD compared with MS controls.[47] IL-6 promotes survival of a plasmablast population responsible for secreting anti-AQP4 antibodies, likely contributing to increased anti-AQP4 antibody titers.[48]

Tocilizumab

Tocilizumab (Actemra) is a humanized anti-IL-6 receptor monoclonal antibody approved for the treatment of rheumatoid arthritis, giant cell arteritis, juvenile idiopathic arthritis, and cytokine release syndrome. In 2013, several case reports documented the effectiveness of tocilizumab in NMOSD, including patients refractory to rituximab.[49–52] In an open-label pilot study of monthly tocilizumab IV infusions in patients who had experienced multiple relapses in the preceding year on immunosuppressants and corticosteroids, 5 of 7 participants achieved relapse freedom for at least 1 year.[53] In another observational study of 8 patients treated with tocilizumab as an add-on therapy for NMOSD,[54] tocilizumab reduced relapses by 90% compared with baseline, with most relapses occurring in patients receiving lower dosing or extended treatment intervals. An open-label randomized phase 2 trial (TANGO) included 118 patients with active NMOSD who were randomized 1:1 to either tocilizumab, 8 mg/kg, monthly IV infusions or azathioprine, 2 to 3 mg/kg, oral daily.[4] Analysis of the primary outcome of time to first relapse favored tocilizumab over azathioprine with a median of 78.9 weeks for tocilizumab versus 56.7 weeks for azathioprine. In the per-protocol analysis, 89% of tocilizumab-treated patients were relapse-free versus 52% on azathioprine at 60 weeks, an 81.2% risk reduction. Adverse events were mostly mild and observed at lower rates in the tocilizumab arm. A single death occurred in each arm of the study. Prescribing information includes warnings regarding the risk of tuberculosis, invasive fungal infections, and opportunistic infections, but these have been mostly reported in conditions that are commonly treated with multiple concurrent immunosuppressants. Gastrointestinal perforation may be a concern in at-risk patients, as IL-6 prevents apoptosis of the intestinal epithelium,[55] but has not been reported in NMOSD. Although studies on the effectiveness of tocilizumab in NMOSD used the IV preparation of the drug, a recent case series suggested that subcutaneous administration of tocilizumab was similarly efficacious[56] and has the advantage of at-home administration.

Satralizumab

Satralizumab (Enspryng) is a humanized anti-IL6 monoclonal antibody, which has been studied in 2 phase III randomized clinical trials for NMOSD, SAkuraSky, and SAkuraStar. In SAkuraSky, adolescents and adults with an EDSS less than or equal to 6.5 (bilateral crutches or better) were randomized 1:1 to receive either satralizumab, 120 mg, subcutaneously or placebo as add-on to baseline immunosuppression (azathioprine, mycophenolate, or glucocorticoids).[57] During the 96-week trial, there was a 62% relative reduction in relapses in the treated group, with 89% of patients remaining relapse-free on satralizumab compared with 66% in the placebo arm. Efficacy was more pronounced in seropositive participants, with a 79% relative risk reduction, compared with a 34% risk reduction in seronegative NMOSD. SAkuraStar tested satralizumab as monotherapy versus placebo for adults with active NMOSD and EDSS less than or equal to 6.5 and demonstrated a 55% relapse relative risk reduction compared with placebo,[7] with higher efficacy—a 74% relative risk reduction—when restricting the analysis to AQP4 seropositive participants, suggesting different pathophysiology in seronegative patients. Neither SAkuraSky nor SAkuraStar found a significant effect of satralizumab on secondary outcome measures of pain or fatigue. In SAkuraSky and SAkuraStar, overall infection rates, including serious infection and neoplasm rates, were similar in both arms. Injection reactions occurred in 12% to 13% of satralizumab-treated patients and 5% to 16% of placebo patients. There was no anaphylaxis and no mortalities in either trial.

Satralizumab is approved to treat adults and children with NMOSD in Japan and AQP4-positive adults in the United States. It is contraindicated in patients with hepatitis B and active or untreated latent tuberculosis. It is administered subcutaneously at weeks 0, 2, and 4, then monthly, with instructions on holding treatment in the event of active infection, elevated liver enzymes, or neutropenia.[58]

DISEASE-MODIFYING THERAPIES: COMPLEMENT INHIBITORS

Neuropathological analysis of acute lesions in NMO has shown extensive complement activation in a perivascular pattern.[59] These observations predated the discovery of a pathogenic autoantibody and led to the dual hypotheses that CNS vasculature may be an early and specific target of NMOSD and that complement activation plays an important role in the pathogenesis of the disease.[59] Both of these hypotheses were confirmed with the discovery of an NMOSD-specific autoantibody directed to an antigen on the blood-brain barrier—the AQP4 Ab—and demonstration of the spectacular efficacy of complement inhibitors in preventing relapses of NMOSD.

Eculizumab

Eculizumab (Soliris) is a humanized monoclonal antibody that binds plasma C5 and thereby blocks the formation of the cytotoxic membrane-attack complex and the generation of a proinflammatory C5a paracrine factor. An open-label study of eculizumab enrolled 14 AQP4 seropositive patients with NMOSD who collectively suffered 55 attacks in the 2 years preceding the trial (despite treatment in 10 of the patients).[60] During the 12-month on-trial period, 12 of the patients had no attacks and 2 patients had possible attacks but without worsening disability scores. Within 1 year of stopping eculizumab in the clinical trial, 5 patients experienced a total of 8 relapses despite restarting immunosuppressive therapies. Serious adverse events in treated patients included meningococcal sepsis in a patient who received prior immunization, and a fatal myocardial infarction during follow-up that was deemed unrelated to the study drug.

Following the very encouraging results of the open-label trial, eculizumab was tested in a phase III randomized double-blind, placebo-controlled trial that enrolled adult AQP4-positive patients with NMOSD with EDSS less than or equal to 7 (wheelchair-bound, or better) and highly active disease (at least 2 relapses in the prior year or 3 in the prior 24 months).[61] Patients were randomized 2:1 to eculizumab, 900 mg, IV weekly x 4 doses followed by 1200 mg every 2 weeks or to placebo infusions. All patients were allowed to continue prior oral immunosuppression during the trial. The primary endpoint—an adjudicated clinical relapse— occurred in 3% of patients in the eculizumab group and 43% of patients in the non-eculizumab group, yielding a 94% relative risk reduction. In a subset analysis of patients who were on concomitant immunosuppression, 4% of the eculizumab group and 54% of the non-eculizumab group of patients experienced a relapse. Serious adverse events included one death from pulmonary empyema in a patient on eculizumab and concomitant azathioprine. During the open-label extension trial involving 137 patients (282 patient-years), serious adverse events were reported in 36% of treated patients, including 2 cases of sepsis and 1 case of Neisseria gonorrhea infection[5] but no deaths. All subjects received meningococcal vaccination at the start of the trial, and there were no cases of meningococcal infection during either the trial or open-label follow-up period.

All patients who are starting eculizumab must receive the meningococcal vaccination (MenACWY and MenB) and be enrolled in the Risk Evaluation and Mitigation Strategy program (https://www.solirisrems.com/).[62] Widespread clinical use of this extremely effective medication has so far been limited by concerns about its safety, the need for bimonthly IV infusions, and high cost.

DISEASE-MODIFYING THERAPIES: BROAD-SPECTRUM IMMUNOSUPPRESSANTS

Multiple therapies with broad immunosuppressive properties have been used for NMOSD as monotherapy or in conjunction with low-dose corticosteroids. Low-dose corticosteroids have also been deployed as monotherapy, and there is limited evidence that corticosteroid doses greater than 10 mg/d may be protective against relapses.[63] Retrospective comparisons involving the different therapies are subject to confounding by indication and other biases and have produced mixed results. One study demonstrated the superiority of rituximab and mycophenolate mofetil (MMF) over azathioprine,[64] whereas another, albeit with a small number of azathioprine-treated cases, found that rituximab and azathioprine were more efficacious than MMF.[65] A prospective study of low-dose rituximab, azathioprine, and MMF found the 3 treatments to be of comparable efficacy, but MMF and rituximab were better tolerated.[66] Based on the randomized trials that allowed for oral immunosuppression in the "placebo" arms,[57,61] the efficacy of the older, broad-spectrum oral immunosuppressants is likely less robust compared with that of the more targeted approaches discussed earlier (B-cell depletion, IL-6 blockade, complement inhibition).

Azathioprine

Azathioprine is an antimetabolite, which causes a decrease in lymphocyte proliferation. Azathioprine was efficacious for NMOSD in doses of 2 mg/kg/d when used in conjunction with high-dose prednisone in a small open-label prospective cohort study.[67] In clinical practice, it is often used as monotherapy. Azathioprine has been widely prescribed for NMOSD, especially in resource-poor settings, although it seems to be less effective than rituximab[64,66,68,69] or tocilizumab.[4] Serious adverse events are hepatotoxicity and malignancies: lymphoma was observed in 3% of patients in a large NMOSD series.[70]

Mycophenolate Mofetil

MMF is a noncompetitive inhibitor of an enzyme essential for de novo synthesis of guanosine-5′-monophosphate, a purine nucleotide. MMF inhibits proliferation of lymphocytes and is used for the treatment of autoimmune conditions and the prevention of organ transplant rejection. Following a case report of MMF effectiveness in a patient with NMOSD,[71] a case series of 24 patients with NMOSD documented a decrease from baseline aldosterone-to-renin ratio (ARR) 1.28 to 0.09 posttreatment and stabilization of disability in 63% of patients. One death in a patient with severe NMOSD was recorded during the 29-month median follow-up.[72] A retrospective, multicenter Korean study[73] reported a decrease in the ARR in 88% of patients (median ARR improvement from 1.5 to 0) and EDSS improvement or stabilization in 91%. MMF seems effective in doses of 1750 mg to 2000 mg per day and may be used in conjunction with prednisone.[74] MMF has been associated with increased risk of lymphoma in transplant patients and nonmelanoma skin carcinomas, so routine dermatologic screening in patients on long-term therapy is advisable. Other known adverse events include infections, gastrointestinal symptoms, including ulcers and hemorrhage, and cytopenias. MMF is teratogenic—congenital malformations have been reported in 26% of live births and the risk of first-trimester pregnancy loss is 45% in exposed patients, thus women of childbearing age must be counseled accordingly before starting therapy.[75]

Methotrexate

Methotrexate is a dihydrofolate reductase inhibitor used in weekly oral doses for the treatment of rheumatoid arthritis, Crohn's disease, and other autoimmune diseases. The evidence for methotrexate in NMOSD comes from small observational studies, the largest of which included 14 patients.[76–79] The improvement in ARR ranged from 64% to 100%, and relapse freedom was attained in 22% to 75% of patients.[76,77,79] Patients should be monitored for bone marrow suppression and liver function. Rare serious adverse events include hepatotoxicity, pneumonitis, aplastic anemia, and opportunistic infections. Methotrexate is teratogenic and is not recommended for women of childbearing age when safer options are available.

Tacrolimus

Tacrolimus is an oral immunosuppressant that inhibits the intracellular calcineurin pathway required for T-cell activation and is widely used in organ transplantation and systemic autoimmune diseases. A Japanese retrospective cohort study of patients with NMOSD treated with "induction prednisolone" followed by tapering doses of prednisolone and tacrolimus in 25 patients, dosed 1 to 6 mg/d, achieved relapse freedom in 92%, with relapses only seen in patients with subtherapeutic serum concentrations.[80] A Chinese retrospective study of 25 patients with NMOSD treated with tacrolimus 2 to 3 mg/d (except for one pediatric patient treated with 1 mg/d) and concomitant prednisone in 60% of patients, found that tacrolimus decreased the ARR by 86% and improved the EDSS from 4.5 pretreatment to 2.3 at the last follow-up.[81] One patient died of a serious infection.[81] Tacrolimus prescribing information includes a boxed warning related to an increased risk of serious infections and malignancies.[82]

Mitoxantrone

Mitoxantrone inhibits topoisomerase II, an enzyme crucial in DNA repair, leading to a reduction in B- and T-cell counts. A recently published systematic review[83] of mitoxantrone in NMOSD identified 8 studies with 117 patients. Three of the five studies with pre- and posttreatment ARR reported significant improvement 6 months to 5 years following treatment. A comparison of AQP4 seropositive patients treated with rituximab, azathioprine/prednisolone, or mitoxantrone suggested a greater decrease in relapse rates with rituximab and azathioprine/prednisolone than with mitoxantrone.[84] Mitoxantrone is not widely used due to dose-limiting cardiotoxicity and risk of acute myeloid leukemia (incidence of nearly 1% in a large Italian series of patients with MS).[85] The risk of acute leukemia seems to be higher with a cumulative dose[86] greater than 60 mg/m^2, but acute leukemia was also reported in a patient with NMOSD who received a lower dose.[87]

Cyclophosphamide

Cyclophosphamide is an alkylating agent widely used in oncology. In a nonblinded prospective cohort study[88] of Chinese patients with NMOSD that included 119 patients treated with azathioprine, 38 with MMF, and 41 with IV cyclophosphamide, all in combination with oral steroids, the 3 drugs had a similarly positive effect in decreasing ARR during 15-month follow-up, but cyclophosphamide did not improve EDSS, whereas the other 2 treatments did. However, another group found cyclophosphamide to have poor efficacy; in a cohort of 7 patients treated with cyclophosphamide only 1 (14%) was clinically stable.[89]

AUTOLOGOUS HEMATOPOIETIC STEM CELL TRANSPLANT AS A DISEASE-MODIFYING THERAPY

Autologous hematopoietic stem cell transplant (AHSCT) is under investigation for NMOSD as well as many other autoimmune conditions. Results of the 2 larger studies of AHSCT for NMOSD were discrepant. In the European retrospective AHSCT registry that included 16 patients with NMOSD refractory to immunosuppressants, only 10% remained relapse-free at 5 years.[90] Yet, in the US-based clinical trial of 12 patients with NMOSD treated with AHSCT, 83% were relapse-free at 5 years.[91] Each study recorded one fatality. The differences in outcomes could be partially due to differences in the regimen—European Registry did not use rituximab, whereas the US group did—as well as differences in patient characteristics. Complications of AHSCT include neutropenic fever[91,92] and other serious infections that are estimated to occur at a rate of 0.2 per year per patient[91]; electrolyte abnormalities; blood pressure fluctuations; and emergence of new autoimmune diseases, including myasthenia gravis and hyperthyroidism.[91] Mortality from AHSCT improved considerably over the last several decades: the overall mortality after AHSCT was only 0.2% in 2012 to 2016.[93] Given the uncertainty of benefit and concerns of long-term safety, AHSCT should currently be restricted to carefully selected patients with NMOSD, preferably in the context of a research protocol.[94]

SUMMARY

Discovery of the NMO-specific antibody against AQP4 in 2004 was a watershed event in the history of NMOSD. AQP4-antibody testing allows for earlier diagnosis, redefinition of NMOSD,[1] and easier distinction from MS.[95] Distinguishing NMOSD from MS is critically important, as some of the MS disease-modifying therapies, including interferon β, fingolimod, and natalizumab, are ineffective in NMOSD and may even exacerbate the disease.[96–98] Anti-AQP4 antibody mediates its injurious effect in part through complement-dependent cytotoxicity.[95] Thus, the most effective therapeutic approaches in NMOSD involve depleting B cells, decreasing IL-6, which prolongs survival of AQP4 antibody–secreting cells,[48] and blocking complement activation. These strategies have now been rigorously proved in randomized clinical trials to decrease the relapse rate in NMOSD by 74% to 94%.[6,7,61] The older immunosuppressants and corticosteroids are still widely used for NMOSD, especially in resource-limited settings but will likely be increasingly replaced by the newer, more targeted and likely more efficacious therapies.

The remarkable advances in NMOSD therapeutics coincided with a dramatic decrease in mortality. In a large natural history study from the 1990s, 5-year survival in NMOSD was only 68%,[99] whereas a recent population-based study recorded a mortality of 3%. The success comes at a cost of life-long immunosuppression and increased risk of infections and other complications. The next frontier in NMOSD therapeutics is to move away from the "blunt hammer" of immunosuppression to "precise scalpels" that target the pathogenic AQP4 immunity leaving the rest of the immune system intact.[100] Various stratagems are being tested that involve inverse DNA, autoreactive T cells, dendritic cell vaccines, enhancement of regulatory T and B cell function, oral tolerizations, and others.[101,102] The importance of advancing these targeted immunomodulatory approaches to the clinical arena has never been more acute than at the time when this article is being written, at the height of the global COVID-19 pandemic.

CLINICS CARE POINTS

- There is strong evidence that early treatment with plasmapheresis (typically 5 – 7 courses) is associated with better long-term outcomes in NMOSD.
- Disease-modifying therapies should be deployed early in the disease, preferably after the first attack because they are likely to significantly impact the long term prognosis.
- Review the patient's vaccination history prior to starting lifelong immunosuppressant treatment. Live vaccines (eg. MMR) are not advised during treatment with rituximab, inebilizumab, tocilizumab or satralizumab. Two meningococcal vaccines are recommended prior to starting eculizumab at least 2 weeks prior to the first dose.

DISCLOSURE

Dr A.I. Wallach has received consulting fees from Biogen. She serves as a site investigator for trials by Biogen, Hoffman La-Roche, TG Therapeutics, and MedDay Pharmaceuticals. Dr M. Tremblay has received consulting fees from Biogen and Genentech. Dr I. Kister served on advisory boards for Biogen and Genentech and received consulting fees from Roche and research support for investigator-initiated grants from Sanofi Genzyme, Biogen, EMD Serono, National MS Society, and Guthy-Jackson Charitable Foundation.

REFERENCES

1. Wingerchuk DM, Banwell B, Bennett JL, et al. International consensus diagnostic criteria for neurcmyelitis optica spectrum disorders. Neurology 2015; 85(2):177–89.
2. Flanagan EP, Cabre P, Weinshenker BG, et al. Epidemiology of aquaporin-4 autoimmunity and neuromyelitis optica spectrum. Ann Neurol 2016;79(5): 775–83.
3. Tahara M, Oeda T, Okada K, et al. Safety and efficacy of rituximab in neuromyelitis optica spectrum disorders (RIN-1 study): a multicentre, randomised, double-blind, placebo-controlled trial. Lancet Neurol 2020;19(4):298–306.
4. Zhang C, Zhang M, Qiu W, et al. Safety and efficacy of tocilizumab versus azathioprine in highly relapsing neuromyelitis optica spectrum disorder (TANGO): an open-label, multicentre, randomised, phase 2 trial. Lancet Neurol 2020;19(5):391–401.
5. Wingerchuck DM. Long-term safety and effectiveness of eculizumab in neuromyelitis optica spectrum disorder. Paper presented at: ECTRIMS2019. 11-13 September 2019, Stockholm, Sweden.
6. Cree BAC, Bennett JL, Kim HJ, et al. Inebilizumab for the treatment of neuromyelitis optica spectrum disorder (N-MOmentum): a double-blind, randomised placebo-controlled phase 2/3 trial. Lancet 2019;394(10206):1352–63.
7. Traboulsee A, Greenberg BM, Bennett JL, et al. Safety and efficacy of satralizumab monotherapy in neuromyelitis optica spectrum disorder: a randomised, double-blind, multicentre, placebo-controlled phase 3 trial. Lancet Neurol 2020;19(5):402–12.
8. Kister I, Paul F. Pushing the boundaries of neuromyelitis optica: does antibody make the disease? Neurology 2015;85(2):118–9.
9. Nakamura M, Nakazawa T, Doi H, et al. Early high-dose intravenous methylprednisolone is effective in preserving retinal nerve fiber layer thickness in patients with neuromyelitis optica. Graefes Arch Clin Exp Ophthalmol 2010;248(12): 1777–85.
10. Stiebel-Kalish H, Hellmann MA, Mimouni M, et al. Does time equal vision in the acute treatment of a cohort of AQP4 and MOG optic neuritis? Neurol Neuroimmunol Neuroinflamm 20ˉ9;6(4):e572.
11. Gal RL, Vedula SS, Beck R. Corticosteroids for treating optic neuritis. Cochrane Database Syst Rev 2012;(4):CD001430.
12. Weinshenker BG, O'Brien PC, Petterson TM, et al. A randomized trial of plasma exchange in acute central nervous system inflammatory demyelinating disease. Ann Neurol 1999;46(6):878–86.
13. Kleiter I, Gahlen A, Borisow N, et al. Apheresis therapies for NMOSD attacks: A retrospective study of 207 therapeutic interventions. Neurol Neuroimmunol Neuroinflamm 2018;5(6):e504.
14. Abboud H, Petrak A, Mealy M, et al. Treatment of acute relapses in neuromyelitis optica: Steroids alone versus steroids plus plasma exchange. Mult Scler 2016; 22(2):185–92.
15. Kumawat BL, Choudhary R, Sharma CM, et al. Plasma Exchange as a First Line Therapy in Acute Attacks of Neuromyelitis Optica Spectrum Disorders. Ann Indian Acad Neurol 2019;22(4):389–94.
16. Bonnan M, Cabre P. Plasma Exchange in Severe Attacks of Neuromyelitis Optica. Mult Scler Int 2012;2012:1–9.

17. Mori S, Kurimoto T, Ueda K, et al. Short-term effect of additional apheresis on visual acuity changes in patients with steroid-resistant optic neuritis in neuromyelitis optica spectrum disorders. Jpn J Ophthalmol 2018;62(4):525–30.
18. Srisupa - Olan T, Siritho S, Kittisares K, et al. Beneficial effect of plasma exchange in acute attack of neuromyelitis optica spectrum disorders. Mult Scler Relat Disord 2018;20:115–21.
19. Hacohen Y, Banwell B. Treatment Approaches for MOG-Ab-Associated Demyelination in Children. Curr Treat Options Neurol 2019;21(1):2.
20. Elsone L, Panicker J, Mutch K, et al. Role of intravenous immunoglobulin in the treatment of acute relapses of neuromyelitis optica: experience in 10 patients. Mult Scler 2014;20(4):501–4.
21. Noseworthy JH, O'Brien PC, Petterson TM, et al. A randomized trial of intravenous immunoglobulin in inflammatory demyelinating optic neuritis. Neurology 2001;56(11):1514–22.
22. Roed HG, Langkilde A, Sellebjerg F, et al. A double-blind, randomized trial of IV immunoglobulin treatment in acute optic neuritis. Neurology 2005;64(5):804–10.
23. Beh SC, Kildebeck E, Narayan R, et al. High-dose methotrexate with leucovorin rescue: For monumentally severe CNS inflammatory syndromes. J Neurol Sci 2017;372:187–95.
24. Amatya B, Khan F, Galea M. Rehabilitation for people with multiple sclerosis: an overview of Cochrane Reviews. Cochrane Database Syst Rev 2019;(1):CD012732.
25. Bennett JL, O'Connor KC, Bar-Or A, et al. B lymphocytes in neuromyelitis optica. Neurol Neuroimmunol Neuroinflamm 2015;2(3):e104.
26. Cree BA, Lamb S, Morgan K, et al. An open label study of the effects of rituximab in neuromyelitis optica. Neurology 2005;64(7):1270–2.
27. Nosadini M, Alper G, Riney CJ, et al. Rituximab monitoring and redosing in pediatric neuromyelitis optica spectrum disorder. Neurol Neuroimmunol Neuroinflamm 2016;3(1):e188.
28. Zephir H, Bernard-Valnet R, Lebrun C, et al. Rituximab as first-line therapy in neuromyelitis optica: efficiency and tolerability. J Neurol 2015;262(10):2329–35.
29. Collongues N, Brassat D, Maillart E, et al. Efficacy of rituximab in refractory neuromyelitis optica. Mult Scler 2016;22(7):955–9.
30. Wong E, Vishwanath VA, Kister I. Rituximab in neuromyelitis optica: A review of literature. World J Neurol 2015;5(1):39–46.
31. Damato V, Evoli A, Iorio R. Efficacy and Safety of Rituximab Therapy in Neuromyelitis Optica Spectrum Disorders: A Systematic Review and Meta-analysis. JAMA Neurol 2016;73(11):1342–8.
32. Gao F, Chai B, Gu C, et al. Effectiveness of rituximab in neuromyelitis optica: a meta-analysis. BMC Neurol 2019;19(1):36.
33. Kim S-H, Jeong IH, Hyun J-W, et al. Treatment Outcomes With Rituximab in 100 Patients With Neuromyelitis Optica: Influence of FCGR3A Polymorphisms on the Therapeutic Response to Rituximab. JAMA Neurol 2015;72(9):989–95.
34. Ellrichmann G, Bolz J, Peschke M, et al. Peripheral CD19(+) B-cell counts and infusion intervals as a surrogate for long-term B-cell depleting therapy in multiple sclerosis and neuromyelitis optica/neuromyelitis optica spectrum disorders. J Neurol 2019;266(1):57–67.
35. Yang CS, Yang L, Li T, et al. Responsiveness to reduced dosage of rituximab in Chinese patients with neuromyelitis optica. Neurology 2013;81(8):710–3.

36. Greenberg BM, Graves D, Remington G, et al. Rituximab dosing and monitoring strategies in neuromyelitis optica patients: creating strategies for therapeutic success. Mult Scler 2012;18(7):1022–6.
37. Novi G, Bovis F, Capobianco M, et al. Efficacy of different rituximab therapeutic strategies in patients with neuromyelitis optica spectrum disorders. Mult Scler Relat Disord 2019;36:101430.
38. Ciron J, Audoin B, Bourre B, et al. Recommendations for the use of Rituximab in neuromyelitis optica spectrum disorders. Rev Neurol 2018;174(4):255–64.
39. Perumal JS, Kister I, Howard J, et al. Disease exacerbation after rituximab induction in neuromyelitis optica. Neurol Neuroimmunol Neuroinflamm 2015; 2(1):e61.
40. Dale RC, Brilot F, Duffy LV, et al. Utility and safety of rituximab in pediatric autoimmune and inflammatory CNS disease. Neurology 2014;83(2):142–50.
41. Vollmer BL, Wallach AI, Corboy JR, et al. Serious safety events in rituximab-treated multiple sclerosis and related disorders. Ann Clin Transl Neurol 2020. https://doi.org/10.1002/acn3.51136. Epub ahead of print. PMID: 32767531.
42. Wolf AB, Ryerson LZ, Pandey K, et al. Rituximab-induced serum sickness in multiple sclerosis patients. Mult Scler Relat Disord 2019;36:101402.
43. Parrotta E, Zhovtis Ryerson L, Krupp LB. It's not always an infection: pyoderma gangrenosum of the urogenital tract in two patients with multiple sclerosis treated with rituximab. ACTRIMS Forum. West Palm Beach, FL, February 27, 2020.
44. Chen D, Gallagher S, Monson NL, et al. Inebilizumab, a B Cell-Depleting Anti-CD19 Antibody for the Treatment of Autoimmune Neurological Diseases: Insights from Preclinical Studies. J Clin Med 2016;5(12):107.
45. Uplizna Prescribing Information. 2020. Available at: https://www.uplizna.com/Uplizna_Prescribing_Information.pdf. Accessed August 16, 2020.
46. Uzawa A, Mori M, Ito M, et al. Markedly increased CSF interleukin-6 levels in neuromyelitis optica, but not in multiple sclerosis. J Neurol 2009;256(12): 2082–4.
47. Uzawa A, Mori M, Arai K, et al. Cytokine and chemokine profiles in neuromyelitis optica: significance of interleukin-6. Mult Scler 2010;16(12):1443–52.
48. Chihara N, Aranami T, Sato W, et al. Interleukin 6 signaling promotes anti-aquaporin 4 autoantibody production from plasmablasts in neuromyelitis optica. Proc Natl Acad Sci U S A 2011;108(9):3701–6.
49. Kieseier BC, Stuve O, Dehmel T, et al. Disease amelioration with tocilizumab in a treatment-resistant patient with neuromyelitis optica: implication for cellular immune responses. JAMA Neurol 2013;70(3):390–3.
50. Araki M, Aranami T, Matsuoka T, et al. Clinical improvement in a patient with neuromyelitis optica following therapy with the anti-IL-6 receptor monoclonal antibody tocilizumab. Mod Rheumatol 2013;23(4):827–31.
51. Ayzenberg I, Kleiter I, Schroder A, et al. Interleukin 6 receptor blockade in patients with neuromyelitis optica nonresponsive to anti-CD20 therapy. JAMA Neurol 2013;70(3):394–7.
52. Lauenstein AS, Stettner M, Kieseier BC, et al. Treating neuromyelitis optica with the interleukin-6 receptor antagonist tocilizumab. BMJ Case Rep 2014;2014. bcr2013202939.
53. Araki M, Matsuoka T, Miyamoto K, et al. Efficacy of the anti-IL-6 receptor antibody tocilizumab in neuromyelitis optica: a pilot study. Neurology 2014; 82(15):1302–6.

54. Ringelstein M, Ayzenberg I, Harmel J, et al. Long-term Therapy With Interleukin 6 Receptor Blockade in Highly Active Neuromyelitis Optica Spectrum Disorder. JAMA Neurol 2015;72(7):756–63.

55. Kuhn KA, Manieri NA, Liu TC, et al. IL-6 stimulates intestinal epithelial proliferation and repair after injury. PLoS One 2014;9(12):e114195.

56. Lotan I, Charlson RW, Ryerson LZ, et al. Effectiveness of subcutaneous tocilizumab in neuromyelitis optica spectrum disorders. Mult Scler Relat Disord 2019; 39:101920.

57. Yamamura T, Kleiter I, Fujihara K, et al. Trial of Satralizumab in Neuromyelitis Optica Spectrum Disorder. N Engl J Med 2019;381(22):2114–24.

58. Enspryng Prescribing Information. 2020. Available at: https://www.gene.com/download/pdf/enspryng_prescribing.pdf. Accessed August 16, 2020.

59. Lucchinetti CF, Mandler RN, McGavern D, et al. A role for humoral mechanisms in the pathogenesis of Devic's neuromyelitis optica. Brain 2002;125(Pt 7): 1450–61.

60. Pittock SJ, Lennon VA, McKeon A, et al. Eculizumab in AQP4-IgG-positive relapsing neuromyelitis optica spectrum disorders: an open-label pilot study. Lancet Neurol 2013;12(6):554–62.

61. Pittock SJ, Berthele A, Fujihara K, et al. Eculizumab in Aquaporin-4-Positive Neuromyelitis Optica Spectrum Disorder. N Engl J Med 2019;381(7):614–25.

62. Avasarala J, Sokola BS, Mullins S. Eculizumab package insert recommendations for meningococcal vaccinations: call for clarity and a targeted approach for use of the drug in neuromyelitis optica spectrum disorder. CNS Spectr 2019;1–3 [Epub ahead of print].

63. Watanabe S, Misu T, Miyazawa I, et al. Low-dose corticosteroids reduce relapses in neuromyelitis optica: a retrospective analysis. Mult Scler 2007;13(8): 968–74.

64. Mealy MA, Wingerchuk DM, Palace J, et al. Comparison of relapse and treatment failure rates among patients with neuromyelitis optica: multicenter study of treatment efficacy. JAMA Neurol 2014;71(3):324–30.

65. Poupart J, Giovannelli J, Deschamps R, et al. Evaluation of efficacy and tolerability of first-line therapies in NMOSD. Neurology 2020;94(15):e1645–56.

66. Yang Y, Wang CJ, Wang BJ, et al. Comparison of efficacy and tolerability of azathioprine, mycophenolate mofetil, and lower dosages of rituximab among patients with neuromyelitis optica spectrum disorder. J Neurol Sci 2018;385: 192–7.

67. Mandler RN, Ahmed W, Dencoff JE. Devic's neuromyelitis optica: a prospective study of seven patients treated with prednisone and azathioprine. Neurology 1998;51(4):1219–20.

68. Nikoo Z, Badihian S, Shaygannejad V, et al. Comparison of the efficacy of azathioprine and rituximab in neuromyelitis optica spectrum disorder: a randomized clinical trial. J Neurol 2017;264(9):2003–9.

69. Bichuetti DB, Lobato de Oliveira EM, Oliveira DM, et al. Neuromyelitis optica treatment: analysis of 36 patients. Arch Neurol 2010;67(9):1131–6.

70. Costanzi C, Matiello M, Lucchinetti CF, et al. Azathioprine: tolerability, efficacy, and predictors of benefit in neuromyelitis optica. Neurology 2011;77(7):659–66.

71. Falcini F, Trapani S, Ricci L, et al. Sustained improvement of a girl affected with Devic's disease over 2 years of mycophenolate mofetil treatment. Rheumatology (Oxford) 2006;45(7):913–5.

72. Jacob A, Matiello M, Weinshenker BG, et al. Treatment of neuromyelitis optica with mycophenolate mofetil: retrospective analysis of 24 patients. Arch Neurol 2009;66(9):1128–33.

73. Huh SY, Kim SH, Hyun JW, et al. Mycophenolate mofetil in the treatment of neuromyelitis optica spectrum disorder. JAMA Neurol 2014;71(11):1372–8.

74. Jiao Y, Cui L, Zhang W, et al. Dose effects of mycophenolate mofetil in Chinese patients with neuromyelitis optica spectrum disorders: a case series study. BMC Neurol 2018;18(1):47.

75. Kylat RI. What Is the Teratogenic Risk of Mycophenolate? J Pediatr Genet 2017; 6(2):111–4.

76. Ng ASL, Tan K. Methotrexate is effective for the treatment of neuromyelitis optica spectrum disorders in Asian patients. Clin Exp Neuroimmunol 2015;6(2): 149–53.

77. Kitley J, Elsone L, George J, et al. Methotrexate is an alternative to azathioprine in neuromyelitis optica spectrum disorders with aquaporin-4 antibodies. J Neurol Neurosurg Psychiatry 2013;84(8):918–21.

78. Minagar A, Sheremata WA. Treatment of Devic's Disease with Methotrexate and Prednisone. Int J MS Care 2000;2(4):43–9.

79. Ramanathan RS, Malhotra K, Scott T. Treatment of neuromyelitis optica/neuromyelitis optica spectrum disorders with methotrexate. BMC Neurol 2014;14:51.

80. Tanaka M, Kinoshita M, Tanaka K. Corticosteroid and tacrolimus treatment in neuromyelitis optica related disorders. Mult Scler 2015;21(5):669.

81. Chen B, Wu Q, Ke G, et al. Efficacy and safety of tacrolimus treatment for neuromyelitis optica spectrum disorder. Sci Rep 2017;7(1):831.

82. Highlights of Prescribing Information. Available at: https://www.accessdata.fda. gov/drugsatfda_docs/label/2018/210115s000,050708s047,050709s040lbl.pdf. Accessed April 25, 2020.

83. Enriquez CAG, Espiritu AI, Pasco PMD. Efficacy and tolerability of mitoxantrone for neuromyelitis optica spectrum disorder: A systematic review. J Neuroimmunol 2019;332:126–34.

84. Jarius S, Aboul-Enein F, Waters P, et al. Antibody to aquaporin-4 in the long-term course of neuromyelitis optica. Brain 2008;131(Pt 11):3072–80.

85. Martinelli V, Cocco E, Capra R, et al. Acute myeloid leukemia in Italian patients with multiple sclerosis treated with mitoxantrone. Neurology 2011;77(21): 1887–95.

86. Ellis R, Boggild M. Therapy-related acute leukaemia with Mitoxantrone: what is the risk and can we minimise it? Mult Scler 2009;15(4):505–8.

87. Cabre P, Olindo S, Marignier R, et al. Efficacy of mitoxantrone in neuromyelitis optica spectrum: clinical and neuroradiological study. J Neurol Neurosurg Psychiatry 2013;84(5):511–6.

88. Xu Y, Wang Q, Ren HT, et al. Comparison of efficacy and tolerability of azathioprine, mycophenolate mofetil, and cyclophosphamide among patients with neuromyelitis optica spectrum disorder: A prospective cohort study. J Neurol Sci 2016;370:224–8.

89. Bichuetti DB, Oliveira EM, Boulos Fde C, et al. Lack of response to pulse cyclophosphamide in neuromyelitis optica: evaluation of 7 patients. Arch Neurol 2012;69(7):938–9.

90. Greco R, Bondanza A, Oliveira MC, et al. Autologous hematopoietic stem cell transplantation in neuromyelitis optica: a registry study of the EBMT Autoimmune Diseases Working Party. Mult Scler 2015;21(2):189–97.

91. Burt RK, Balabanov R, Han X, et al. Autologous nonmyeloablative hematopoietic stem cell transplantation for neuromyelitis optica. Neurology 2019;93(18): e1732–41.
92. Aouad P, Li J, Arthur C, et al. Resolution of aquaporin-4 antibodies in a woman with neuromyelitis optica treated with human autologous stem cell transplant. J Clin Neurosci 2015;22(7):1215–7.
93. Muraro PA, Martin R, Mancardi GL, et al. Autologous haematopoietic stem cell transplantation for treatment of multiple sclerosis. Nat Rev Neurol 2017;13(7): 391–405.
94. Sharrack B, Saccardi R, Alexander T, et al. Autologous haematopoietic stem cell transplantation in multiple sclerosis and other immune-mediated neurological diseases: guidelines and recommendations of the European Society for Blood and Marrow Transplantation and the Joint Accreditation Committee of the International Society for Cellular Therapy (4540). Neurology 2020;94(15 Supplement):4540.
95. Jarius S, Wildemann B, Paul F. Neuromyelitis optica: clinical features, immuno-pathogenesis and treatment. Clin Exp Immunol 2014;176(2):149–64.
96. Kim SH, Kim W, Li XF, et al. Does interferon beta treatment exacerbate neuro-myelitis optica spectrum disorder? Mult Scler 2012;18(10):1480–3.
97. Kleiter I, Hellwig K, Berthele A, et al. Failure of natalizumab to prevent relapses in neuromyelitis optica. Arch Neurol 2012;69(2):239–45.
98. Min JH, Kim BJ, Lee KH. Development of extensive brain lesions following fingo-limod (FTY720) treatment in a patient with neuromyelitis optica spectrum disorder. Mult Scler 2012;18(1):113–5.
99. Wingerchuk DM, Hogancamp WF, O'Brien PC, et al. The clinical course of neuromyelitis optica (Devic's syndrome). Neurology 1999;53(5):1107–14.
100. Steinman L, Axtell RC, Barbieri D, et al. Piet Mondrian's trees and the evolution in understanding multiple sclerosis, Charcot Prize Lecture 2011. Mult Scler 2013; 19(1):5–14.
101. Steinman L, Bar-Or A, Behne JM, et al. Restoring immune tolerance in neuromyelitis optica: Part I. Neurol Neuroimmunol Neuroinflamm 2016;3(5):e276.
102. Bar-Or A, Steinman L, Behne JM, et al. Restoring immune tolerance in neuromyelitis optica: Part II. Neurol Neuroimmunol Neuroinflamm 2016;3(5):e277.

Advances and Ongoing Controversies in Patent Foramen Ovale Closure and Cryptogenic Stroke

Joaquin B. Gonzalez, MD[a],*, Fernando D. Testai, MD, PhD[b]

KEYWORDS

- Cryptogenic stroke • Patent foramen ovale • PFO closure
- Embolic stroke of undetermined source

KEY POINTS

- Up to 25% of the general population have a patent foramen ovale (PFO).
- The sole presence of a PFO does not increase the risk of incident stroke.
- The prevalence of PFO is higher in patients with cryptogenic stroke than in those with stroke of known source.
- There is no good evidence to support transcatheter PFO closure in unselected patients with stroke.
- PFO closure should be considered in carefully selected patients with cryptogenic stroke, particularly in those who are young and have atrial septal aneurysm and/or large interatrial shunts.

INTRODUCTION

Cryptogenic stroke (CS) refers to the development of cerebral embolism that is not attributed to lacunar infarction, large-artery atherosclerosis, cardioembolism, or other determined cause after vascular, serologic, and cardiac evaluation.[1] The main drawback of this traditional definition is that the necessary work-up to diagnose CS is not specified. Also, according to the Trial of Org 10172 in Acute Stroke Treatment (TOAST) statement, a stroke can be considered cryptogenic if its origin is unknown despite extensive evaluation, the work-up is incomplete, or more than 1 mechanism can explain it.[1] With these limitations in mind, it is estimated that approximately 30% of

[a] Interventional Cardiology, Department of Cardiology, Advocate Illinois Masonic Medical Center, 3134 North Clark Street, Chicago, IL 60657, USA; [b] Stroke Section, Department of Neurology and Rehabilitation, University of Illinois College of Medicine at Chicago, 912 South Wood Street, Chicago, IL 60612, USA
* Corresponding author.
E-mail address: gonzalezjoamd@gmail.com

Neurol Clin 39 (2021) 51–69
https://doi.org/10.1016/j.ncl.2020.09.013
0733-8619/21/© 2020 Elsevier Inc. All rights reserved.

all strokes are cryptogenic.[2] In the Oxford Vascular Study, the prevalence of traditional atherosclerotic risk factors or comorbid atherosclerotic disease, represented by myocardial infarction, peripheral vascular disease, and carotid artery occlusive disease, is lower in CS than in individuals with other defined causes. In addition, up to 63% of the recurrent events in patients with CS remained cryptogenic after extensive work-up.[3] These observations suggest that CS is a defined stroke subtype that may require targeted preventive strategies.

During normal fetal development, a foramen ovale is necessary for the shunting of placental oxygenated blood from the right atrium to the left atrium, bypassing the high-resistance pulmonary circulation. Shortly after birth, the lungs expand and the resistance in the pulmonary circuit and right atrium decreases. As the blood starts to circulate through the lungs and the cardiac shunting decreases, different biochemical pathways cause the septum primum and the septum secundum to fuse. By the end of this process, the interatrial septum closes, leaving a remnant called foramen ovale. Autopsy studies have shown that in nearly 25% of the general population the closure of the foramen ovale is incomplete. The resultant atrial septal abnormality, called patent foramen ovale (PFO), functions as a valve that allows right-to-left shunting. Most PFOs are small and become apparent only after provocative maneuvers such Valsalva or cough. The prevalence of PFO in patients less than 55 years old with CS is higher than in those with stroke of known cause (40% vs 15%; $P<.001$). Although less pronounced, this also holds true for patients greater than or equal to 55 years old (28% for CS vs 12% for non-CS; $P<.001$).[4] Based on these observations, it was suggested that some CS could be caused by paradoxic embolism through a PFO and that stroke recurrence could be prevented by percutaneous PFO closure. An influential observational study that included 581 patients with stroke of unknown origin showed that PFO alone does not affect the rate of recurrent cerebrovascular events.[5] In comparison, a meta-analysis of 48 observational studies showed that the rate of recurrent neurologic events after CS or transient ischemic attack (TIA) is almost 6 times higher with medical therapy compared with percutaneous PFO closure.[6] These apparent discordant results could be explained, at least in part, by patient selection. In addition, several anatomic characteristics, including shunt severity, atrial septum hypermobility, and associated atrial septal aneurysm (ASA), increase the risk of stroke recurrence in patients with PFO. ASA, in particular, is far less common than PFO. ASA is defined as a greater than 10-mm to 15-mm bulging of the atrial septum into the right atrium, left atrium, or both caused by redundant atrial septal tissue. ASA is often found incidentally in healthy individuals. However, observational studies showed that the association of PFO with ASA increases 5 times the odds of initial stroke and almost 24 times the risk of recurrent stroke.[5,7,8] The pathogenesis of embolism in ASA has been attributed to paradoxic embolism through a coexistent PFO, associated atrial arrhythmias, and thrombus formation in the aneurysmal sac.

Six randomized clinical trials shed light on the role of percutaneous PFO closure in patients with CS (**Table 1**). This article reviews the methodologies used for the diagnosis and characterization of PFO, the evidence supporting percutaneous PFO closure in CS, and the characteristics of patients that may benefit from these interventions.

PATENT FORAMEN OVALE CLOSURE VERSUS MEDICAL TREATMENT

- The CLOSURE I Trial (Evaluation of the STARFlex Septal Closure System in Patients With a Stroke or TIA Due to the Possible Passage of a Clot of Unknown

Table 1
Randomized clinical trials comparing patent foramen ovale closure with medical treatment in the prevention of recurrent stroke in patients with cryptogenic cerebral ischemia

Study	n	Major Inclusion Criteria	Interventions	Primary Outcome	Average Follow-up (y)	Results HR or Relative Risk (95% CI)	Safety
CLOSURE[9]	909	• 18–60 y • CS or TIA • PFO	• PFO closure with STARFlex device • Antithrombotics (antiplatelet agents and/or anticoagulation)	Stroke or TIA, death from any cause during 30 d of the procedure or neurologic death	2	PFO closure: 23 events (5.5%) Antithrombotics: 29 events (6.8%) 0.78 (0.45–1.35); $P = .37$[a]	AF PFO closure: 5.7% Antithrombotics: 0.7% ($P<.001$)
PC[10]	414	• <60 y • CS or peripheral thromboembolism • PFO	• PFO closure with Amplatzer PFO Occluder • Antithrombotics (antiplatelet agents or anticoagulation)	Death, nonfatal stroke, TIA, or peripheral embolism	4.1	PFO closure: 9 events (3.4%) Antithrombotics: 18 events (5.2%) 0.63 (0.24–1.62); $P = .34$[a]	AF PFO closure: 2.9% Antithrombotics: 1.0% ($P = .16$)
RESPECT[11]	980	• 18–60 y • Cryptogenic ischemic stroke • PFO identified by transesophageal echocardiography	• PFO closure with Amplatzer PFO Occluder • Antithrombotics (antiplatelet agents or anticoagulation)	Nonfatal ischemic stroke, fatal ischemic stroke, or early death after randomization	2.6	PFO closure: 9 events (0.66 events per 100 patient-years) Antithrombotics: 16 events (1.38 events per 100 patient-years) 0.49 (0.22–1.11); $P = .08$[a]	AF PFO closure: 3.0% Antiplatelet: 1.5% ($P = .13$)
RESPECT Long-term outcomes[12]	—	—	—	—	5.9	PFO closure: 18 events (0.58 events per 100 patient-years) Antiplatelet: 28 events (1.07 events per 100 patient-years) 0.55 (0.31–0.999); $P = .046$[a]	—

(continued on next page)

Table 1
(continued)

Study	n	Major Inclusion Criteria	Interventions	Primary Outcome	Average Follow-up (y)	Results HR or Relative Risk (95% CI)	Safety
REDUCE[14]	664	• 18–59 y • Cryptogenic ischemic stroke within 180 d • PFO with a right-to-left shunt	• PFO closure with Helex Septal Occluder or Cardioform Septal Occluder • Antiplatelet alone	• Clinical ischemic stroke • New brain infarction (clinical or silent brain infarction on brain imaging)	3.2	Clinical ischemic stroke PFO closure: 6 strokes (1.4%) Antiplatelet: 12 strokes (5.4) 0.23 (0.09–0.62); *P* = .002[a] New brain infarction PFO closure: 22 events (5.7%) Antiplatelet: 20 events (11.3%) 0.51 (0.29–0.91); *P* = .04[b]	AF or flutter PFO closure: 6.6% Antiplatelet: 0.4% *P*<.001
CLOSE[16]	663	• 16–60 y • CS • PFO with associated ASA or large interatrial shunt[d]	• PFO closure with any device approved by the Interventional Cardiology Committee • Antiplatelet alone • Anticoagulation (warfarin [INR 2–3] or direct oral anticoagulants)	Fatal or nonfatal stroke	5.3	Closure vs antiplatelet PFO closure: no strokes (0%) Antiplatelet: 14 strokes (4.9%) 0.03 (0–0.26); *P*<.001[a] Anticoagulation vs antiplatelet Anticoagulation: 3 strokes (1.5%) Antiplatelet: 7 strokes (3.8%) 0.44 (0.11–1.48); *P* = .17[a]	AF or flutter PFO closure: 4.6% Antiplatelet: 0.9% *P* = .02 Major risk of fatal bleeding Anticoagulation: 5.3% Antiplatelet: 2.3% *P* = .18

Study	Sample	Inclusion Criteria	Intervention	Primary Outcome	HR	Results
DEFENSE-PFO[17]	120	• No age limit (mean age: 52 y) • CS • High-risk PFO (ASA, hypermobility of the atrial septum, or large PFO)[e]	• PFO closure with Amplatzer PFO Occluder • Antithrombotics (antiplatelet agents or anticoagulation)	Stroke, vascular death, or major bleeding	2.8	Primary outcome: PFO closure: no events (0%) Antithrombotics: 6 events (12.9%) P<.013[c] Ischemic stroke PFO closure: no events (0%) Antithrombotics: 5 events (10.5%) P<.023[c] AF or flutter PFO closure: 2 event (2.2%) Antiplatelet: none P = not provided Major risk of fatal bleeding Anticoagulation: 0% Antiplatelet: 2 events (2.5%) P = .15

Abbreviations: CLOSE, The PFO Closure or Anticoagulants Versus Antiplatelet Therapy to Prevent Stroke Recurrence; CLOSURE, Evaluation of the STARFlex Septal Closure System in Patients with a Stroke or TIA Due to the Possible Passage of a Clot of Unknown Origin Through a PFO; DEFENSE-PFO, Device Closure Versus Medical Therapy for CS Patients With High-Risk PFO; HR, hazard ratio; PC, PFO and Cryptogenic Embolism; REDUCE, The GORE Septal Occluder Device for PFO Closure in Stroke Patients; RESPECT, Randomized Evaluation of Recurrent Stroke Comparing PFO Closure to Established Current Standard of Care Treatment.

[a] Results expressed as HR (95% CI).

[b] Results expressed as RR (95% CI).

[c] HR not provided because of early termination resulting in smaller sample size than originally planned.

[d] Large shunt defined as more than 30 microbubbles on transthoracic echocardiogram or transesophageal echocardiography detected either spontaneously or during provocation maneuvers.

[e] Large PFO defined as greater than or equal to 2 mm.

Origin Through a PFO) was a multicenter, randomized, open-label trial that compared percutaneous closure plus medical therapy with medical therapy alone for the prevention of recurrent stroke in patients 18 to 60 years of age.[9] The study included 909 patients with recent CS or TIA, and the follow-up extended for 2 years. Subjects in the medical group were treated with aspirin (81 mg or 352 mg daily), warfarin (International Normalized Ratio [INR] 2.0–3.0), or both. The antithrombotic treatment was left at the discretion of the treating physician at each site. The closure group underwent treatment with the STAR-Flex Septal Occluder plus clopidogrel 75 mg daily for 6 months and aspirin 81 mg or 325 mg daily for 2 years. The primary outcome of stroke or TIA occurred in 5.5% in the closure group and 6.8% in the medical group (adjusted hazard ratio [HR], 0.78; 95% confidence interval [CI], 0.45–1.35; $P = .37$). The investigators concluded that PFO closure plus aspirin was not different to medical therapy alone for the prevention of stroke or TIA in patients with CS. The study had several caveats that are worth mentioning. The rate of atrial fibrillation (AF) was 5.7% in the closure group and 0.7% in the medical treatment group ($P<.0001$). More than half of the cases of AF in the closure group were periprocedural, suggesting that the procedure itself could predispose to AF. The rate of effective PFO closure was 86% and left atrial thrombus was observed in 1.1% of the patients in this group. Also, the evaluation of CS was not standardized and the enrollment in the study was hindered by patients' and physicians' preferences in favor of PFO closure. More importantly, almost a quarter of the strokes in the closure group occurred within the first 30 days after the procedures, suggesting that the events could represent a periprocedural complication associated with the device placement.

- The PC (Patent Foramen Ovale and Cryptogenic Embolism) trial was a randomized, open-label study that compared medical treatment with percutaneous closure of PFO for the prevention of recurrent stroke in patients with ischemic stroke, TIA, or peripheral thromboembolism of unknown origin.[10] The selection of antithrombotic in the medical group was left at the discretion of the treating team and could have included antiplatelet agents or anticoagulants. Subjects in the interventional group underwent closure with the Amplatzer PFO Occluder device and received treatment with acetylsalicylic acid (100–325 mg daily) as well as ticlopidine 250 to 500 mg daily or clopidogrel 75 to 150 mg daily for 6 months. A total of 414 subjects aged less than 60 years were randomized to PFO closure or medical treatment and followed for approximately 4 years. The primary efficacy end point of death, nonfatal stroke, TIA, or peripheral embolism occurred in 3.4% of the patients in the closure group and 5.2% of those in the medical group (HR, 0.63; 95% CI, 0.24–1.62; $P = .34$). The rate of stroke, which is a harder end point than TIA, was lower in the closure arm (1.5%) than in the medical arm (2.4%); however, this difference did not reach statistical significance ($P = .14$). Based on these findings, the investigators concluded that PFO closure is not superior to medical treatment in the prevention of recurrent embolism or death. The rate of new-onset AF was 2.9% in the closure group and 1.0% in the medical group ($P = .16$). In general, the study was limited by increased attrition and slow recruitment. In addition, there was indirect evidence that mild TIAs were more likely to be reported in the medical arm, raising the question of selective reporting bias.
- The RESPECT (Randomized Evaluation of Recurrent Stroke Comparing PFO Closure to Established Current Standard of Care Treatment) trial was a randomized, open-label study with blinded adjudication that compared PFO closure

with medical treatment in the prevention of recurrent stroke in patients with CS.[11] The primary outcome of the study was a composite of nonfatal ischemic stroke, fatal ischemic stroke, or early death after randomization. A total of 980 subjects aged 18 to 60 years were randomized to PFO closure or medical treatment. The average follow-up extended for 2.6 years. The medical arm allowed the use of antiplatelet agents and warfarin but the selection of antithrombotic treatment was not dictated by protocol. Subjects in the closure arm underwent PFO closure with the Amplatzer PFO Occluder device and received treatment with aspirin 81 to 325 mg daily plus clopidogrel for 1 month followed by aspirin alone for 5 months. In the intention-to-treat analysis, the rate of recurrent stroke was 0.66 per 100 patient-years in the closure arm and 1.38 per 100 patient-years in the medical arm (HR, 0.49; 95% CI, 0.22–1.11; P = .08). It is worth mentioning that 3 of the 9 strokes in the closure arm occurred without the device in place. Thus, in the prespecified per-protocol analysis, 6 strokes occurred in the closure arm and 16 in the medical arm (HR, 0.37; 95% CI, 0.14–0.96; P = .03). Also, in the as-treated analysis, 5 strokes occurred in the closure arm and 16 in the medical arm (HR, 0.27; 95% CI, 0.10–0.75; P = .007). Although the intention-to-treat analysis did not reach statistical significance, the overall results of the study suggested superiority of closure compared with medical treatment, particularly in individuals with ASA as well as those with large PFOs. In addition, the event rates in both arms were nonsymmetric, suggesting a trend for superiority in the PFO closure arm. Thus, the US Food and Drug Administration (FDA) requested additional long-term follow-up data before considering the approval of the Amplatzer Occluder for PFO closure. In 2017, the investigators published the results of the long-term outcomes. In the median follow-up of 5.9 years, the rate of recurrent stroke was 0.58 per 100 patient-years in the closure arm and 1.07 per 100 patient-years in the medical arm (HR, 0.55; 95% CI, 0.31–0.99; P = .046).[12] Also, the rate of recurrent CS adjudicated using the TOAST criteria was 0.03 per 100 patient-years in the closure arm and 0.41 per 100 patient-years in the medical arm (HR, 0.08; 95% CI, 0.01–0.58; P = .01). The rates of serious adverse events, including AF, were similar in both arms. RESPECT became a landmark study that showed the superiority of PFO closure with the Amplatzer PFO Occluder device compared with medical treatment in the prevention of recurrent stroke in patients with CS younger than 60 years. Based on these results, the FDA approved the use of Amplatzer Occluder for young patients with CS and PFO.[13] It is important to mention that, in a post hoc analysis, almost a third of the recurrent strokes were deemed to be unrelated to the PFO. This observation highlights the importance of patient selection, which should include comprehensive neurologic and cardiologic evaluation to exclude other stroke mechanisms.

- The REDUCE (The GORE Septal Occluder Device for PFO Closure in Stroke Patients) trial was a randomized, open-label study with blinded adjudication that compared transcatheter PFO closure plus medical treatment with medical treatment alone for the prevention of recurrent stroke in patients with cryptogenic cerebral ischemia.[14] A total of 664 subjects younger than 60 years were included in the study, and the follow-up extended for a minimum of 2 years and a maximum of 5 years. Compared with previous studies, the antithrombotic treatment in the medical arm was restricted to antiplatelet agents only. Subjects in the PFO closure arm received clopidogrel 75 mg daily for 3 days after the procedure. The subsequent antiplatelet treatment was not dictated by protocol. The only device permitted in the study was the Helex Septal Occluder, which, because of design refinements, was replaced by the Cardioform Septal Occluder. Patients were not eligible to participate in the study if they had uncontrolled vascular risk factors or a specific indication for anticoagulation. The coprimary end points were recurrent clinical ischemic stroke and incidence of new brain infarction, which was defined as clinical ischemic stroke or silent brain infarction detected on imaging. During the median follow-up period of 3.2 years, the rate of ischemic stroke was 1.4% in the PFO closure arm and 5.4% in the medical arm (effect size [ES], 0.23; 95% CI, 0.09 to 0.62; $P = .002$). Also, new brain infarction occurred in 5.7% of the subjects assigned to the PFO closure arm and 11.3% of those receiving antiplatelet treatment (ES, 0.51; 95% CI, 0.29–0.91; $P = .04$). In terms of safety, the rate of AF or atrial flutter was higher in the PFO group than in the medical group (6.6% vs 0.4%; $P<.001$). Almost 80% of the events occurred within 45 days of the PFO closure and about 60% resolved within 2 weeks of onset. In addition, 1.4% of the subjects in the PFO closure group had serious device-associated adverse events, including device dislocation and thrombosis. Based on the results of REDUCE, the FDA approved the GORE Cardioform Septal Occluder device for the prevention of recurrent stroke in patients between the ages of 18 to 60 years with PFO and CS presumed to be caused by paradoxic embolism.[15]

- The CLOSE (Patent Foramen Ovale Closure or Anticoagulants Versus Antiplatelet Therapy to Prevent Stroke Recurrence) trial was a 3-arm randomized, open-label study that compared PFO closure, antiplatelet treatment alone, and oral anticoagulation for the prevention of recurrent stroke in patients aged 16 to 60 years with CS.[16] Compared with previous studies, this trial included only subjects with PFO who had associated ASA, defined as aneurysm greater than or equal to 15 mm and excursion greater than 10 mm on transesophageal echocardiogram (TEE), or large interatrial shunt, defined as more than 30 microbubbles on transthoracic echocardiogram (TTE) or TEE detected in the left atrium either spontaneously or during provocative maneuvers. The antiplatelet arm received aspirin, clopidogrel, or aspirin plus extended-released dipyridamole. Subjects in the oral anticoagulant arm could be treated with vitamin K antagonist (target INR of 2–3) or direct oral anticoagulants. Subjects in the PFO closure arm were treated with aspirin 75 mg daily plus clopidogrel 75 mg daily for 3 months followed by single antiplatelet treatment. Although the particular occluder was not dictated by protocol, only medical devices approved by the Interventional Cardiology Committee were allowed in this study. A total of 664 patients were enrolled in the study, and the mean follow-up was 5.3 years. The primary outcome of fatal or nonfatal stroke occurred in 14 of the subjects assigned to the antiplatelet-only group, with a 5-year cumulative stroke risk of 4.9%. In comparison, there were no strokes in the PFO closure group (HR, 0.03; 95% CI, 0.00–0.26; $P<.001$). In the intention-to-treat analysis, there were 3 strokes in the anticoagulation arm and 7 in the antiplatelet arm, resulting in 5-year cumulative stroke risks of 1.5% and 3.8% for each arm, respectively. Despite the trend toward superiority in favor of anticoagulation rather than antiplatelet agents, the investigators did not pursue additional statistical analysis because they considered that the study was underpowered to compare these two groups. In terms of safety, the rate of AF was 4.6% in the closure arm and 0.9% in the antiplatelet arm. The slow recruitment, open-label nature of the study, and low number of primary events are important limitations of this trial. However, the results confirmed the superiority PFO closure compared with antiplatelet treatment in the prevention of stroke in young patients with CS and an associated ASA or large interatrial shunt. However, questions remain in relation to the superiority of anticoagulation compared with antiplatelet agents for the prevention of stroke in patients with this stroke subtype.

- In the DEFENSE-PFO (Device Closure Versus Medical Therapy for Cryptogenic Stroke Patients With High-Risk Patent Foramen Ovale) study, patients with CS with high-risk PFO were randomized to percutaneous PFO closure with the Amplatzer PFO Occluder or antithrombotic treatment.[17] High-risk PFO included PFO with associated ASA, hypermobile interatrial septum (excursion into either atrium of at least 10 mm), or size of the interatrial shunt at least 2 mm on TEE. The selection of the optimal antithrombotic treatment in the medical arm, including antiplatelet agents or warfarin, was left at the discretion of the treating group. Based on power analysis, the study planned to include 210 subjects. However, because of the positive results of the other aforementioned studies, recruitment was terminated early for patient safety and the final sample size was 120. In the 2-year follow-up, the primary outcome of stroke, vascular death, or major bleeding occurred in 6 subjects in the medical arm (2-year event rate of 12.9%) but there were no events in those randomized to PFO closure ($P = .013$). In subgroup analysis, there were 5 ischemic strokes in the medical arm (2-year event rate of 10.5%) but no strokes were reported in the PFO arm ($P = .023$). In terms of safety, 2 events of AF were identified in the PFO closure arm and none in the medical arm. In addition to slow recruitment, low number of participating centers, and early termination, which undermined power, DEFENSE-PFO has a few additional caveats that are worth mentioning. Compared with the other trials, older age was not an exclusionary criterion. Nonetheless, most of the randomized patients were young and the mean age was 51.8 years. Baseline characteristics in the control and treatment groups were comparable. However, patients in the PFO closure arm were, on average, 5 years younger than in the medical arm. In contrast, smoking and hypercholesterolemia were more frequent in the medical arm. Despite these limitations, the results of DEFENSE-PFO support the use of PFO closure in young patients with CS, particularly in those with high-risk features.

- Meta-analyses of randomized trials: a meta-analysis of the randomized trials mentioned earlier (n = 3440) showed that the rate of recurrent stroke in patients with CS and PFO is 2.0% after closure and 4.5% in those treated medically (relative risk [RR], 0.43; 95% CI, 0.21–0.90; $P = .024$).[18] In comparison, the rates of TIA and mortality were similar in both groups. Despite the substantial reduction in the RR of stroke of 51.5% in favor of PFO closure, the absolute risk reduction was modest (2.1%) and the number of procedures necessary to prevent 1 stroke in 3.7 years was 47.[19] In addition, new-onset AF or flutter was more common in the closure arm (4.3%) than in the medical arm (0.7%; $P<.001$).[18] In subgroup analysis, the superiority of PFO closure compared with medical treatment was greater in patients with substantial shunt (RR, 0.23; 95% CI, 0.11–0.48; $P<.001$) than in those without substantial shunt (RR, 0.94; 95% CI, 0.46–1.95; $P = .874$). Similarly, the effect of closure was more robust in patients with associated ASA (RR, 0.17; 95% CI, 0.06–0.53; $P = .002$) than in those without ASA (RR, 0.85; 95% CI, 0.43–1.68; $P = .65$). Most of the studies that investigated the role of anticoagulation for the prevention of stroke in patients with CS and PFO were not adequately powered. Three studies compared PFO closure with mixed antiplatelet and anticoagulation treatment (n = 2303), 1 study compared PFO closure with anticoagulation (n = 353), and 3 studies compared anticoagulation with antiplatelet agents (n = 503). A meta-analysis including these studies showed that anticoagulation may be equally effective to PFO closure and probably superior to antiplatelet agents for the prevention of stroke in patients with CS or TIA. However, anticoagulants confer a higher risk of hemorrhage than the other two approaches.[20]

DIAGNOSIS AND CHARACTERIZATION OF PATENT FORAMEN OVALE

PFO does not result in left-to-right shunt-related complications and is rarely associated with other diseases, such as stroke, migraine, platypnea-orthodeoxia, or provoked exercise desaturation. However, several factors increase the risk of stroke in patients with PFO. These factors include the presence of a hypermobile septum primum, known as ASA, increased shunt size, and anatomic characteristic, including a prominent eustachian valve or Chiari network. The likelihood of a PFO being related to an embolic event is also influenced by volume status and hemodynamic fluctuations that occur in relation to respirations and changes in intrathoracic pressures.

The diagnosis of a PFO can be done in different ways. A guidewire or catheter crossing the interatrial septum from the right atrium to the left atrium is the most accurate method for confirming the presence of a communication between the 2 chambers. This initial step is fundamental when treating these defects with percutaneous closure devices. However, despite its accuracy, cardiac angiography does not provide sufficient details for planning the procedure, including the type of defect or anatomic characteristics. Therefore, ancillary studies, such as TTE, TEE, cardiac computed tomography (CT), or cardiac MRI, are typically required.[21]

CLINICS CARE POINTS

> • Cardiac angiography does not typically provide sufficient details for planning the PFO closure.

TEE with color Doppler and agitated saline injection (bubble study) is considered the gold standard for the diagnosis of PFO. This technique permits evaluating the anatomy, size, and specific location of the defect as well as the presence of pulmonary shunts or an atrial septal defect, which can sometimes coexist with the PFO. The shunt size, in particular, can be estimated by direct measurement of the PFO length or by counting the number of microbubbles that cross from the right atria to the left atria after 3 to 6 cardiac cycles. The crossing of microbubbles, and the diagnosis of the PFO, can be enhanced by provocative maneuvers that can transiently increase the pressure in the right atrium, such as the Valsalva maneuver and cough. Different criteria have been used to quantify PFO size. However, in general, PFOs measuring more than 2 mm and those associated with more than 20 microbubbles in the left atrium after opacification of the right atrium are considered large.[22] The presence of a large PFO, ASA, prominent eustachian valve, or Chiari network are easily confirmed with TEE. All these details have risk stratification value and allow the planning of the therapeutic procedure, including the selection of the type, size, and number of devices. Studies comparing TEE with right heart catheterization for the detection of PFO have confirmed that TEE has a sensitivity of 91% to 100% and an accuracy of 88% to 97%. In comparison, TTE with bubble study has a sensitivity of approximately 50%. In addition, TTE lacks the ability to provide the anatomic details that could be obtained from a properly done TEE.[23]

CLINICS CARE POINTS

- PFOs more than 2 mm in size and those associated with more than 20 microbubbles are considered large.

Transcranial Doppler (TCD) with injection of agitated saline (bubble study) is another noninvasive tool that can be used for the diagnosis of right-to-left shunts. TCD has high sensitivity and low cost. However, it does not allow determining the exact location of the shunt (intracardiac vs extracardiac), nor does it give any anatomic information that could guide its definite treatment.[23,24]

Other imaging modalities that are worthwhile mentioning are cardiac CT and cardiac MRI. Both techniques are noninvasive and have excellent accuracy. However, they are not routinely used because they are more costly and, in the case of cardiac CT, expose patients to radiation and intravenous contrast with the consequent risk of nephrotoxicity.[22]

The authors believe that TEE is the study of choice if a PFO is suspected and its identification could change management. There is a variety of algorithms proposed by different groups and institutions, and some recommend using noninvasive and less expensive tests first, such as TTE. However, because of its low sensitivity and limited anatomic resolution, TTEs have to be complemented with a second modality, usually a TEE.[22,23] Thus, it is our opinion that TEE with color Doppler and bubble study is the study of choice because it is safe, highly accurate, and provides interventionists key information for planning the closure of the defect.

PATIENT SELECTION

Taken together, the results of the randomized clinical trials discussed earlier confirm that PFO closure is effective for the prevention of recurrent stroke in patients with CS and PFO. However, the enthusiasm generated by these studies is tempered by different methodological factors, which are summarized in **Box 1**. In addition, the negative results of CLOSURE and PC, the more stringent patient selection used in the positive studies (anticoagulants were not allowed in REDUCE and high-risk PFOs were required for CLOSE and DEFENSE-PFO), and the modest beneficial effect of PFO closure, highlighted by the number needed to treat of 47, raised concerns about the cost/benefit ratio of transcatheter interventions in unselected populations.

Box 1
Limitations of randomized clinical trials that have investigated the role of patent foramen ovale closure in cryptogenic stroke

- Open-label design
- Low number of primary outcomes
- Variable requirements to make the diagnosis of CS
- Short follow-up (particularly in CLOSURE I and RESPECT)
- Increased attrition
- Differential dropout rates in the interventional and the control groups
- Slow recruitment
- Early termination (DEFENSE-PFO)

Furthermore, albeit rare, PFO closure is not free of complications (**Box 2**). The most commonly reported complication is new-onset AF. Most studies have shown that AF is transient and resolves within weeks of the intervention. However, long-term studies addressing the potential recurrence of AF have not been performed. Thus, the detractors of transcatheter interventions claim that, albeit beneficial, PFO closure may replace a stroke risk factor with another that is potentially more severe. In this context, the appropriate selection of candidates for closure is of paramount importance.

The first step is the accurate diagnosis of cryptogenic embolism. Patients are usually young, lack typical vascular risk factors, and have a negative work-up for defined causes of stroke, including cardioembolism, artery-to-artery embolism, or lacunar infarction. Previous history of deep venous thrombosis or pulmonary embolism as well as onset of symptoms after a recent travel or Valsalva further increase the possibility of paradoxic embolism through a PFO. In contemporary medical practice, there is no consensus on what constitutes a reasonable work-up for CS. A 3-tier diagnostic algorithm has been proposed (**Fig. 1**); however, because CS is a diagnosis of exclusion, uncertainties exist in relation to the yield and cost-effectiveness of pursuing these extensive evaluations in all patients.[25] A new construct called embolic stroke of undetermined source (ESUS) was coined in 2014.[2] Compared with CS, where the diagnostic work-up is not specified, ESUS requires brain CT or brain MRI showing a nonlacunar infarct, precordial echocardiography, cardiac monitoring for at least 24 hours, and imaging of the extracranial and intracranial cerebral arteries. TEE is not required to diagnose ESUS. Thus, the left atrium is partially characterized and the aortic arch is not assessed. Despite this limitation, ESUS constitutes a subset of patients with CS who had a reasonable minimal work-up to exclude major causes of stroke.

CLINICS CARE POINTS

- The accurate diagnosis of cryptogenic stroke and careful patient selection are fundamental steps to determine eligibility for PFO closure.

The second step in patient selection requires addressing whether the PFO constitutes a pathogenic or an incidental finding. Several factors predict the risk of recurrent stroke in patients with PFO (**Table 2**).[26] The Risk of Paradoxical Embolism (RoPE) score is a screening tool that was developed and validated to estimate the likelihood of a PFO being associated with the pathogenesis of the CS. The RoPE score is composed of 6 variables and ranges from 0 to 10 points, with higher scores denoting

---

Box 2
Complications associated with patent foramen ovale closure

- AF and flutter
- Device migration and erosion
- Cardiac thrombosis
- Hematoma at the puncture site
- Periprocedural embolism
- Incomplete occlusion

Tier 1	
Brain imaging	MRI brain
	CT of the brain
Neurovascular imaging	MRA of head/neck
	CTA of head/neck
	Carotid duplex
	Transcranial Doppler ultrasonography
Cardiac assessment	Transthoracic echocardiography
	Transesophageal echocardiography
	12-lead electrocardiogram
	Inpatient cardiac telemetry
	24h Holter monitoring
Hematologic workup	Complete blood count
	Thrombin time/INR
	Partial thromboplastin time

 Negative work-up

Tier 2	
Neurovascular imaging	Catheter angiography
	Transcranial Doppler with microemboli detection
	Workup for vasculitis
Cardiac assessment	Prolonged (2–4 wk) cardiac monitoring
Hematologic workup	Hypercoagulable assessment

 Negative work-up

Tier 3	
Genetic testing	Mitochondrial diseases
	Fabry disease
	Cerebral autosomal dominant arteriopathy with subcortical infarcts and leukoencephalopathy (CADASIL)
	Other genetics causes of stroke
Cardiac assessment	Cardiac CT
	Cardiac MR
	Prolonged (1–3 y) loop recording
Hematologic workup	Workup for occult malignancy

 Negative work-up

Cryptogenic Stroke

Fig. 1. Proposed work-up for the diagnosis of CS. CTA, CT angiography. (*Data from* Saver JL. CLINICAL PRACTICE. cryptogenic stroke. *N Engl J Med*. 2016;374(21):2065-2074.)

Table 2
Predictors of recurrent cryptogenic stroke in patients with patent foramen ovale[26]

Variable	N	Number of Studies	Odds or HR (95% CI)
Older age	2171	4	1.47 (1.2–1.8)
ASA	630	5	3.0 (1.8 4.8)
Aspirin vs oral anticoagulants	1235	5	2.5 (1.1–6.1)
Coagulation disorders	258	2	2.75 (1.2–6.5)
Stroke at index	367	2	3.0 (1.4–6.5)
PFO size	334	2	3.0 (1.9–4.6)

Data from Pristipino C, Sievert H, D'Ascenzo F, et al. European position paper on the management of patients with patent foramen ovale. general approach and left circulation thromboembolism. *Eur Heart J.* 2018.

increased likelihood of the stroke being caused by the PFO (**Table 3**). Based on the analysis of a cohort of 3674 patients with CS, it was estimated that the PFO-attributable fraction for the index stroke increases from 0% for scores 0 to 3 to 88% for scores 9 to 10 (**Fig. 2**).[27] The exact cutoff to identify patients with CS in whom transcatheter closure is indicated has not been clearly identified. However, data obtained in a small cohort suggest that closure in patients with RoPE scores less than 7 should be carefully weighted.[28]

The 2019 European position statement on the management of PFO in patients with CS recommends estimating the probability that the PFO has a causal role in the occurrence of stroke and the risk of stroke recurrence before deciding on PFO closure versus medical management. It also stresses the importance of investigating for defined causes of stroke, in particular paroxysmal AF (**Table 4**). Furthermore, both the European position statement on the management of PFO and the 2019 consensus statement of the Society for Cardiovascular Angiography and Interventions recommend using a multidisciplinary approach for the optimal selection of candidates for PFO closure. This multidisciplinary team should include, at minimum, an interventional cardiologist skilled in the percutaneous treatment of cardiac structural defects and a neurologist with experience in the care of patients with stroke.[22] The

Table 3
Risk of paradoxical embolism score

Patient Characteristic	Points
No history of hypertension	1
No history of diabetes mellitus	1
No history of previous stroke or TIA	1
Nonsmoker	1
Cortical infarct on imaging	1
Age (y)	
18–29	5
30–39	4
40–49	3
50–59	2
60–69	1
≥70	0

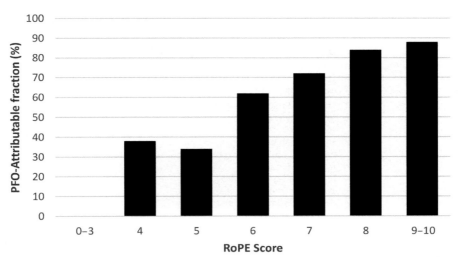

Fig. 2. PFO-attributable fraction for the index stroke based on the RoPE score. (*Data from* Kent DM, Ruthazer R, Weimar C, et al. An index to identify stroke-related vs incidental patent foramen ovale in cryptogenic stroke. *Neurology.* 2013;81(7):619-625.)

treatment of these patients should be individualized and counseling should include discussions about risks and benefits of percutaneous interventions as well as alternative approaches. **Fig. 3** shows a recommended algorithm for the selection of candidates for PFO closure based on the randomized studies discussed in this article.

Table 4
Highlights of the 2019 European position statement on the management of patients with patent foramen ovale[26]

General management	1. Interdisciplinary assessment and decision making are recommended
	2. Active involvement of the patient in the decision-making process is mandatory
	3. The decision making should take into account:
	a. Probability of a causal role of the PFO in the stroke
	b. Risk of stroke recurrence
	4. Risk stratification should take into account clinical, anatomic, and imaging characteristics
PFO diagnosis	1. The most sensitive technique should be used as a first line for the diagnosis of PFO
	2. TCD ultrasonography has a higher sensitivity than transthoracic echocardiography to detect right-to-left shunting
	3. Transesophageal echocardiography should be performed to stratify risk
Estimating the probability of a causal role of the PFO in the stroke	1. No single clinical, anatomic, or imaging characteristics are sufficient to quantify the probability of a PFO causal role
	2. PFO is more likely to have a causal role when patients are young and lack other stroke risk factors; however, the presence of vascular risk factors does not exclude a causative role of PFO
	3. ASA, shunt severity, and atrial septal hypermobility are associated with a causal role of PFO

(continued on next page)

Table 4 (*continued*)	
	4. Simultaneous pulmonary embolism and/or deep vein thrombosis suggest a causal role of PFO 5. The RoPE score should only be part of a comprehensive individual evaluation

Estimating stroke recurrence	1. The risk of recurrent embolism in unselected patients with PFO is low
	2. No single variable is sufficient to quantify the probability of stroke recurrence
	3. Some variables are associated with higher risk of recurrent stroke in patients with PFO (see **Table 2**)
	  a. Older age
	  b. ASA and/or PFO diameter
	  c. Aspirin vs oral anticoagulants
	  d. Coagulation disorders
	  e. Stroke at index
	  f. D-dimer >1000 at admission

AF rule-out strategy	1. All patients should undergo routine 12-lead electrocardiogram and either in-patient cardiac telemetry or 24-h Holter monitoring 2. In patients >65 y old with negative routine monitoring, it is reasonable to consider implantable cardiac monitoring before deciding on PFO closure or permanent oral anticoagulation 3. In patients 55–64 y old at risk for AF with negative routine monitoring, it is reasonable to consider implantable cardiac monitoring before deciding on PFO closure or permanent oral anticoagulation 4. In patients <55 y old with ≥2 high-risk factors for AF with negative routine monitoring, it is reasonable to consider implantable cardiac monitoring before deciding on PFO closure or permanent oral anticoagulation[a]
Position statements	1. Perform percutaneous closure of a PFO in carefully selected patients aged from 18 to 65 y with a confirmed CS, TIA, or systemic embolism and an estimated high probability of a causal role of the PFO as assessed by clinical, anatomic, and imaging features 2. Percutaneous closure of a PFO must be proposed to each patient evaluating the individual probability of benefit based on an assessment of both the role of the PFO in the thromboembolic event and the expected results and risks of lifelong medical therapy 3. The choice of device should take into consideration that most available evidence has been obtained with the AMPLATZER PFO Occluder or the GORE CARDIOFORM Septal Occluder. The use of the latter should be balanced against a lower complete closure rate and a higher risk of AF compared with medical therapy
Drug therapy after PFO closure	1. The choice of the type of antiplatelet drug in the follow-up is currently empiric 2. It is reasonable to use dual antiplatelet therapy for 1–6 mo after PFO closure 3. The authors suggest a single antiplatelet therapy be continued for at least 5 y

[a] High-risk factors include uncontrollable hypertension, structural heart abnormalities (left ventricular hypertrophy, left atrial enlargement), uncontrollable diabetes, and congestive heart failure.

Data from Pristipino C, Sievert H, D'Ascenzo F, et al. European position paper on the management of patients with patent foramen ovale. general approach and left circulation thromboembolism. *Eur Heart J.* 2018.

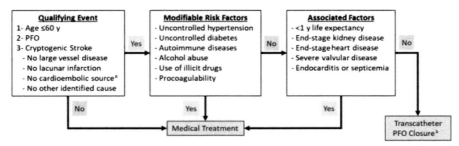

Fig. 3. Algorithm for PFO closure in patients with CS. [a] Consider performing extended cardiac monitoring to evaluate for paroxysmal AF or atrial flutter. [b] Enhanced reasons for PFO closure include large PFO with substantial shunt and associated ASA.

CLINICS CARE POINTS

- A multidisciplinary team composed, at least, by an interventional cardiologist and a vascular neurologist is recommended to determine if PFO closure is indicated.

SUMMARY

PFO is common in the general population and its sole presence does not increase the risk of incident stroke. There is no good evidence to support the closure of the heart defect in unselected patients. However, PFO closure should be given consideration rather than antiplatelet treatment in the prevention of recurrent stroke in young individuals with cryptogenic ischemia, particularly in those with high-risk PFOs.

DISCLOSURE

The authors have nothing to disclose.

REFERENCES

1. Adams HP Jr, Bendixen BH, Kappelle LJ, et al. Classification of subtype of acute ischemic stroke. definitions for use in a multicenter clinical trial. TOAST. trial of org 10172 in acute stroke treatment. Stroke 1993;24(1):35–41.
2. Hart RG, Diener HC, Coutts SB, et al. Embolic strokes of undetermined source: The case for a new clinical construct. Lancet Neurol 2014;13(4):429–38.
3. Li L, Yiin GS, Geraghty OC, et al. Incidence, outcome, risk factors, and long-term prognosis of cryptogenic transient ischaemic attack and ischaemic stroke: A population-based study. Lancet Neurol 2015;14(9):903–13.
4. Handke M, Harloff A, Olschewski M, et al. Patent foramen ovale and cryptogenic stroke in older patients. N Engl J Med 2007;357(22):2262–8.
5. Mas JL, Arquizan C, Lamy C, et al. Recurrent cerebrovascular events associated with patent foramen ovale, atrial septal aneurysm, or both. N Engl J Med 2001; 345(24):1740–6.
6. Agarwal S, Bajaj NS, Kumbhani DJ, et al. Meta-analysis of transcatheter closure versus medical therapy for patent foramen ovale in prevention of recurrent neurological events after presumed paradoxical embolism. JACC Cardiovasc Interv 2012;5(7):777–89.
7. Mas JL, Zuber M. Recurrent cerebrovascular events in patients with patent foramen ovale, atrial septal aneurysm, or both and cryptogenic stroke or transient

ischemic attack. french study group on patent foramen ovale and atrial septal aneurysm. Am Heart J 1995;130(5):1083–8.

8. Piechowski-Jozwiak B, Bogousslavsky J. Stroke and patent foramen ovale in young individuals. Eur Neurol 2013;69(2):108–17.

9. Furlan AJ, Reisman M, Massaro J, et al. Closure or medical therapy for cryptogenic stroke with patent foramen ovale. N Engl J Med 2012;366(11):991–9.

10. Meier B, Kalesan B, Mattle HP, et al. Percutaneous closure of patent foramen ovale in cryptogenic embolism. N Engl J Med 2013;368(12):1083–91.

11. Carroll JD, Saver JL, Thaler DE, et al. Closure of patent foramen ovale versus medical therapy after cryptogenic stroke. N Engl J Med 2013;368(12):1092–100.

12. Saver JL, Carroll JD, Thaler DE, et al. Long-term outcomes of patent foramen ovale closure or medical therapy after stroke. N Engl J Med 2017;377(11):1022–32.

13. FDA approves new device for prevention of recurrent strokes in certain patients. 2016. Available at: https://www.fda.gov/news-events/press-announcements/fda-approves-new-device-prevention-recurrent-strokes-certain-patients. Accessed July 02, 2019.

14. Sondergaard L, Kasner SE, Rhodes JF, et al. Patent foramen ovale closure or antiplatelet therapy for cryptogenic stroke. N Engl J Med 2017;377(11):1033–42.

15. GORE® CARDIOFORM septal occluder - P050006/S060. 2018. Available at: https://www.fda.gov/medical-devices/recently-approved-devices/gorer-cardioform-septal-occluder-p050006s060. Accessed July 02, 2019.

16. Mas JL, Derumeaux G, Guillon B, et al. Patent foramen ovale closure or anticoagulation vs. antiplatelets after stroke. N Engl J Med 2017;377(11):1011–21.

17. Lee PH, Song JK, Kim JS, et al. Cryptogenic stroke and high-risk patent foramen ovale: The DEFENSE-PFO trial. J Am Coll Cardiol 2018;71(20):2335–42.

18. Lattanzi S, Brigo F, Cagnetti C, et al. Patent foramen ovale and cryptogenic stroke or transient ischemic attack: To close or not to close? A systematic review and meta-analysis. Cerebrovasc Dis 2018;45(5–6):193–203.

19. Ntaios G, Papavasileiou V, Sagris D, et al. Closure of patent foramen ovale versus medical therapy in patients with cryptogenic stroke or transient ischemic attack: Updated systematic review and meta-analysis. Stroke 2018;49(2):412–8.

20. Mir H, Siemieniuk RAC, Ge LC, et al. Patent foramen ovale closure, antiplatelet therapy or anticoagulation in patients with patent foramen ovale and cryptogenic stroke: A systematic review and network meta-analysis incorporating complementary external evidence. BMJ Open 2018;8(7). https://doi.org/10.1136/bmjopen-2018-023761.

21. Hara H, Virmani R, Ladich E, et al. Patent foramen ovale: Current pathology, pathophysiology, and clinical status. J Am Coll Cardiol 2005;46(9):1768–76.

22. Horlick E, Kavinsky CJ, Amin Z, et al. SCAI expert consensus statement on operator and institutional requirements for PFO closure for secondary prevention of paradoxical embolic stroke: The american academy of neurology affirms the value of this statement as an educational tool for neurologists. Catheter Cardiovasc Interv 2019;93(5):859–74.

23. Mojadidi MK, Winoker JS, Roberts SC, et al. Accuracy of conventional transthoracic echocardiography for the diagnosis of intracardiac right-to-left shunt: A meta-analysis of prospective studies. Echocardiography 2014;31(9):1036–48.

24. Mahmoud AN, Elgendy IY, Agarwal N, et al. Identification and quantification of patent foramen ovale-mediated shunts: Echocardiography and transcranial doppler. Interv Cardiol Clin 2017;6(4):495–504.

25. Saver JL. Clinical practice. cryptogenic stroke. N Engl J Med 2016;374(21): 2065–74.
26. Pristipino C, Sievert H, D'Ascenzo F, et al. European position paper on the management of patients with patent foramen ovale. general approach and left circulation thromboembolism. Eur Heart J 2018. https://doi.org/10.1093/eurheartj/ehy649.
27. Kent DM, Ruthazer R, Weimar C, et al. An index to identify stroke-related vs incidental patent foramen ovale in cryptogenic stroke. Neurology 2013;81(7):619–25.
28. Prefasi D, Martinez-Sanchez P, Fuentes B, et al. The utility of the RoPE score in cryptogenic stroke patients. Int J Stroke 2016;11(1):NP7–8.

Advances and Future Directions of Neuromodulation in Neurologic Disorders

Matthew R. Burns, MD, PhD, Shannon Y. Chiu, MD,
Bhavana Patel, DO, Sotiris G. Mitropanopoulos, MD,
Joshua K. Wong, MD, Adolfo Ramirez-Zamora, MD*

KEYWORDS

- Deep brain stimulation • Epilepsy • Chronic pain • Dystonia • Chorea
- Tourette syndrome • Essential tremor • Parkinson disease

KEY POINTS

- Deep brain stimulation is a safe and effective therapy for a growing number of neurologic conditions.
- Neuromodulation advances include the development of directional leads, new programming and stimulation paradigms, closed loop capabilities, as well as an increasing number of controllable variables.
- New anatomic targets for neuromodulation are being explored for the treatment of complex neuropsychiatric conditions.

INTRODUCTION

Deep brain stimulation (DBS) is a safe and innovative neuromodulatory therapy applied in multiple neurologic disorders including movement disorders, dementia, epilepsy, neuropsychiatric conditions, and pain.[1] Although the mechanism of action of DBS is not entirely understood, advances in biomedical technology, neuroimaging, neuroanatomy, and neurophysiology have propelled research and adoption of neuromodulation in other conditions. Historically, DBS emerged as an alternative therapy to traditional neurosurgical lesioning treatments based on improved safety with bilateral procedures and reversible side effects.[2,3] In this review, the authors highlight some of the most current insights and advances in this rapidly evolving field.

The Fixel Institute for Neurological Diseases, Department of Neurology, The University of Florida, 3009 Williston Road, Gainesville, FL 32608, USA
* Corresponding author.
E-mail address: Adolfo.Ramirez-Zamora@neurology.ufl.edu

Neurol Clin 39 (2021) 71–85
https://doi.org/10.1016/j.ncl.2020.09.004
0733-8619/21/© 2020 Elsevier Inc. All rights reserved.

ADVANCES IN UNDERSTANDING OF MECHANISM OF ACTION

Since the introduction of DBS, a complete understanding of mechanisms of action has been elusive. Several hypotheses have been proposed despite our incomplete knowledge of related brain physiology.[4,5] The "inhibition" hypothesis proposes that DBS exerts a dampening effect on overactive neurons in the basal ganglia. DBS is thought to decouple local cell body activity from downstream axonal activity via a "functional lesion,"[6] and computational models reveal that DBS exerts local neuronal suppression as previously observed but also results in increased action potential propagation to downstream axons.[7] These ideas are based on animal studies showing excessive inhibition of the pallidum in Parkinson disease (PD) and a decrease in neuronal firing of the subthalamic (STN) nucleus with high-frequency stimulation (HFS),[8] leading to improvements in bradykinesia and rigidity.[9–12] The "jamming" hypothesis suggests that DBS disrupts the normal communication pathways of the basal ganglia, extending its effect beyond the regions immediately adjacent to the lead contacts. Observations on the physiologic responses to DBS over various stimulation frequencies, effects on neighboring neurons, and complex interactions based on physiologic recordings at multiple locations serve as the foundation for this hypothesis.[11,13–15]

In addition, recent studies of STN DBS in PD animal models have detected high-fidelity antidromic action potentials to the cortex along with preserved downstream activation of the globus pallidus (GPi).[16,17] Updates in computational modeling have led to an increase in model components, and the complexity of interactions between them suggests that DBS alters the real-time dynamics of neurotransmitter flow in the form of synaptic suppression at different brain network levels. As our understanding of these complex mechanisms continues to evolve, direct application in clinical practice or development of newer technology is expected.

PARKINSON DISEASE

PD is a progressive neurodegenerative disorder characterized by resting tremor, rigidity, bradykinesia, and postural instability. DBS has emerged as an effective therapy in PD for symptomatic management of medically refractory tremor, motor fluctuations, and/or troublesome dyskinesia superior to medical therapy alone.[18–20]

Briefly, suitable candidates include patients with diagnosis of idiopathic PD of at least 5 years, clear motor fluctuations with robust levodopa response without prominent cognitive impairment or neuropsychiatric symptoms.[21] DBS target selection should be individualized for every patient,[21,22] and several comparative, prospective, randomized studies have shown comparable motor benefit and quality of life between Gpi and STN targets.[22] Nonetheless, a variety of new therapeutic targets are currently under investigation in PD for treatment of freezing of gait, refractory tremor, or associated nonmotor symptoms (**Table 1**).

Recent technological advances in DBS include the development of DBS leads capable of current shaping or steering. DBS side effects occur when undesired tissues/pathways are stimulated (eg, muscle pulling from internal capsule stimulation or sensory changes related to stimulation of medial lemniscus). With traditional leads, complex programming strategies including bipolar or interleaving settings are used to minimize stimulation-induced side effects but may provide suboptimal symptomatic control. Newer DBS leads offer directional stimulation, avoiding undesired tissues/pathways while directing stimulation toward therapeutic regions. In addition, newer devices provide an expanded range of features to reduce side effects including lower pulse widths, shaping of stimulation using multiple independent current control,

Table 1
Emerging neuromodulation targets in Parkinson disease

Target	Indication
Centromedian and parafascicular thalamic complex	Refractory tremor[91]
Nucleus basalis of Meynert	PD dementia[92]
Pedunculopontine nucleus (PPN)	Freezing of gait,[93] sleep[94,95]
Substantia nigra pars reticulate (SNr)	Freezing of gait[96]
Spinal cord stimulation	Freezing of gait[97]
Caudal zona incerta	Refractory tremor[98]
Combined subthalamic nucleus and SNr	Freezing of gait[99]

anodic stimulation, newer leads designs, and programming using constant current versus voltage (**Table 2**).

New research shows promise improving motor outcomes using alternative pulse shapes such as patterned stimulation algorithms (eg, bursts of 0.1-s duration repeated at 5 Hz with an impulse width of 60 μs[23]) or square biphasic pulses to enhance the therapeutic window.[24,25] In addition, the development of adaptive closed-loop DBS has emerged as a promising new tool for motor and paroxysmal symptoms in PD.[4] Adaptive closed-loop approaches use individual patient's electrophysiological signature and pathology status to delivering customized stimulation, providing therapeutic benefit with fewer side effects and prolonging battery life. Research has identified abnormal brain coupling in the phase of activity in beta-frequency band (13–35 Hz) as a physiologic biomarker in PD that correlates with parkinsonian symptoms, and it is modulated by either dopaminergic treatment or DBS. Additional electrophysiologic biomarkers currently being investigated include narrowband gamma oscillation in the motor cortex between 60 and 90 Hz associated with dyskinesia,[5] the use of patterned stimulation using neural activity phase rather than just local field potentials (LFP),[8] or disruption of longer bursts of hypersynchronized beta activity (more pervasive oscillatory synchronization within the neural circuit).[9] Biomarker detection using machine learning control algorithms might be required and may need to adapt over time to compensate for neuroplasticity seen with disease progression. Development of external sensing devices and algorithms for tremor control[10] or freezing of gait and using stimulation-induced signals such as evoked resonant neural activity in STN DBS for programming and placement of DBS leads are under investigation as well.[10] Short-term studies of adaptive DBS in PD are promising thus far[7,26,27]; however, more studies are needed to evaluate long-term efficacy of adaptive DBS in PD, particularly addressing additional treatment-refractory symptoms such as postural instability, dysarthria, cognitive, and mood dysfunction.

ESSENTIAL TREMOR

Essential tremor (ET) is one of the most common adult-onset movement disorders, affecting nearly 10 million Americans.[28] ET classically involves postural and kinetic tremors of the hands and arms but can involve the head, voice, trunk, or legs. Approximately 50% of patients develop medication-refractory tremor and/or intolerable side effects from medications. For these patients, surgical therapy, primarily DBS of the ventral intermediate (VIM) nucleus of the thalamus, is an effective option.[11,29,30]

Table 2
Comparison of commercially available deep brain stimulation systems in the United States

System Features	Boston Scientific	Medtronic	Abbott
Number of lead contacts	1-3-3-1 segmented with current steering and multiple independent current control; 8 contacts/lead	1-1-1 segmented not available; 4 contacts/lead	1-3-3-1 segmented current shaping lead; 8 contacts/lead
Programming platform	Bionic Navigator software on touch screen interface with tissue activation, volume visualization, multiple independent current control, anodic stimulation	Samsung Galaxy tablet	iOS software wireless platform with Apple mobile digital devices as programming platforms
Programming features	Programmer connects through a wireless IR link	Wireless through Medtronic wireless close-range communicator	Wireless through Apple devices
Parameter control	2–250 Hz; 20–450 PW; 12.7 mA/contact max or 20 mA total max; up to 4 independent freq. ctrl/program	2–250 Hz; 60–450 PW; 10.5 V/25.5 mA max. No independent freq. ctrl	2–240 Hz; 20–500 PW, 12.75 mA max. up to 2 independent freq. ctrl
Battery	Dual-chamber Vercise primary cell and rechargeable Vercise Gevia	Single-chamber Activa SC and dual-chamber PC; rechargeable activa RC	Dual-chamber Abbott Infinity
Sensing	Not commercially available	NEXUS, PRECEPT, advanced sensing platform in development	Not commercially available
Wireless capability	3 feet	Not available	3–6 feet
MRI compatibility	Unavailable	Conditionally compatible	Conditionally compatible

Abbreviation: PW, pulse width.

Although some studies report decrease in tremor benefit over time, it remains unclear whether these longitudinal changes are due to disease progression, effects of atrophy, side effects from long-term stimulation, and/or due to disruption of neuronal oscillatory pathways within the tremor network.[12,13]

Although VIM DBS remains the primary target for ET, the posterior subthalamic area/caudal zona incerta (PSA/cZI) region has been proposed as an alternative target for stimulation in ET.[14] Few studies, however, have directly compared the efficacy of VIM versus PSA/cZI.[15,26,31] The proposed advantage of PSA/cZI stimulation relies on the notion that more effective stimulation can be delivered to compact, bundled white matter projections from the cerebellum before reaching the VIM, potentially improving axial symptoms as well.[27] Alternative surgical targets for neuromodulation of both ET and other complex, refractory tremor syndromes include dual lead placement in VIM and thalamic ventralis oralis anterior and posterior (Voa/Vop), STN, and GPi.[7] As a pallidal receiving area, Voa/Vop stimulation in conjunction with VIM has been used in the treatment of postural-action tremors alone or as a rescue lead for severe, refractory tremor.[16]

Newer technology including segmented electrodes may improve steering of current away from unintended tissue/pathways in the thalamus and toward VIM efferent and afferent projections for tremor suppression.[17] Meanwhile, the application of closed-loop DBS has been used in conjunction with central or peripheral sensors that detect abnormal brain activity during tremor states, thus delivering customized stimulation only at tremor onset.[6,32] Thalamic DBS for tremor has seen marked advances in technology with new methods to direct lead placement and connectivity assessments including anatomic (diffusion tensor imaging and tractography) and functional techniques (electrocardiogram, functional MRI, and invasive neurophysiological techniques including microelectrode recordings, LFPs, and electrocorticography). A combination of advances in both technology and lead localization has the potential to translate into further improvements in clinical outcomes.[33]

DYSTONIA

Dystonia is a movement disorder characterized by sustained or intermittent muscle contractions causing abnormal, often repetitive, movements, postures, or both. Several randomized blinded sham-controlled studies have demonstrated safety and efficacy of pallidal DBS in focal and segmental dystonia in children and adults.[34–36] The extent of benefit from DBS may depend on an individual's unique genetic background and phenotype.[37] Although posteroventral lateral GPi is currently the most common DBS target,[38] recent evidence supports efficacy in STN,[39–41] along with early reports stimulating the sensorimotor thalamus.[42] At present time, there are no comparative studies available, and unique side effects have been reported with evolving targets such as generalized dyskinesia with STN DBS and gait difficulties or weight gain with thalamic stimulation. There is enormous interest in identifying specific neurophysiological biomarkers for dystonia to aid with DBS programming and implantation, as programming is challenging, slow, and not standardized. A few series and reports point to possible abnormal electrophysiologic signals, primarily a high theta band activity in both deep basal ganglia structures and cortex.[43,44] Given the delayed but sustainable effects of long-term DBS stimulation in dystonia, even when DBS is turned off, the field has begun to examine the potential symptomatic and disease-modifying effect of earlier DBS intervention for dystonia. More research is needed in all these areas of dystonia research.

TOURETTE SYNDROME

Tourette syndrome (TS) is characterized by motor and phonic tics often associated with comorbid obsessive-compulsive disorder, attention-deficit hyperactivity disorder, impulsivity, depression, and anxiety.[45] Most of the individuals with TS experience an improvement in tics during late adolescence; however, tics may persist or become debilitating in about 20% of individuals.[46] For refractory, severe, or disabling tics DBS can be an effective treatment option. Thalamic DBS was first introduced as a treatment option for TS in 1999, and various targets have since been proposed and evaluated by expert centers worldwide with promising outcomes.[47,48] The most commonly used target is the medial thalamus (centromedian nucleus, parafascicular nucleus, ventralis oralis nucleus), but additional targets include anteromedial or posterior ventrolateral GPi, anterior internal capsule, nucleus accumbens, subthalamic nucleus, fields of Forel (H1), and globus pallidus externus.[49–57] A recent meta-analysis revealed decreased tic severity among all thalamic and pallidal targets, with a greater than 20% improvement in YGTSS scores. A greater than 50% improvement in tic severity scores was observed in 64% of individuals. Traditionally, DBS therapy for TS delivers continuous stimulation; however, adaptive DBS is of particular interest in disorders with paroxysmal symptoms such as TS. Newer technology might be needed to successfully deliver adaptive stimulation in TS; improved sensing capabilities, biomarkers, real-timer recording, and signal synchronization of DBS devices would be essential. In 2012 the International TS DBS Registry and Database was launched in association with the Tourette Association of America to create a worldwide registry to help answer these questions.[48,58] Currently there are 33 participating centers with 277 individuals with DBS for TS registered [https://tourettedeepbrainstimulationregistry.ese.ufhealth.org].

TARDIVE DYSKINESIA AND CHOREA

Chorea is defined as an irregular, nonstereotyped, involuntary movement that flow to adjacent body regions and is caused by a variety of neurodegenerative, drug-induced, autoimmune, vascular, and metabolic causes.[59–61] Medically refractory chorea has been managed primarily with pallidal DBS stimulation, although there are few reports of thalamic stimulation as well.[59] In Huntington disease, long-term benefit (up to 4 years) in chorea has been reported with a mean improvement in the Unified Huntington's Disease Rating Scale chorea subscore of 59.8% in single-case reports.[62,63] Additional case reports and small open-label studies suggest sustained and marked efficacy with pallidal DBS in chorea with DBS in other neurodegenerative conditions causing refractory chorea including neuroacanthocytosis.[64,65] Prolonged use of dopamine receptor-blocking agents can produce a variable syndrome of chorea, dystonia, and parkinsonism called tardive dyskinesia (TD). DBS has been evaluated in patients with refractory TD in a prospective, multicenter, double-blind, study showing adequate safety, tolerability, and efficacy using pallidal DBS in 10 patients with severe TD.[66] Long-term outcomes of the original cohort with the addition of 10 more cases were recently reported showing persistent safety and efficacy.[66]

DEMENTIA

Alzheimer disease (AD) is a neurodegenerative cognitive and memory disorder characterized by progressive pathologic accumulation of beta-amyloid plaques, neurofibrillary tangles of tau proteins, and neuronal cell death. Evidence implicates disruption of neural networks in the pathophysiology of disease,[67,68] and as a result, research efforts have begun to focus on DBS applications in AD attempting to modulate and disrupt aberrant signals that might contribute to neurodegeneration. Anatomic targets currently in clinical trials include the Fornix,[69,70] nucleus basalis of Meynert,[71,72] and ventral capsule/ventral striatum.[73] Preliminary evidence has shown that DBS of the fornix has possible benefit in patients older than 65 years in early stages, and new clinical trials are undergoing ADVANCE-2 (NCT03622905). Early, preliminary studies are investigating the role of DBS in other dementias.

EPILEPSY

Neurostimulation is primarily indicated in epilepsy when the patient meets criteria for drug-resistant epilepsy, defined by failure of rational polytherapy of at least 2 well-tolerated and appropriately chosen antiseizures drugs, and is a poor candidate for traditional surgical treatments.[74] There are a variety of neuromodulatory approaches to epilepsy, but the main modalities include DBS, responsive neurostimulation, and vagal nerve stimulation. Other emerging modalities for the treatment of epilepsy include repetitive transcranial magnetic stimulation, transcranial direct current stimulation, and external trigeminal nerve stimulation.

In the Electrical Stimulation of the Anterior Nucleus of Thalamus for treatment of refractory Epilepsy (SANTE) trial, the anterior nuclei (AN) of the thalami were selected as targets based on data showing at least a 50% reduction in seizure frequency.[75] The AN connect to the superior frontal and temporal lobe structures, which are areas involved in seizure onset and propagation. At 3 months, the stimulated group had a 29% reduction in seizure frequency over the control group (40.4% vs 14.5%).[75] At 2 years, 102 participants remained in the study and had a 56% median percent reduction in seizure frequency, of which 54% had at least a 50% reduction. The procedure was safe with no intracranial bleeding or infection, but the treatment arm included complaints of decreased mood and memory issues. At 5 years postimplantation, 75 participants remained active in the study, and the median improvement was 69%.[76] Eleven subjects reported seizure-free intervals of 6 months. Subgroup analysis based on seizure onset zone yielded a 76%, 59%, and 68% reduction in seizures from temporal lobe, frontal lobe, and other onset locations, respectively, at 5 years.[75] Other targets in DBS for epilepsy include the centromedian nucleus of the thalamus, the subthalamic nucleus, the hippocampus, and the cerebellum showing potential benefit with modulation of different nodes in the epileptic network; however, most studies were small with uncontrolled designs.[77]

PAIN

DBS has been applied to a variety of pain syndromes ranging from poststroke pain, spinal cord injury, brachial plexus injury, and headache.[78] There are 3 commonly targeted structures for neuromodulation of pain: (1) the thalamus, specifically the ventral posterolateral nucleus and ventral posteromedial nucleus (VPL/VPM), (2) the periventricular and periaqueductal gray (PVG/PAG), and (3) the anterior cingulate cortex (ACC). Neuromodulation of the VPL/VPM and PVG/PAG have been the most well established in the literature.[79–81] One longitudinal study of VPL/VPM and PVG/PAG DBS for various pain conditions revealed 59% of patients experienced significant acute pain relief.[81] After approximately 80 months of follow-up, 31% of patients continued to experience pain relief. In another study with up to 15 years of follow-up after VPL/VPM or PVG/PAG DBS for various pain syndromes, 62% of patients continued to experience adequate pain relief.[82] A meta-analysis of DBS for pain reported that modulation of the PVG/PAG alone or PVG/PAG with VPL/VPM or internal capsule was more effective than VPL/VPM alone. In addition, overall 58% of patients achieved pain relief. DBS was most effective in treating intractable low back pain and least successful in treating central thalamic pain/poststroke pain. Although central thalamic pain syndrome has historically been difficult to treat, Franzini and colleagues[83] recently investigated DBS of the posterior limb of the internal capsule in 4 patients. Three of four patients achieved long-term pain relief post-DBS. After a mean follow-up of 5.88 years, the average reduction in pain was 38% based on the 10-point visual analog scale.

Inspired by lesional therapies for cancer-related pain, ACC DBS has emerged as the newest potential target for pain.[84,85] Spooner and colleagues[86] published the first

Table 3
Other neurologic and psychiatric disorders managed with neuromodulation under investigation

Indication	Potential DBS Target	Trial[a]
Tinnitus	Auditory pathways Area LC VIM	Phase I–II
Major depression	SCC NAc Habenula Medial forebrain bundle VC/VS ITP BNST	Phase I–III
Obsessive-compulsive disorder	NAc STN BNST ITP ALIC VC/VS	Phase I–IV
Schizophrenia	Temporal cortex NAc VTA SCC	Preclinical/Phase I
Addiction	NAc STN	Phase I–III
Anorexia nervosa	SCC NAc ALIC	Phase I
Obesity	Lateral hypothalamus NAc	Phase I

This table lists some additional indications and targets not previously mentioned in this review.

Abbreviations: ALIC, anterior limb of the capsula interna; Area LC, locus of caudate neurons; BNST, bed nucleus of stria terminalis; ITP, inferior thalamic peduncle; NAc nucleus accumbens; VC/VS, ventral capsule/ventral striatum; VIM, ventral intermediate nucleus of the thalamus; SCC, subgenual cingulate cortex; STN, subthalamic nucleus; VTA, ventral tegmental area.

[a] Refer to clinicaltrials.gov for more details.

Data from Clinicaltrials.gov; and Budman et al. Potential Indications for Deep Brain Stimulation in Neurological Disorders: An Evolving Field. Eur J Neurol. 2018 Mar;25(3):434-e30; and Lee et al. Current and Future Directions of Deep Brain Stimulation for Neurological and Psychiatric Disorders. J Neurosurg. 2019 Aug 1;131(2):333-342; and Lozano et al. Deep Brain Stimulation: Current Challenges and Future Directions. Nat Rev Neurol. 2019 Mar;15(3):148-160.

case report of ACC DBS in 2007 in a patient with medically refractory neuropathic pain from a complete C4 spinal cord injury. At 3 months post-DBS implantation, the patient reported a 3 out of 10 on the pain visual analog scale compared with 10 out of 10 with DBS off. Since then, several other case reports have described success in ACC DBS for medically refractory neuropathic pain.[87–89] One recent study has showed some efficacy of ACC DBS for central thalamic pain.[90] In this study, 5 patients with medically refractory central thalamic pain syndrome underwent simultaneous bilateral ACC DBS. The investigators reported an average of 38% and 35% improvement of pain at 6- and 18-months post-DBS implantation, respectively.

DISCUSSION AND FUTURE DIRECTIONS

Recent advances in our understanding of brain neurophysiology in neurologic disorders, coupled with improved signal acquisition and delivery of neurostimulation, have propelled growing interest in the study and use of neuromodulation in neurologic and psychiatric conditions (**Table 3**). As detailed in previous sections, new research continues to shape the practice and future of neuromodulation in neurology. Collaborative, long-term, controlled trials are necessary to establish long-term safety, define appropriate candidates, and persistent efficacy. In response to issues arising from the development and application of DBS and other neurotechnologies, incorporating ethical principles and guidelines to research will continue to be crucial. The future is bright, and neuromodulation techniques will continue to increase our understating of pathologic brain states while helping patients around the globe.

ACKNOWLEDGMENTS

MRB acknowledges salary and research support from the Parkinson's; BP acknowledges salary and research support from the American Academy of Neurology. Also JKW's research is supported by R25 NS108939.

DISCLOSURE

There are no disclosures relevant to the content of this paper. Unrelated to the content of the paper, in the past year.

REFERENCES

1. Budman E, Deeb W, Martinez-Ramirez D, et al. Potential indications for deep brain stimulation in neurological disorders: an evolving field. Eur J Neurol 2018; 25(3):434–434.e30.
2. Hariz MI, Hariz GM. Therapeutic stimulation versus ablation. Handb Clin Neurol 2013;116:63–71.
3. Laitinen LV, Bergenheim AT, Hariz MI. Leksell's posteroventral pallidotomy in the treatment of Parkinson's disease. J Neurosurg 1992;76(1):53–61.
4. Little S, Pogosyan A, Neal S, et al. Adaptive deep brain stimulation in advanced Parkinson disease. Ann Neurol 2013;74(3):449–57.
5. Swann NC, de Hemptinne C, Miocinovic S, et al. Gamma Oscillations in the Hyperkinetic State Detected with Chronic Human Brain Recordings in Parkinson's Disease. J Neurosci 2016;36(24):6445–58.
6. Herron JA, Thompson MC, Brown T, et al. Chronic electrocorticography for sensing movement intention and closed-loop deep brain stimulation with wearable sensors in an essential tremor patient. J Neurosurg 2017;127(3):580–7.

7. Ramirez-Zamora A, Okun MS. Deep brain stimulation for the treatment of uncommon tremor syndromes. Expert Rev Neurother 2016;16(8):983–97.

8. Pina-Fuentes D, van Dijk JMC, Drost G, et al. Direct comparison of oscillatory activity in the motor system of Parkinson's disease and dystonia: A review of the literature and meta-analysis. Clin Neurophysiol 2019;130(6):917–24.

9. Tinkhauser G, Pogosyan A, Little S, et al. The modulatory effect of adaptive deep brain stimulation on beta bursts in Parkinson's disease. Brain 2017;140(4): 1053–67.

10. Ramirez-Zamora A, Giordano JJ, Gunduz A, et al. Evolving Applications, Technological Challenges and Future Opportunities in Neuromodulation: Proceedings of the Fifth Annual Deep Brain Stimulation Think Tank. Front Neurosci 2017;11:734.

11. Baizabal-Carvallo JF, Kagnoff MN, Jimenez-Shahed J, et al. The safety and efficacy of thalamic deep brain stimulation in essential tremor: 10 years and beyond. J Neurol Neurosurg Psychiatry 2014;85(5):567–72.

12. Favilla CG, Ullman D, Wagle Shukla A, et al. Worsening essential tremor following deep brain stimulation: disease progression versus tolerance. Brain 2012;135(Pt 5):1455–62.

13. Martinez-Ramirez D, Morishita T, Zeilman PR, et al. Atrophy and other potential factors affecting long term deep brain stimulation response: a case series. PLoS One 2014;9(10):e111561.

14. Blomstedt P, Sandvik U, Fytagoridis A, et al. The posterior subthalamic area in the treatment of movement disorders: past, present, and future. Neurosurgery 2009; 64(6):1029–38 [discussion: 1038–42].

15. Hamel W, Herzog J, Kopper F, et al. Deep brain stimulation in the subthalamic area is more effective than nucleus ventralis intermedius stimulation for bilateral intention tremor. Acta Neurochir (Wien) 2007;149(8):749–58 [discussion: 758].

16. Yamamoto T, Katayama Y, Kano T, et al. Deep brain stimulation for the treatment of parkinsonian, essential, and poststroke tremor: a suitable stimulation method and changes in effective stimulation intensity. J Neurosurg 2004;101(2):201–9.

17. Keane M, Deyo S, Abosch A, et al. Improved spatial targeting with directionally segmented deep brain stimulation leads for treating essential tremor. J Neural Eng 2012;9(4):046005.

18. Benabid AL, Pollak P, Gervason C, et al. Long-term suppression of tremor by chronic stimulation of the ventral intermediate thalamic nucleus. Lancet 1991; 337(8738):403–6.

19. Pollak P, Benabid AL, Gross C, et al. [Effects of the stimulation of the subthalamic nucleus in Parkinson disease]. Rev Neurol (Paris) 1993;149(3):175–6.

20. Siegfried J, Lippitz B. Bilateral chronic electrostimulation of ventroposterolateral pallidum: a new therapeutic approach for alleviating all parkinsonian symptoms. Neurosurgery 1994;35(6):1126–9 [discussion: 1129–30].

21. Almeida L, Deeb W, Spears C, et al. Current Practice and the Future of Deep Brain Stimulation Therapy in Parkinson's Disease. Semin Neurol 2017;37(2): 205–14.

22. Ramirez-Zamora A, Ostrem JL. Globus Pallidus Interna or Subthalamic Nucleus Deep Brain Stimulation for Parkinson Disease: A Review. JAMA Neurol 2018; 75(3):367–72.

23. Horn MA, Gulberti A, Gülke E, et al. A New Stimulation Mode for Deep Brain Stimulation in Parkinson's Disease: Theta Burst Stimulation. Mov Disord 2020;35(8): 1471.

24. De Jesus S, Almeida L, Shahgholi L, et al. Square biphasic pulse deep brain stimulation for essential tremor: The BiP tremor study. Parkinsonism Relat Disord 2018;46:41–6.
25. Akbar U, Raike RS, Hack N, et al. Randomized, Blinded Pilot Testing of Nonconventional Stimulation Patterns and Shapes in Parkinson's Disease and Essential Tremor: Evidence for Further Evaluating Narrow and Biphasic Pulses. Neuromodulation 2016;19(4):343–56.
26. Barbe MT, Reker P, Hamacher S, et al. DBS of the PSA and the VIM in essential tremor: A randomized, double-blind, crossover trial. Neurology 2018;91(6): e543–50.
27. Ramirez-Zamora A, Smith H, Kumar V, et al. Evolving Concepts in Posterior Subthalamic Area Deep Brain Stimulation for Treatment of Tremor: Surgical Neuroanatomy and Practical Considerations. Stereotact Funct Neurosurg 2016;94(5): 283–97.
28. Louis ED, Ottman R. How many people in the USA have essential tremor? Deriving a population estimate based on epidemiological data. Tremor Other Hyperkinet Mov (N Y) 2014;4:259.
29. Pahwa R, Lyons KE, Wilkinson SB, et al. Long-term evaluation of deep brain stimulation of the thalamus. J Neurosurg 2006;104(4):506–12.
30. Benabid AL, Pollak P, Gao D, et al. Chronic electrical stimulation of the ventralis intermedius nucleus of the thalamus as a treatment of movement disorders. J Neurosurg 1996;84(2):203–14.
31. Eisinger RS, Wong J, Almeida L, et al. Ventral Intermediate Nucleus Versus Zona Incerta Region Deep Brain Stimulation in Essential Tremor. Mov Disord Clin Pract 2018;5(1):75–82.
32. Tan H, Debarros J, He S, et al. Decoding voluntary movements and postural tremor based on thalamic LFPs as a basis for closed-loop stimulation for essential tremor. Brain Stimul 2019;12(4):858–67.
33. Ramirez-Zamora A, Giordano J, Boyden ES, et al. Proceedings of the Sixth Deep Brain Stimulation Think Tank Modulation of Brain Networks and Application of Advanced Neuroimaging, Neurophysiology, and Optogenetics. Front Neurosci 2019;13:936.
34. Krauss JK, Pohle T, Weber S, et al. Bilateral stimulation of globus pallidus internus for treatment of cervical dystonia. Lancet 1999;354(9181):837–8.
35. Volkmann J, Mueller J, Deuschl G, et al. Pallidal neurostimulation in patients with medication-refractory cervical dystonia: a randomised, sham-controlled trial. Lancet Neurol 2014;13(9):875–84.
36. Kupsch A, Benecke R, Müller J, et al. Pallidal deep-brain stimulation in primary generalized or segmental dystonia. N Engl J Med 2006;355(19):1978–90.
37. Jinnah HA, Alterman R, Klein C, et al. Deep brain stimulation for dystonia: a novel perspective on the value of genetic testing. J Neural Transm (Vienna) 2017; 124(4):417–30.
38. Moro E, LeReun C, Krauss JK, et al. Efficacy of pallidal stimulation in isolated dystonia: a systematic review and meta-analysis. Eur J Neurol 2017;24(4):552–60.
39. Ostrem JL, Racine CA, Glass GA, et al. Subthalamic nucleus deep brain stimulation in primary cervical dystonia. Neurology 2011;76(10):870–8.
40. Gupta A. Subthalamic stimulation for cervical dystonia. Acta Neurochir 2020; 162(8):1879.
41. Hua X, Zhang B, Zheng Z, et al. Predictive factors of outcome in cervical dystonia following deep brain stimulation: an individual patient data meta-analysis. J Neurol 2020. https://doi.org/10.1007/s00415-020-09765-9.

42. Pauls KA, Hammesfahr S, Moro E, et al. Deep brain stimulation in the ventrolateral thalamus/subthalamic area in dystonia with head tremor. Mov Disord 2014;29(7): 953–9.

43. Miocinovic S, de Hemptinne C, Qasim S, et al. Patterns of Cortical Synchronization in Isolated Dystonia Compared With Parkinson Disease. JAMA Neurol 2015; 72(11):1244–51.

44. Miocinovic S, Swann NC, de Hemptinne C, et al. Cortical gamma oscillations in isolated dystonia. Parkinsonism Relat Disord 2018;49:104–5.

45. Robertson MM. The Gilles de la Tourette syndrome: the current status. Br J Psychiatry 1989;154:147–69.

46. Cath DC, Hedderly T, Ludolph AG, et al. European clinical guidelines for Tourette syndrome and other tic disorders. Part I: assessment. Eur Child Adolesc Psychiatry 2011;20:155–71.

47. Vandewalle V, van der Linden C, Groenewegen HJ, et al. Stereotactic treatment of Gilles de la Tourette syndrome by high frequency stimulation of thalamus. Lancet 1999;353:724.

48. Deeb W, Rossi PJ, Porta M, et al. The International Deep Brain Stimulation Registry and Database for Gilles de la Tourette Syndrome: How Does It Work? Front Neurosci 2016;10:170.

49. Cavanna AE, Eddy CM, Mitchell R, et al. An approach to deep brain stimulation for severe treatment-refractory Tourette syndrome: the UK perspective. Br J Neurosurg 2011;25:38–44.

50. Dehning S, Mehrkens JH, Muller N, et al. Therapy-refractory Tourette syndrome: beneficial outcome with globus pallidus internus deep brain stimulation. Mov Disord 2008;23:1300–2.

51. Massano J, Sousa C, Foltynie T, et al. Successful pallidal deep brain stimulation in 15-year-old with Tourette syndrome: 2-year follow-up. J Neurol 2013;260:2417–9.

52. Flaherty AW, Williams ZM, Amirnovin R, et al. Deep brain stimulation of the anterior internal capsule for the treatment of Tourette syndrome: technical case report. Neurosurgery 2005;57:E403 [discussion: E403].

53. Kuhn J, Lenartz D, Mai JK, et al. Deep brain stimulation of the nucleus accumbens and the internal capsule in therapeutically refractory Tourette-syndrome. J Neurol 2007;254:963–5.

54. Martinez-Torres I, Hariz MI, Zrinzo L, et al. Improvement of tics after subthalamic nucleus deep brain stimulation. Neurology 2009;72:1787–9.

55. Piedimonte F, Andreani JC, Piedimonte L, et al. Behavioral and motor improvement after deep brain stimulation of the globus pallidus externus in a case of Tourette's syndrome. Neuromodulation 2013;16:55–8 [discussion: 58].

56. Maciunas RJ, Maddux BN, Riley DE, et al. Prospective randomized double-blind trial of bilateral thalamic deep brain stimulation in adults with Tourette syndrome. J Neurosurg 2007;107:1004–14.

57. Neudorfer C, El Majdoub F, Hunsche S, et al. Deep Brain Stimulation of the H Fields of Forel Alleviates Tics in Tourette Syndrome. Front Hum Neurosci 2017; 11:308.

58. Martinez-Ramirez D, Jimenez-Shahed J, Leckman JF, et al. Efficacy and Safety of Deep Brain Stimulation in Tourette Syndrome: The International Tourette Syndrome Deep Brain Stimulation Public Database and Registry. JAMA Neurol 2018;75(3):353–9.

59. Edwards TC, Zrinzo L, Limousin P, et al. Deep brain stimulation in the treatment of chorea. Mov Disord 2012;27:357–63.

60. Barton B, Zauber SE, Goetz CG. Movement disorders caused by medical disease. Semin Neurol 2009;29(2):97–110.

61. Bhidayasiri R, Truong DD. Chorea and related disorders. Postgrad Med J 2004; 80:527–34.

62. Gonzalez V, Cif L, Biolsi B, et al. Deep brain stimulation for Huntington's disease: long-term results of a prospective open-label study. J Neurosurg 2014;121(1): 114–22.

63. Biolsi B, Cif L, Fertit HE, et al. Long-term follow-up of Huntington disease treated by bilateral deep brain stimulation of the internal globus pallidus. J Neurosurg 2008;109:130–2.

64. Li P, Huang R, Song W, et al. Deep brain stimulation of the globus pallidus internal improves symptoms of chorea-acanthocytosis. Neurol Sci 2012;33(2):269–74.

65. Wang KL, Hess CW, Xu D, et al. High Frequency Bilateral Globus Pallidus Interna Deep Brain Stimulation Can Improve Both Chorea and Dysarthria in Chorea-acanthocytosis. Parkinsonism Relat Disord 2019;62:248–50.

66. Pouclet-Courtemanche H, Rouaud T, Thobois S, et al. Long-term efficacy and tolerability of bilateral pallidal stimulation to treat tardive dyskinesia. Neurology 2016;86:651–9.

67. Greicius MD, Srivastava G, Reiss AL, et al. Default-mode network activity distinguishes Alzheimer's disease from healthy aging: evidence from functional MRI. Proc Natl Acad Sci U S A 2004;101(13):4637–42.

68. Sperling RA, Dickerson BC, Pihlajamaki M, et al. Functional alterations in memory networks in early Alzheimer's disease. Neuromolecular Med 2010;12:27–43.

69. Laxton AW, Tang-Wai DF, McAndrews MP, et al. A phase I trial of deep brain stimulation of memory circuits in Alzheimer's disease. Ann Neurol 2010;68:521–34.

70. Lozano AM, Fosdick L, Chakravarty MM, et al. A Phase II Study of Fornix Deep Brain Stimulation in Mild Alzheimer's Disease. J Alzheimers Dis 2016;54:777–87.

71. Hardenacke K, Hashemiyoon R, Visser-Vandewalle V, et al. Deep Brain Stimulation of the Nucleus Basalis of Meynert in Alzheimer's Dementia: Potential Predictors of Cognitive Change and Results of a Long-Term Follow-Up in Eight Patients. Brain Stimul 2016;9:799–800.

72. Kuhn J, Hardenacke K, Shubina E, et al. Deep Brain Stimulation of the Nucleus Basalis of Meynert in Early Stage of Alzheimer's Dementia. Brain Stimul 2015;8: 838–9.

73. Bittlinger M, Muller S. Opening the debate on deep brain stimulation for Alzheimer disease - a critical evaluation of rationale, shortcomings, and ethical justification. BMC Med Ethics 2018;19:41.

74. Kwan P, Arzimanoglou A, Berg AT, et al. Definition of drug resistant epilepsy: consensus proposal by the ad hoc Task Force of the ILAE Commission on Therapeutic Strategies. Epilepsia 2010;51:1069–77.

75. Fisher R, Salanova V, Witt T, et al. Electrical stimulation of the anterior nucleus of thalamus for treatment of refractory epilepsy. Epilepsia 2010;51:899–908.

76. Salanova V, Witt T, Worth R, et al. Long-term efficacy and safety of thalamic stimulation for drug-resistant partial epilepsy. Neurology 2015;84:1017–25.

77. Klinger N, Mittal S. Deep brain stimulation for seizure control in drug-resistant epilepsy. Neurosurg Focus 2018;45:E4.

78. Farrell SM, Green A, Aziz T. The Current State of Deep Brain Stimulation for Chronic Pain and Its Context in Other Forms of Neuromodulation. Brain Sci 2018;8. https://doi.org/10.3390/brainsci8080158.

79. Richardson DE, Akil H. Pain reduction by electrical brain stimulation in man. Part 1: Acute administration in periaqueductal and periventricular sites. J Neurosurg 1977;47:178–83.
80. Mazars G, Roge R, Mazars Y. [Results of the stimulation of the spinothalamic fasciculus and their bearing on the physiopathology of pain]. Rev Neurol (Paris) 1960;103:136–8.
81. Levy RM, Lamb S, Adams JE. Treatment of chronic pain by deep brain stimulation: long term follow-up and review of the literature. Neurosurgery 1987;21:885–93.
82. Kumar K, Toth C, Nath RK. Deep brain stimulation for intractable pain: a 15-year experience. Neurosurgery 1997;40:736–46 [discussion: 746–7].
83. Franzini A, Messina G, Levi V, et al. Deep brain stimulation of the posterior limb of the internal capsule in the treatment of central poststroke neuropathic pain of the lower limb: case series with long-term follow-up and literature review. J Neurosurg 2019;1–9. https://doi.org/10.3171/2019.5.JNS19227.
84. Viswanathan A, Harsh V, Pereira EA, et al. Cingulotomy for medically refractory cancer pain. Neurosurg Focus 2013;35(3):E1.
85. Pereira EA, Paranathala M, Hyam JA, et al. Anterior cingulotomy improves malignant mesothelioma pain and dyspnoea. Br J Neurosurg 2014;28(4):471–4.
86. Spooner J, Yu H, Kao C, et al. Neuromodulation of the cingulum for neuropathic pain after spinal cord injury. Case report. J Neurosurg 2007;107(1):169–72.
87. Boccard SGJ, Prangnell SJ, Pycroft L, et al. Long-Term Results of Deep Brain Stimulation of the Anterior Cingulate Cortex for Neuropathic Pain. World Neurosurg 2017;106:625–37.
88. Boccard SG, Pereira EA, Moir L, et al. Deep brain stimulation of the anterior cingulate cortex: targeting the affective component of chronic pain. Neuroreport 2014;25:83–8.
89. Boccard SG, Fitzgerald JJ, Pereira EA, et al. Targeting the affective component of chronic pain: a case series of deep brain stimulation of the anterior cingulate cortex. Neurosurgery 2014;74:628–35 [discussion: 635–7].
90. Levi V, Cordella R, D'Ammando A, et al. Dorsal anterior cingulate cortex (ACC) deep brain stimulation (DBS): a promising surgical option for the treatment of refractory thalamic pain syndrome (TPS). Acta Neurochir (Wien) 2019;161:1579–88.
91. Mazzone P, Stocchi F, Galati S, et al. Bilateral Implantation of Centromedian-Parafascicularis Complex and GPi: A New Combination of Unconventional Targets for Deep Brain Stimulation in Severe Parkinson Disease. Neuromodulation 2006;9(3):221–8.
92. Freund H-J, Kuhn J, Lenartz D, et al. Cognitive Functions in a Patient With Parkinson-Dementia Syndrome Undergoing Deep Brain Stimulation. Arch Neurol 2009;66(6):781–5.
93. Thevathasan W, Debu B, Aziz T, et al. Pedunculopontine nucleus deep brain stimulation in Parkinson's disease: A clinical review. Mov Disord 2018;33(1):10–20.
94. Romigi A, Placidi F, Peppe A, et al. Pedunculopontine nucleus stimulation influences REM sleep in Parkinson's disease. Eur J Neurol 2008;15(7):e64–5.
95. Lim AS, Moro E, Lozano AM, et al. Selective enhancement of rapid eye movement sleep by deep brain stimulation of the human pons. Ann Neurol 2009;66(1):110–4.

96. Weiss D, Walach M, Meisner C, et al. Nigral stimulation for resistant axial motor impairment in Parkinson's disease? A randomized controlled trial. Brain 2013; 136(7):2098–108.
97. Samotus O, Parrent A, Jog M. Spinal Cord Stimulation Therapy for Gait Dysfunction in Advanced Parkinson's Disease Patients. Mov Disord 2018;33(5):783–92.
98. Plaha P, Ben-Shlomo Y, Patel NK, et al. Stimulation of the caudal zona incerta is superior to stimulation of the subthalamic nucleus in improving contralateral parkinsonism. Brain 2006;129(Pt 7):1732–47.
99. Valldeoriola F, Muñoz E, Rumià J, et al. Simultaneous low-frequency deep brain stimulation of the substantia nigra pars reticulata and high-frequency stimulation of the subthalamic nucleus to treat levodopa unresponsive freezing of gait in Parkinson's disease: A pilot study. Parkinsonism Relat Disord 2019;60:153–7.

Advances in Treatments in Muscular Dystrophies and Motor Neuron Disorders

Bhaskar Roy, MBBS, MMST[a],*, Robert Griggs, MD[b]

KEYWORDS

- Gene therapy • Muscular dystrophies • Motor neuron disorders
- Neuromuscular diseases • Neurotherapeutics

KEY POINTS

- New Food and Drug Administration–approved drugs in muscular dystrophies and motor neuron disorders.
- New advances in gene therapy in muscular dystrophies and motor neuron disorders.
- Ongoing clinical trials in muscular dystrophies and motor neuron disorders.

INTRODUCTION

Until the past 3 years, treatments had relatively little benefit so that supportive care was the only option for management of muscular dystrophies and motor neuron disorders (MNDs).[1] Advances in molecular genetics that have developed new targets and enabled treatment strategies, coupled with the Orphan Drug Act approved by the United States, in 1983, and orphan medicinal product regulation brought by the European Parliament, in 2000, have led to a new era of treatment of MNDs.[2–4] Soon it will be possible to address the underlying pathology and, in some cases, alter the natural course of disease progression.[5–8]

Given the rapid evolution of gene therapy and its potential application in many muscular dystrophies and MNDs in the future, the major approaches in gene therapies are reviewed briefly before going into the details of recent advances in therapeutic options.

APPROACHES IN GENE THERAPY

Antisense Oligonucleotides

Antisense oligonucleotides (ASOs) are synthetic, single-stranded, nucleic acid sequences (8–20 nucleotides in length), which can bind to selected RNA sequences,

[a] Department of Neurology, Yale School of Medicine, PO Box: 208018, New Haven, CT 06510, USA; [b] Center for Health + Technology, University of Rochester Medical Center, Rochester, NY 14642, USA
* Corresponding author.
E-mail address: bhaskar.roy@yale.edu

Neurol Clin 39 (2021) 87–112
https://doi.org/10.1016/j.ncl.2020.09.005
0733-8619/21/© 2020 Elsevier Inc. All rights reserved.

based on standard Watson-Crick base pairing, and regulate gene expression.[9,10] Modifications of chemical structure has created ASOs with increased stability, affinity, and potency and reduced immune activation.[9,11] Gapmers, which currently are used, are engineered hybrid ASOs, with a central gap region of unmodified nucleotides that still can activate ribonuclease-H (RNase-H), and flanking regions with 20-O-methoxyethyl nucleotides that protect the central region block from nuclease degradations. Peptide nucleic acids and phosphorodiamidate morpholino oligomers, the third-generation ASOs, are product of combined modifications of phosphate, ribose, and nucleoside.[12,13]

ASOs can restore protein expression, reduce expression of a toxic protein, and modify functional effects of a mutant protein.[9,10] Silencing of the causative gene can be a useful strategy for gain of function mutations,[10,14] whereas splice modulation can be used to restore function of a mutant protein or to compensate for its action.[14]

Mechanism of Action

mRNA knock down
Binding of ASO with DNA activates RNase-H, an endonuclease, leading to degradation of mRNA cleavage products, and inhibits protein translation.[15]

Splice site switching/alteration of splicing
ASOs can target splice sites, exons or introns, leading to exclusion or inclusion of a targeted exon. This strategy can help in restoring a normal transcript, removing disease-causing mutation to adjust the reading frame, or switching to a less toxic protein isoform (**Figs. 1** and **2**).[14,16–18]

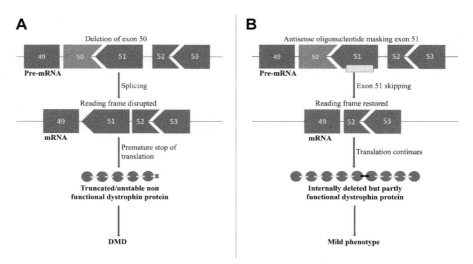

Fig. 1. Exon 51 skipping in DMD. (*A*) The open-reading frame of the dystrophin pre-mRNA is disrupted in most patients DMD. This figure shows how deletion of exon 50 disrupts reading frame and leads to synthesis of a truncated nonfunctional or unstable dystrophin. (*B*) ASO directed against exon 51 can lead to skipping of exon 51 and restore the open reading frame. The generated dystrophin is deleted internally but partly functional. (*Adapted from* Echevarria L, Aupy P, Goyenvalle A. Exon-skipping advances for Duchenne muscular dystrophy. *Hum Mol Genet.* 2018;27(R2):R163-R172; with permission.)

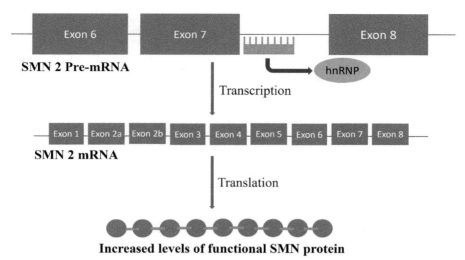

Increased levels of functional SMN protein

Fig. 2. ASO binding to a splicing silencer region on SMN2 pre-mRNA which displaces a heterogenous ribonucleoprotein (hnRNP). This leads to increases incorporation of exon 7 in the mRNA transcript, which ultimately results in increased levels of full-length SMA mRNA and fully functional SMN protein. (*Adapted from* Rao VK, Kapp D, Schroth M. Gene Therapy for Spinal Muscular Atrophy: An Emerging Treatment Option for a Devastating Disease. J Manag Care Spec Pharm. 2018;24(12-a Suppl):S3-S16, https://doi.org/10.18553/jmcp.2018. 24.12-a.s3; with permission.)

Adeno-associated Viral Vectors–Delivered Gene Therapy

Adeno-associated viral (AAVs) vectors are engineered from naturally replication defective, nonpathogenic, nonenveloped parvovirus, in which the viral coding sequences are replaced with a gene expression cassette.[19] The skeletal muscles are repaired by satellite cells fusion and/or myotubes splitting without myonuclei mitosis, and the turnover is slow. As a result, the skeletal muscles expression of a particular gene can be modified for a long period (usually at least decade) even without stem cell transduction or chromosomal integration.[20]

Mechanism of Action

Gene replacement

Gene replacement is the most straightforward strategy, applicable for monogenetic, recessive disorders, where the gene of interest can fit into the delivery vector. This method has been used in packaging of microdystrophin into the delivery vector in DMD.[20,21]

Gene replacement therapy may not be suitable for a dominant disease trait with a large gene size, and in such cases a disease-modifying gene can be delivered by AAVs.[20] Expression of micro-utrophin in DMD is an example of modifier gene expression.[20]

In gene knockdown, AAV-mediated delivery of ASOs, short hairpin RNA (shRNA), or miRNA can be useful in dominant negative gain-of-function diseases.[22–25] AAV-mediated delivery of anti-double homeobox protein 4 (DUX4) miRNAs was reported to prevent the development of facioscapulohumeral muscular dystrophy (FSHD) in a vector-induced mouse model.[24]

The most commonly used strategies for gene editing are clustered regularly interspaced short palindromic repeats (CRISPR)-based direct genome editing and ASO-based exon skipping at the RNA level.

1. CRISPR-associated (Cas) proteins are a class of enzymes that are capable of direct genome cleavage utilizing CRISPR sequences. Sections of DNA can be removed through nonhomologous end joining, or sections of DNA can be added or replaced through homology-directed repair. This technique can be extended for exon skipping with a single, destructive cut at a splicing acceptor site.[20,a]
2. Exon skipping is similar to splice site switching/alteration of splicing by ASOs, where the ASOs are delivered by an AAV vector.[20,26,27]

X-LINKED DYSTROPHIES

1. **Duchenne muscular dystrophy (DMD)** is an X-linked dystrophy caused by mutations in the dystrophin gene on chromosome Xp21, leading to absent or insufficient dystrophin, an essential cytoskeletal protein for strength, stability, and functionality of myofibers.[28,29] Deletions of 1 or more exons of the dystrophin gene account for approximately 65% of cases, and the rest are secondary to duplications, insertions, point mutations, or splicing mutations.[28–30]

Prevalence of DMD is between 16 and 20 per 100,000 live male births, based on reports from the United Kingdom and the United STates.[28] In DMD, compromised cytoskeleton to extracellular matrix link leads to instability of muscle membrane and cell necrosis. Progressive muscular damage results in muscle weakness and delayed motor milestones along with respiratory and cardiac involvement. Patients become nonambulatory at a mean age of 9 years, and, without intervention, mean survival is approximately 19 years.[28,29,31] A multidisciplinary approach ensuring appropriate respiratory, cardiological, orthopedic, psychosocial, and nutritional care is mandatory, and, along with corticosteroids, has increased survival even into the third or fourth decade.[28,32–35]

The corticosteroids prednisone and deflazacort improve muscle strength and function, preserve upper extremity strength, and delay loss of ambulation.[7,28,31,36] Other long-term benefit of glucocorticoids include preserved respiratory function and avoidance of scoliosis surgery.[28,37] Recent studies have reported benefits of early initiation of glucocorticoids before significant physical decline.[28,38] Despite proved benefit, side effects of long-term glucocorticoid use, in particular behavioral disturbance, weight gain, growth restriction, pubertal delay, cataract, osteoporosis, and increased risk of vertebral fracture, are concerning. Efforts to reduce such side effects have led to many alternative regimens with lower and/or alternative day dosing.[28,31,38,39] Although deflazacort has shown delayed loss of ambulation and no weight gain compared with prednisone, it was associated with higher frequency of growth delay, cushingoid appearance, and cataracts.[31,40,41] The best corticosteroid regime still is unclear, and an ongoing international study, FOR-DMD (NCT01603407), comparing 3 most frequent regimes, will provide some insight regarding the optimal corticosteroid dosing.[7,42]

Eteplirsen is a phosphorodiamidate morpholino oligomer, which targets the splice-donor region of exon 51 and induces the cellular machinery to skip over exon 51,

---

[a] Further details of the CRISPR technology are beyond the scope of this review. Interested readers can follow published reviews on this technology.

resulting in reading frame restoration and production of internally truncated but functional dystrophin protein (see **Fig. 1**). The first study (NCT00844597), with 19 ambulatory DMD patients, showed mild improvement in dystrophin production in 7 patients.[43] A randomized, placebo-controlled, double-blind study (NCT01396239) over 24 weeks recruited 12 ambulatory DMD patients amenable to exon 51 skipping. The open-label extension of the study (NCT01540409), where every participant received either 30-mg/kg or 50-mg/kg weekly infusion, showed slower rate of decline in 6-minute walk test (6MWT), lower incidence of loss of ambulation, and relatively stable respiratory function at 36 months compared with historical controls.[7,44] Eteplirsen was not approved by the Committee for Medicinal Products for Human Use, part of European Medicines Agency (EMA). It received conditional approval from the FDA, however, to treat DMD patients amenable to exon skipping in September 2016 (**Table 1**). A phase 3 study is ongoing, and Sarepta Therapeutics (Cambridge, MA), the company that developed Eteplirsen, should provide further functional data to the FDA by 2021, as a condition of the accelerated approval.[51]

Point mutations introducing a premature stop codon into mRNA leading to translation of a truncated and nonfunctional protein are responsible for 10% to 15% of DMD. Ataluren binds to the ribosomal RNA subunits and impedes the recognition of premature stop codons, thus promotes read through of a nonsense mutation to produce a full-length functional protein. An initial open-label phase 2a (NCT00264888) study showed an increase in dystrophin expression in 23/68 patients with nonsense mutation.[52] A randomized, double-blind, placebo-controlled, phase 2b trial in ambulatory male greater than or equal to 5 years of age (NCT00592553) reported slowed decline in 6MWT and timed physical function tests after 48 weeks.[53] In August 2014, ataluren received conditional approval from EMA to treat ambulatory DMD patients aged 5 years or older with nonsense mutation, and additional data confirming the functional efficacy were requested. ACT DMD, a multicenter, randomized, double-blind, placebo-controlled, phase 3 trial (NCT01826487), recruited ambulatory DMD boys, ages 7 years to 16 years, with nonsense mutation, baseline 6MWD greater than or equal to 150 m, and 80% or less of the predicted normal value for age and height. The primary endpoint was in favor of ataluren in the intent-to-treat population analysis but did not reach statistical significance.[54] Statistical significance was noted in the prespecified subgroup with baseline 6MWD between 300 m and 400 m. A clinical trial assessing the long-term outcome of ataluren is ongoing (NCT03179631) and expected to be completed by December 2021. Preliminary data from the first international drug registry for ataluren suggested long-term benefit. Children and adolescents receiving this drug, walked longer than untreated patients, and were physically more able.[7,55] Based on the positive results in children between 2 years to 5 years of age from the phase 2 study, EMA has extended the indication of ataluren from age 2.[7]

Other exon skipping therapies—golodirsen (SRP-4053), exon 53 skipping, and casimersen (SRP-4045), exon 45 skipping—are being investigated in a phase 3 trial (NCT02500381), which is expected to be completed by May 2023 (**Table 2**). Golodirsen received conditional FDA approval in December 2019.[45] Viltolarsen, another exon 53 skipping ASO, has shown positive result in a phase 2 trial, and a phase 3 (NCT04060199) trial is ongoing. SRP-5051, an exon 51 skipping treatment, currently is under phase 2 clinical trial (NCT04004065). Trial

Table 1
Food and Drug Administration–approved drugs in muscular dystrophies and motor neuron disorders

Drug	Mechanism of Action	Results in Support of Approval	Food and Drug Administration Approval
DMD			
Eteplirsen[43,44]	ASO, exon 51 skipping	Increased dystrophin in some patients. Slower rate of decline in 6MWT and lower incidence of loss of ambulation compared with historical control	Conditional approval in September 2016
Deflazacort[40,41]	Corticosteroid	One trial showed improved and maintained muscle strength with deflazacort. Another trial showed delayed loss of ambulation with deflazacort.	February 2017
Golodirsen[45,46]	Exon 53 skipping	Increased dystrophin level from baseline to 48 wk of treatment	Conditional approval in December 2019
SMA			
Risdipalm[141]	Small molecule modulating SMN2 gene splicing	Increased mRNA levels of SMN2. 41% of treated infants were able to sit unassisted for 5 seconds or more. Most of the treated patients (81%) did not require tracheostomy or permanent ventilation.	August 2020
Nusinersen[47,48]	ASO that modifies pre-mRNA splicing of SMN2	Improved motor milestones and motor functioning in treated patients	June 2017
Onasemnogene abeparvovec-xioi[49]	AAV9 vector carrying SMN1 complimentary recombinant DNA	Treated patients demonstrated significant improvement in their ability to reach developmental motor milestones compared with natural history controls.	May 2019
ALS			
Edaravone[50]	Antioxidant, free radical scavenger of peroxyl radicals and peroxynitrite	Slowed disease progression at 24 mo in a subset of treated patients	May 2017

Table 2
Promising therapies under clinical trials

Drug	Mechanism of Action	Preliminary Results	Status
DMD			
Casimersen[56]	Exon 45 skipping	Increased dystrophin level from baseline to 48 wk of treatment	Phase 3 trial ongoing
Viltolarsen[57]	Exon 53 skipping	Increased dystrophin production after 20–24 wk of treatment and possible clinical benefit	Positive phase 2 data, and phase 3 trial ongoing
SMA			
ALS			
Tofersen[58]	ASO inhibiting SOD1 expression	Interim analysis showed decreased production of SOD1 protein in cerebral spinal fluid and possibly slowed disease progression.	Phase 3 study ongoing

with suvodirsen (WVE-210201), a stereo-pure oligonucleotide (NCT03907072), was terminated due to lack of efficacy.[59,60] Multiexon skipping therapeutics, targeting exon 45 to 55, a major hot spot for mutations in DMD, has been investigated in animal models, but further studies are needed to assess their safety and efficacy.[61–63]

For AAV-based gene therapies, currently, a phase 1 study is looking at the dose, safety, and tolerability of single intravenous infusion of PF-06939926, an AAV9-mediated transfer of microdystrophin (NCT03362502). Another open-label phase 1/2 trial (NCT03375164) will be examining the safety of intravenous infusion of rAAVrh74.MHCK7.micro-dystrophin. AAV9 vector–based microdystrophin transfer through SGT-001 also is being examined (NCT03368742).

Several other approaches, aiming at reduction of inflammation and fibrosis, muscle growth and regeneration, and calcium homeostasis, are undergoing. More details of some of these trials are provided in **Table 3**.

Multidisciplinary care is warranted in DMD. Timely immunization, frequent assessment of respiratory function (at least every 6 months), assisted cough and nocturnal ventilation, and addition of daytime ventilation can have a significant impact on quality of life and life expectancy.[28,32] Similarly, annual cardiac assessment and initiation of angiotensin-converting enzyme inhibitors or angiotensin receptor blocker by age 10 is recommended.[28,32] A phase 3 study (NCT02354352) has demonstrated noninferiority of spironolactone to eplerenone in preserving contractile cardiac function in DMD patients with initially preserved left ventricular ejection fraction.[68] To maintain bone health, regular physical activity, calcium and vitamin D supplementation, and periodic assessments of bone health are recommended.[28,32] Zoledronic acid, a bisphosphonate therapy, showed better spine bone mineral density z score at 12 months compared with baseline (NCT00799266).[69] One trial has examined the safety of mild-intensity to moderate–intensity exercise training (NCT02421523) and another trial

Table 3
Other approaches and ongoing trials in Duchenne muscular dystrophy

Name of the Drug	Mechanism of Action	Phase	Study Design	Primary Outcome Measure
Reduction of inflammation and fibrosis				
Anti-inflammatory				
Valmorolone (NCT03439670)	Anti-inflammatory	2b	Randomized, double-blind, placebo and active-controlled (prednisolone) study in ambulatory boys	1. Time to stand test 2. Body size, measured by body mass index z score
Antifibrotic				
Givinostat[64] (NCT02851797)	HDAC inhibitor	3	Randomized, double-blind, parallel group, placebo-controlled study in ambulatory boys	Mean change in 4 standard stairs climb
Pamrevlumab (NCT2606136)	Monoclonal antibody to connective tissue growth factor	2	Open-label trial in nonambulatory DMD patients	Annual change in percent predicted annual FVC
Nuclear factor κB inhibitors				
Edasalonexent[65] (NCT03703882)	Nuclear factor κB inhibitor	3	Randomized, double-blind, placebo-controlled	Change from baseline in North Star Ambulatory Assessment
Muscle growth and regeneration				
Cell-based therapies				
Myoblasts transplant (NCT02196467)		1/2	Randomized, double-blind, single-group study	Safety and tolerability
Cardiosphere-derived cells: CAP-1002[66] (NCT02485938)	Anti-inflammatory, antifibrotic, and regenerative	1/2 (completed)	Randomized, controlled, open-label trial	Safety and tolerability Significant scar size reduction and improvement in systolic thickening

Myostatin inhibition

RO7239361 (NCT02515669)	Myostatin inhibitor	1/2	Randomized, placebo-controlled, double-blind	Safety and tolerability
Other medications				
Tamoxifen[67] (NCT03354039)	Selective estrogen receptor regulator, antioxidant, regulation of calcium homeostasis	3	Randomized, double-blind, parallel, placebo-controlled	Reduction of disease progression (based on motor function measure D1 subscore)
Rimeporide (NCT02710591) (completed)	Sodium/proton type 1 exchanger inhibitor	1b	Open-label study	Safety and tolerability
Respiratory care				
Idebenone (NCT03603288)	Antioxidant	3	Open-label extension study (SIDEROS-E) to assess the long-term safety and efficacy	Incidence and severity of adverse events
Cosyntropin (MNK-1411) (NCT03400852)	Anti-inflammatory, melanocortin receptor agonist	2	Randomized, double-blind, parallel group, placebo controlled, in ambulatory boys	10-m walk/run
Cardiac care				
Bisoprolol (NCT03779646)	β-Blocker	2/3	Randomized, controlled	Change of left ventricle global longitudinal strain in cardiac magnetic resonance from baseline to 12 mo
Nebivolol (NCT01648634)	β-Blocker	3	Randomized, double-blind, placebo-controlled	Delay in the development of left ventricular systolic dysfunction (ejection fraction <45%)
Ifetroban (NCT03340675)	thromboxane and prostaglandin H2 receptor antagonist	2	Randomized, placebo-controlled, double-blind, dose-ranging	Safety and tolerability

(NCT04173234) is examining the effect of aerobic and home exercise program in DMD.[70]

2. **Becker muscular dystrophy (BMD)** is an allelic disorder to DMD with mutations in the dystrophin gene.[71,72] In BMD, the reading frame usually is maintained and variable amount of partially functional protein is expressed.[73] BMD generally is milder than DMD; however, it can present with a wide range of severity. Half of the affected boys demonstrate symptom of muscle weakness by age 10. They can present as mild DMD or with any permutation of the following symptoms: asymptomatic hyperCKemia, myalgia with exertion, and/or calf hypertrophy. Loss of ambulation in BMD usually is delayed and may not occur until third or fourth decade.[63,71,73] Cardiomyopathy usually is common; however, age of onset may depend on the structure of the residual dystrophin protein.[74]

Givinostat, a histone deacetylase (HDAC) inhibitor, with antifibrotic effects, increases cross-sectional area of myofibers.[64] A phase 2, randomized, double-blind, placebo-controlled trial (NCT03238235) is investigating the microscopic and macroscopic effect of givinostat in BMD, along with safety and tolerability. The primary outcome is mean change in cross-sectional area in muscle biopsies. A phase 1/2a trial with follistatin gene therapy was conducted in 6 BMD patients, and, overall, there were some trends of benefit and it was well tolerated.[75] Another open-label phase 2 study (NCT04054375) is evaluating the safety and efficacy of weekly steroid in BMD along with changes in functional outcome measures, muscle magnetic resonance imaging, bone density study, and lean mass percentage as secondary outcome measures.[76]

LIMB-GIRDLE MUSCULAR DYSTROPHIES

Limb-girdle muscular dystrophies (LGMDs) are a heterogenous group of genetic muscle disorders, predominantly affecting the proximal limb muscles. In some cases, distal muscles also can be affected, and cardiac involvement may occur.[77–79] Based on the pattern of inheritance, LGMD historically is classified into type 1, or autosomal dominant inheritance, and type 2, or autosomal recessive inheritance. Considerable variability within the LGMDs, in terms of age of onset, severity of clinical symptoms, and disease progression, frequently is observed.[43,78,79] As of 2018, there are 8 subtypes of LGMD1 and 26 subtypes of LGMD2, and discussion on the emerging therapy on each of them is beyond the scope of this review. Moreover, there is no specific approved therapy for any of the LGMD, and the majority of research still is in the preclinical phase.[77,78] This reviews focuses on some particular genetic abnormalities and treatment strategies.

Dysferlinopathy

Dysferlinopathies, such as LGMD2B and Miyoshi myopathy, are rare muscle diseases with mutation in the dysferlin gene.[80] Dysferlin is abundant in skeletal and cardiac muscles and plays an essential role in membrane repair.[81] AAV-mediated transfer of dysferlin gene has shown promising data in animal model, and a phase 1 trial (NCT02710500) is ongoing.[82] In-frame mutations in exon 32, or even larger deletions, usually are associated with a milder disease course.[80] This suggested the possibility of application of exon skipping technology in dysferlinopathies, and it was performed successfully in preclinical model.[83] Moreover, recent study reported that exons 26-27 and 28-29 may act as the target for multiexon skipping.[80]

Sarcoglycanopathies

AAV-mediated transfer of full length α-sarcoglycan in LGMD2D has shown sustained expression of α-sarcoglycan in 5 out of 6 patients.[84] An open-label, phase 1 trial (NCT03652259) is investigating the safety and tolerability of systemic gene delivery (SRP-9003) in β-sarcoglycan deficient LGMD2E. Similar AAV-mediated transfer of Y-sarcoglycan in 9 nonambulatory LGMD2C patients showed expression of Y-sarco-glycan in 5/9 participants 30 days after gene transfer.[85] Deletion of a single thymine in a string of 5 thymine nucleotides in exon 6 is the most common mutation in LGMD2C. Skipping of exons 4, 5, 6, and 7 can produce a functional protein, named Mini-Gamma, and has shown positive result in patient fibroblast and myotube using modified ASO.[63,86]

Dystroglycanopathies

LGMD2I is associated with mutation in fukutin-related protein (FKRP) gene leading to abnormal glycosylation and α-dystroglycan dysfunction. A randomized, placebo-controlled, double-blind phase 3 study (NCT03783923) is evaluating the safety and efficacy of deflazacort in LGMD2I.

FACIOSCAPULOHUMERAL MUSCULAR DYSTROPHY

FSHD, the third most common muscular dystrophy, is an autosomal dominant, gradually progressive muscular dystrophy, often affecting facial muscles, shoulder girdles, and upper arms. With disease progression, trunk muscles and lower extremity muscles also are affected.[87] A majority (>97%) of patients have FSHD1, with deletion of large repeated elements of the long arm of chromosome 4q (the D4Z4 region). On the other hand, FSHD2 is caused by a deletion-independent mechanism. Ultimately, both lead to inappropriate expression of the transcription factor double homeobox protein 4 (DUX4), which results in the disease through toxic gain of function.[87]

Gene Therapy Approaches

Several gene therapy approaches targeting the DUX4-coding mRNA, such as RNA interference-based approaches; exon skipping strategies to prevent polyadenylation; gene-editing approaches with CRISPR/Cas9; and inhibition of DUX4-mRNA expression, transcriptional initiation, or transcriptional silencing, are going through preclinical research.[88]

Other Therapies Under Trial

Losmapimod is an inhibitor of p38α/β mitogen-activated protein kinases, with the potential to modulate DUX4 expression. A randomized, double-blind, placebo-controlled phase 2 study (NCT04003974) and an open-level pilot study (NCT04004000) are examining the safety and tolerability of losmapimod and initial data are promising.[89] A phase 1 study (NCT03123913) is examining the safety and tolerability of recombinant human growth hormone and testosterone in FSHD.

MOTOR NEURON DISEASES
Spinal Muscular Atrophy

Spinal muscular atrophies (SMAs) are a group of genetic disorders characterized by alpha motor neuron degeneration in the spinal cord leading to progressive muscle weakness and atrophy.[90] The most common form of SMA or 5q proximal SMA results from homozygous deletions or other mutations in the survival motor neuron (SMN) 1 gene localized to 5q11.2-q13.3.[91] The range of phenotypic severity of SMA, based on maximal functional status achieved, can be divided into 4 broad clinical subtypes: very weak infants unable to sit unsupported (type 1), nonambulant patients able to sit independently (type 2), patients who are able to walk (type 3), and adult-onset mild disease (type 4).[90,92]

Patients with 5q proximal SMA carry homozygous deletions or mutations of SMN1 but maintain at least 1 copy of SMN2, a paralogous gene. SMN2 harbors a silent transition within exon 7 leading to altered splicing of the mRNA and production of an unstable, truncated protein (SMN-Δ7), along with a some correctly spliced transcripts of full-length, functional protein (approximately 10%). SMN2 copy number is the most important modifier of the disease, with higher SMN2 copy number associated with more benign evolution of the disease.[7,93,94] In the past decade, some innovative and effective therapies were discovered, which potentially may change the natural course of the disease.[7]

Survival motor neuron 2 modulation

Nusinersen, an antisense-oligonucleotide, binds to the SMN2 pre-mRNA downstream of exon 7 and promotes its incorporation into the mRNA, which leads to the translation of a fully functional SMN protein (see **Fig. 2**). Given its inability to cross the blood-brain barrier, it is injected intrathecally, but several clinical trials have proved the safety and efficacy of nusinersen.[47,48,95] ENDEAR was a phase 3, randomized, double-blind, sham procedure, controlled study assessing the clinical efficacy and safety of nusinersen in infantile-onset SMA. Interim analysis showed better motor-milestone responses in the treated group (41%) vs. 0% in the control group, respectively) leading to early termination of the trial on ethical consideration. Moreover, the likelihood of event-free survival (death or use of permanent ventilation) was higher in the treated group.[47] CHERISH was a similar phase 3 trial in later-onset SMA. The primary outcome measure, change in the Hammersmith Functional Motor Scale–Expanded (HFMSE) score after 15 months of treatment, improved by a mean of 4 points in the treated group versus deteriorated by a mean of 1.9 groups in the control group, at interim analysis. Similar to ENDEAR, this trial was terminated early based on ethical consideration.[48] Enrolled patients continued treatment in an open-label extension study (SHINE).[96] Interim analysis from the ongoing NARTURE study, an open-label study examining the safety and efficacy of nusinersen in genetically diagnosed presymptomatic SMA patients, younger than 6 weeks old, showed delayed symptom onset and better achievements of motor milestones.[97] Extension study from the ISIS-396443-CS12, examining safety of nusinersen in later-onset SMA patients, also showed improved HFMSE score. Upper limb module score, 6MWT distance, and mean compound motor action potential remained relatively stable.[98] Nusinersen received FDA approval in December 2016, and EMA approval in June 2017.[99]

AAV9 vector carrying SMN1 complementary recombinant DNA (onasemnogene abeparvovec-xioi) also has shown encouraging results. A single intravenous administration can lead to systemic expression of the SMN1 protein. The first trial included 15 SMA type 1 cases with homozygous SMN1 exon 7 deletion and 2 copies of SMN2, excluding patients with the c.859G→C disease modifier in exon 7 of SMN2.[49] A majority of the patients in the high-dose group achieved several motor milestones, including head control, sitting unsupported, and rolling, and 2 patients were able to walk unsupported. At 20 months, none of the treated patients required permanent assisted ventilation.[49,95] A long-term outcomes study on a larger cohort is pending.[100] Onasemnogene abeparvovec-xioi received FDA approval in May 2019.[101]

Small molecules that modulate SMN2 gene splicing have the advantage of oral route administration. Risdiplam is such a highly specific molecule that is being examined now in several clinical trials.[95,102] A phase 1 study has reported increased mRNA levels of SMN2 in a dose-dependent manner. Three ongoing phase 2 trials are assessing the safety and efficacy in different SMA patient cohort: (1) SUNFISH (a 2-part trial) for nonambulatory SMA 2 and SMA 3 patients between ages 2 years and 25 years[103]; (2) FIREFISH (a 2-part trial) recruiting SMA1 patients between age 1 month and 7 months of age, with 2 copies of SMN[104]; (3) JEWELFISH an open-label exploratory study on SMA patients who previously were enrolled in SMN2-targeted treatments.[105] Interim analysis, as reported by the developing company, showed that treated SMA1 infants met developmental milestones (19/21 were alive), and none required tracheostomy or permanent ventilation. Data from SMA2 and SMA3 patients showed greater than 2-fold increase in SMN protein levels and improvement in motor function. No drug-related safety reports were reported.[106] Another orally administered molecule, branaplam, also is going through a phase 1/2 open-label clinical trial (NCT02268552) to evaluate safety, tolerability, and efficacy in type 1 SMA with 2 copies of SMN2.

Other approaches

1. Among neuroprotective therapies, olesoxime, a novel cholesterol-like compound, was evaluated in a phase 2 randomized, double-blind adaptive, placebo-controlled, 3-stage study in SMA2 or nonambulatory SMA3 patients. The primary aim of improvement in functional domains 1 and 2 of the motor function measure was not achieved. A significantly higher percentage of treated patients, however, showed improvement or remained stable. An open-label extension study (NCT02628743) is ongoing.[107]
2. Among muscle-enhancing therapies, SRK-015 promotes growth and differentiation of muscles cells by inhibiting latent myostatin. A phase 1 trial confirmed safety and a phase 2 study (NCT03921528) is ongoing.[108]

Reldesemtiv, intended to slow the rate of calcium release from the regulatory troponin complex of fast skeletal muscle fibers, has shown safety in phase 1 trial. A phase 2 trial (NCT02644668) also has shown statistically significant concentration dependent increase in changes from baseline in 6MWT distance, a submaximal exercise test of aerobic capacity, and endurance.[109]

Amyotrophic Lateral Sclerosis

Amyotrophic lateral sclerosis (ALS) is the most common motor neuron disorder in adults.[110] It is a fatal neurodegenerative disease with progressive degeneration of the upper and lower motor neurons. ALS usually starts with insidious-onset focal weakness, which eventually spreads to most muscles, including diaphragm. Survival from the time of symptom onset is approximately 3 years to 5 years, and respiratory failure is the leading cause of death.[111] Despite decades of research and several clinical trials, there is no cure for ALS to date. Two FDA-approved drugs, riluzole and edaravone, provide only mild clinical benefit.[50,112–114] Meta-analysis examining the effect of riluzole showed a survival benefit of 1.7 months.[112]

Oxidative stress biomarkers are higher in ALS patients compared with controls without ALS, and oxidative stress might play an important role in the disease progression of ALS.[50,115,116]

1. Edaravone is a free-radical scavenger of peroxyl radicals and peroxynitrite, which underwent a randomized, double-blind, parallel-group, placebo-controlled phase 3 trial. Although the original study did not fulfill primary endpoint, post hoc analysis of the data suggested slowed progression in a small subset of patient with early-stage

ALS.[50] It did not show any benefit, however, in patients with advanced ALS.[117] A follow-up 24-week active-treatment extension study showed no concern regarding the safety of edaravone.[114] Predictive modeling suggested benefit of continuous use of edaravone during the extension study compared with the projected disease progression from the first 24 weeks of data from the placebo group.[113] Edaravone received FDA approval in the United States in May 2017; however, it is not approved by the EMA.[118,119] An ongoing phase 3 study is examining the long-term safety and tolerability of oral edaravone (NCT04165824).

With the evolution of gene mapping and DNA analysis technologies, more than 30 genes have been attributed to increased risk of ALS, accounting for 15% of the sporadic and 70% of the familial ALS.[10,120] With the rapid advances of gene therapy in the past decade, new genetic therapies are emerging.

1. ASOs: First causative mutation of ALS was described in the SOD1 gene, which is found in approximately 12% of patients with familial ALS. Most of these mutations generally are point mutations, leading to toxic gain of function. The p.A4V mutation, the most common variant in North America, is associated with extremely rapid progression and survival of no more than 12 months.[121] ISIS SOD1Rx, an ASO designed to inhibit SOD1 expression, has shown safety in phase 1 clinical trial.[122] A phase 3 trial examining the efficacy, safety, and tolerability of BIB067 (tofersen, renamed molecule) is ongoing (NCT02623699). An interim analysis showed decreased production of SOD1 protein in Cerebrospinal fluid and possibly slowed disease progression.[58]

   A hexonucleotide repeat expansion in the first intron of the C9orf72 is associated with 40% of familial ALS and approximately 25% of sporadic ALS. BIIB078, an allele-specific ASO for C9orf72, selectively targets mutant specific transcripts for degradation is going through a phase 1 trial (NCT03626012). Other ASOs targeting upstream or downstream of the C9orf72 expanded repeat have been investigated in animal models.[10]

2. Several AAV-mediated gene therapies have shown promise in the preclinical phase, and some of them potentially may go into early-phase clinical trials.[10,123–125]

Stem Cell Therapy transplantation may counteract the multifaceted pathogenesis in ALS by replacing lost or diseased cells, immunomodulation, or by providing neuroprotective factors. Safety of intrathecal autologous adipose-derived mesenchymal stromal cells (MSCs) in patients with ALS has been demonstrated in a phase 1 clinical trials, and a phase 2 trial (NCT03268603) is ongoing.[126] Other phase 1/2 clinical trials have reported safety of intrathecal transplant of bone marrow–derived MSCs and slowed rate of decline of ALS-functional rating scale (FRS).[127,128] Stability of FVC was noted in 1 of those clinical trial.[128] MSCs secreting neurotrophic factor transplantation intrathecally and/or intramuscularly also showed safety and slowed rate of disease progression and decline in FVC in a phase 1/2 trial.[129]

Several other approaches for ALS are undergoing clinical trials. **Table 4** provides a summary of such approaches.

FUTURE DIRECTIONS

Emergence of new therapeutics, along with their potential benefits, also has created new challenges. Collaborative efforts in the coming years may help to make these disease-modifying and potentially life-saving therapies available to all in need. Some of the barriers are discussed briefly.

Table 4
Ongoing clinical trials in amyotrophic lateral sclerosis

Name of the Drug (National Clinical Trial Identifier)	Mechanism of Action	Phase	Study Design	Primary Outcome Measure
Anti-inflammatory and antioxidant				
RNS60 (NCT03456882)	Anti-inflammatory	2	Randomized, double-blind, placebo-controlled, parallel group, add-on phase II trial	Effect of RNS60 treatment on selected pharmacodynamic biomarkers
Vitamin E (NCT04140136)	Antioxidant	2	Randomized, double-blind, placebo-controlled	Mean change of revised ALS-FRS at baseline and 6 mo between treatment groups
Betamethasone in FUS-related ALS (NCT03707795)	Antioxidant	1	Nonrandomized, single group	Betamethasone plasma level
IPL344 (NCT03652805)	Activation of the Pi3k/Akt signaling pathway	1/2	Open-label, dose-escalating Study	Safety and tolerability
DNL 747 (NCT03757351)	Inhibitor of RIPK1, anti-inflammatory	1	Randomized, placebo-controlled, double-blind, crossover study	Safety and tolerability
Neuroprotective				
Masitinib (NCT03127267)	Oral tyrosine kinase inhibitor	3	Randomized, double-blind, placebo-controlled, parallel groups	Change in ALS-FRS–R in 48 wk
Tauroursodeoxycholic Acid (NCT03800524)	Hydrophilic bile acid, antiapoptotic	3	Randomized, placebo-controlled, double blind	Identification of the responder patients defined as those showing an improvement of at least 20% in the ALS-FRS–R slope
Biotin (high dose) (NCT03427086)	Neuroprotective	2	Double-blind, placebo-controlled, randomized 2:1 study	Safety and tolerability
Vitamin B$_{12}$ (ultrahigh dose) (NCT03548311)[130]	Neuroprotective	3	Randomized, double-blind, placebo-controlled	Drop in ALS-FRS–R

(continued on next page)

Table 4
(continued)

Name of the Drug (National Clinical Trial Identifier)	Mechanism of Action	Phase	Study Design	Primary Outcome Measure
Recombinant Human erythropoietin (NCT03835507)[131]	Neuroprotective	1/2	Randomized, double-blind, placebo-controlled	Changes in ALS–FRS–R score from baseline to 12 mo
Deferiprone (NCT03293069)	Iron chelator	2/3	Randomized, placebo-controlled, double-blind study	Combined assessment of function and survival score based on changes in ALS–FRS–R total scores and time to death from baseline to 12 mo
Cannabinoids (NCT03690791)[132]	Activation of endocannabinoid system	3	Randomized, double-blind	Difference in mean ALS-FRS–R total score between groups at the end of treatment
L-Serine (NCT03580616)[133]	Prevents BMAA misincorporation into neuroproteins	2	Open-label, single group	Tolerability, change in ALS-FRS–R scale
Ranolazine (NCT03472950)	Inhibits the late Na^+ current and intracellular Ca^{2+} accumulation	2	Open-label	Safety, dose-related toxicities
Fasudil (NCT03792490)	Inhibition of Rho kinase	2	Randomized, double-blind, placebo-controlled	Safety and tolerability, survival time
Memantine (NCT02118727)	NMDA receptor antagonist	2	Double-blind, placebo-controlled	Disease progression as measured by the number of points lost on the ALS-FRS–R
AMX-0035 combination of sodium phenylbutyrate and taurourso-deoxycholic acid (NCT03127514)[134]	Targets mitochondrial and endoplasmic reticulum stress system	2	Randomized, double-blind	ALS-FRS–R slope over 24 wk, incidence of adverse events
Fixed dose ciprofloxacin/ celecoxib (NCT04090684)	Neuroprotective	1	Open level, single group	Safety and tolerability

Metformin (NCT04220021)	Reduces toxic proteins produced from the C9orf72 repeat expansion	2	Open label study	Safety and tolerability
Targeting SOD1				
AP-101 (NCT03981536)	Human monoclonal antibody targeting superoxide dismutase-1	1	Open-label, single-ascending dose study to evaluate safety, tolerability, and pharmacokinetics	Safety
Cu(II)ATSM (NCT04082832) [NCT02870634, NCT03136809]	Inhibits activity of misfolded SOD1	2/3	Randomized, double-blind, placebo-controlled	Revised ALS-FRS-R total score, Edinburgh Cognitive and Behavioral ALS Screen
Other approaches				
Levosimendan (ODM-109) (NCT03505021)[135]	Calcium sensitizer	3	Randomized, placebo-controlled	Supine slow vital capacity (change from baseline to 12 wk)
Reldesemtiv (NCT03160898)	Fast skeletal muscle troponin activator	2	Multicenter, double-blind, randomized, dose-ranging, placebo-controlled study	Change from baseline to wk 12 in the percent predicted slow vital capacity
Pimozide (NCT03272503)	Neuroleptic	2	Randomized, placebo-controlled, double-blind	Change in ALS-FRS-R
Arimoclomol (NCT03491462)[136]	Heat shock protein coinducer promoting nascent protein folding	3	Randomized, placebo-controlled	Combined assessment of function and survival at 76 wk
Colchicine (NCT03693781)	Enhanced expression of heat shock protein B8 and blocking TDP-43 accumulation	2	Randomized, placebo-controlled, double-blind	Decrease in disease progression measured by ALS-FRS-R from baseline to wk 30
BIB100 (NCT03945279)	Inhibitor of exportin 1, a protein that mediates export of many proteins and RNA species from the cell nucleus	1	Double-blind, placebo-controlled	Safety and tolerability

Abbreviations: ALS-FRS-R, Revised Amyotrophic Lateral Sclerosis Functional Rating Scale; BMAA, β-methylamino-L-alanine; TDP-43, TAR DNA binding protein 43.

1. Newborn screening: early diagnosis and timely intervention may prevent a lifetime of chronic disability and can be lifesaving. The initiation of treatment in the pre-symptomatic state has been shown to improve clinical outcomes in SMA, DMD, and Pompe disease.[137] Newborn screening for Pompe and SMA already is approved by the US Department of Health and Human Services–endorsed Recommended Uniform Screening Panel, although the final implementation of such screening depends on the state-level approval. SMA newborn screening is not available routinely in most of the European countries yet, and it was rejected by the UK national screening committee.[138]
2. Economic burden: most of the recently approved orphan drugs are expensive and can cost several hundred thousand dollars per patient. The price of several molecules was raised after obtaining the orphan designation. Moreover, there is a significant price difference between countries.[139,140] The fairness of such pricing has been questioned, and attempts are ongoing to make these drugs more affordable. With only a handful of newly approved drugs, the health care cost is rising rapidly and significantly affecting the national health care budget. Without the implementation of new financial policies, it would be impossible to handle the cost burden of such therapies when more drugs will be approved in the future.
3. Durability of response: the newly approved therapies are promising; however, long-term follow-up data are required to fully understand the durability of response to genetic therapies. If the response is not durable, then repeated treatments will be required, adding to the total cost burden. Durability of response should be a focus of future research.

SUMMARY

Exon skipping therapeutics in DMD have led to successful expression of dystrophin protein with potential clinical benefits. Other therapies, now under clinical trial, may improve the quality of life in DMD. Altered splicing of SMN2 and AAV9-mediated gene therapy have transformed SMA from a disease that is fatal by 2 years of age to one where early treatment promises near-normal growth and development. Similar approaches in other muscular dystrophies and genetic ALS are under investigation, and there is potential for more therapies in the future. The current breakthroughs and most of the soon-to-be-developed life-saving treatments, however, will not reach the patients in need without wide implementation of newborn screening and structured health policy to address the economic burden of such therapies.

DISCLOSURE

Dr B. Roy has served as a consultant/advisor for Alexion Pharmaceuticals. Dr R. Griggs has received grant funding from Muscular Dystrophy Association (MDA), Muscular Dystrophy Association (NIH), Parent Project Muscular Dystrophy (PPMD), PTC therapeutics (PTC), and Sarepta BioPharma. He also has served as a consultant for PTC, Sarepta, and Strongbridge Biopharma, and on a Data and Safety Monitoring Board (DSMB) for Solid Biosciences.

REFERENCES

1. Boycott KM, Vanstone MR, Bulman DE, et al. Rare-disease genetics in the era of next-generation sequencing: discovery to translation. Nat Rev Genet 2013; 14(10):681–91.
2. Asbury CH. The Orphan Drug Act. The first 7 years. JAMA 1991;265(7):893–7.

3. Joppi R, Bertele V, Garattini S. Orphan drugs, orphan diseases. The first decade of orphan drug legislation in the EU. Eur J Clin Pharmacol 2013;69(4):1009–24.
4. Herder M. What Is the Purpose of the Orphan Drug Act? PLoS Med 2017;14(1).
5. Al-Zaidy SA, Mendell JR. From Clinical Trials to Clinical Practice: Practical Considerations for Gene Replacement Therapy in SMA Type 1. Pediatr Neurol 2019; 100:3–11. https://doi.org/10.1016/j.pediatrneurol.2019.06.007.
6. High KA, Roncarolo MG. Gene Therapy. N Engl J Med 2019;381(5):455–64.
7. Vita G, Vita GL, Musumeci O, et al. Genetic neuromuscular disorders: living the era of a therapeutic revolution. Part 2: diseases of motor neuron and skeletal muscle. Neurol Sci 2019;40(4):671–81.
8. Vita G, Vita GL, Stancanelli C, et al. Genetic neuromuscular disorders: living the era of a therapeutic revolution. Part 1: peripheral neuropathies. Neurol Sci 2019; 40(4):661–9.
9. Goyal N, Narayanaswami P. Making sense of antisense oligonucleotides: A narrative review. Muscle Nerve 2018;57(3):356–70.
10. Klim JR, Vance C, Scotter EL. Antisense oligonucleotide therapies for Amyotrophic Lateral Sclerosis: Existing and emerging targets. Int J Biochem Cell Biol 2019;110:149–53.
11. Deleavey GF, Damha MJ. Designing Chemically Modified Oligonucleotides for Targeted Gene Silencing. Chem Biol 2012;19(8):937–54.
12. Bennett CF, Swayze EE. RNA Targeting Therapeutics: Molecular Mechanisms of Antisense Oligonucleotides as a Therapeutic Platform. Annu Rev Pharmacol 2010;50:259–93.
13. Kurreck J. Antisense technologies - Improvement through novel chemical modifications. Eur J Biochem 2003;270(8):1628–44.
14. Evers MM, Toonen LJ, van Roon-Mom WM. Antisense oligonucleotides in therapy for neurodegenerative disorders. Adv Drug Deliv Rev 2015;87:90–103.
15. Lima WF, De Hoyos CL, Liang XH, et al. RNA cleavage products generated by antisense oligonucleotides and siRNAs are processed by the RNA surveillance machinery. Nucleic Acids Res 2016;44(7):3351–63.
16. Du LT, Pollard JM, Gatti RA. Correction of prototypic ATM splicing mutations and aberrant ATM function with antisense morpholino oligonucleotides. Proc Natl Acad Sci U S A 2007;104(14):6007–12.
17. Evers MM, Tran HD, Zalachoras I, et al. Ataxin-3 protein modification as a treatment strategy for spinocerebellar ataxia type 3: Removal of the CAG containing exon. Neurobiol Dis 2013;58:49–56.
18. Singh NK, Singh NN, Androphy EJ, et al. Splicing of a critical exon of human survival motor neuron is regulated by a unique silencer element located in the last intron. Mol Cell Biol 2006;26(4):1333–46.
19. Dunbar CE, High KA, Joung JK, et al. Gene therapy comes of age. Science 2018;359(6372):eaan4672.
20. Crudele JM, Chamberlain JS. AAV-based gene therapies for the muscular dystrophies. Hum Mol Genet 2019;28(R1):R102–7.
21. Ramos JN, Hollinger K, Bengtsson NE, et al. Development of Novel Microdystrophins with Enhanced Functionality. Mol Ther 2019;27(3):623–35.
22. Bisset DR, Stepniak Konieczna EA, Zavaljevski M, et al. Therapeutic impact of systemic AAV-mediated RNA interference in a mouse model of myotonic dystrophy. Hum Mol Genet 2015;24(17):4971–83.
23. Furling D, Doucet G, Langlois MA, et al. Viral vector producing antisense RNA restores myotonic dystrophy myoblast functions. Gene Ther 2003;10(9): 795–802.

24. Wallace LM, Saad NY, Pyne NK, et al. Pre-clinical Safety and Off-Target Studies to Support Translation of AAV-Mediated RNAi Therapy for FSHD. Mol Ther Methods Clin Dev 2018;8:121–30.

25. Grunewald J, Zhou RH, Garcia SP, et al. Transcriptome-wide off-target RNA editing induced by CRISPR-guided DNA base editors. Nature 2019;569(7756): 433–7.

26. Newswire P. Audentes Therapeutics announces expansion of AAV technology platform and pipeline with new development programs for Duchennemuscular dystrophy and myotonic dystrophy 2019 Available at: https://www.prnewswire. com/news-releases/audentes-therapeutics-announces-expansion-of-aav-techn ology-platform-and-pipeline-with-new-development-programs-for-duchenne-m uscular-dystrophy-and-myotonic-dystrophy-300825843.html. Accessed: October 3, 2020.

27. Vulin A, Barthelemy I, Goyenvalle A, et al. Muscle function recovery in golden retriever muscular dystrophy after AAV1-U7 exon skipping. Mol Ther 2012; 20(11):2120–33.

28. Birnkrant DJ, Bushby K, Bann CM, et al. Diagnosis and management of Duchenne muscular dystrophy, part 1: diagnosis, and neuromuscular, rehabilitation, endocrine, and gastrointestinal and nutritional management. Lancet Neurol 2018;17(3):251–67.

29. Messina S, Vita GL. Clinical management of Duchenne muscular dystrophy: the state of the art. Neurol Sci 2018;39(11):1837–45.

30. Chamberlain JR, Chamberlain JS. Progress toward Gene Therapy for Duchenne Muscular Dystrophy. Mol Ther 2017;25(5):1125–31.

31. Guglieri M, Bushby K, McDermott MP, et al. Developing standardized corticosteroid treatment for Duchenne muscular dystrophy. Contemp Clin Trials 2017; 58:34–9.

32. Birnkrant DJ, Bushby K, Bann CM, et al. Diagnosis and management of Duchenne muscular dystrophy, part 2: respiratory, cardiac, bone health, and orthopaedic management. Lancet Neurol 2018;17(4):347–61.

33. Birnkrant DJ, Bushby K, Bann CM, et al. Diagnosis and management of Duchenne muscular dystrophy, part 3: primary care, emergency management, psychosocial care, and transitions of care across the lifespan. Lancet Neurol 2018;17(5):445–55.

34. Passamano L, Taglia A, Palladino A, et al. Improvement of survival in Duchenne Muscular Dystrophy: retrospective analysis of 835 patients. Acta Myol 2012; 31(2):121–5.

35. Saito T, Kawai M, Kimura E, et al. Study of Duchenne muscular dystrophy long-term survivors aged 40 years and older living in specialized institutions in Japan. Neuromuscul Disord 2017;27(2):107–14.

36. Matthews E, Brassington R, Kuntzer T, et al. Corticosteroids for the treatment of Duchenne muscular dystrophy. Cochrane Database Syst Rev 2016;(5):CD003725.

37. Lebel DE, Corston JA, McAdam LC, et al. Glucocorticoid treatment for the prevention of scoliosis in children with Duchenne muscular dystrophy: long-term follow-up. J Bone Joint Surg Am 2013;95(12):1057–61.

38. Lamb MM, West NA, Ouyang L, et al. Corticosteroid Treatment and Growth Patterns in Ambulatory Males with Duchenne Muscular Dystrophy. J Pediatr 2016; 173:207–13.e3.

39. Griggs RC, Herr BE, Reha A, et al. Corticosteroids in Duchenne muscular dystrophy: major variations in practice. Muscle Nerve 2013;48(1):27–31.

40. Bello L, Gordish-Dressman H, Morgenroth LP, et al. Prednisone/prednisolone and deflazacort regimens in the CINRG Duchenne Natural History Study. Neurology 2015;85(12):1048–55.
41. Griggs RC, Miller JP, Greenberg CR, et al. Efficacy and safety of deflazacort vs prednisone and placebo for Duchenne muscular dystrophy. Neurology 2016; 87(20):2123–31.
42. Crow RA, Hart KA, McDermott MP, et al. A checklist for clinical trials in rare disease: obstacles and anticipatory actions-lessons learned from the FOR-DMD trial. Trials 2018;19(1):291.
43. Cirak S, Arechavala-Gomeza V, Guglieri M, et al. Exon skipping and dystrophin restoration in patients with Duchenne muscular dystrophy after systemic phosphorodiamidate morpholino oligomer treatment: an open-label, phase 2, dose-escalation study. Lancet 2011;378(9791):595–605.
44. Mendell JR, Goemans N, Lowes LP, et al. Longitudinal effect of eteplirsen versus historical control on ambulation in Duchenne muscular dystrophy. Ann Neurol 2016;79(2):257–71.
45. Golodirsen FDA approval. Available at: https://www.fda.gov/news-events/press-announcements/fda-grants-accelerated-approval-first-targeted-treatment-rare-duchenne-muscular-dystrophy-mutation. Accessed December 19, 2019.
46. Muntoni F, Frank D, Sardone V, et al. Golodirsen Induces Exon Skipping Leading to Sarcolemmal Dystrophin Expression in Duchenne Muscular Dystrophy Patients With Mutations Amenable to Exon 53 Skipping. Neurology 2018;90(15 Supplement).
47. Finkel RS, Mercuri E, Darras BT, et al. Nusinersen versus Sham Control in Infantile-Onset Spinal Muscular Atrophy. N Engl J Med 2017;377(18):1723–32.
48. Mercuri E, Darras BT, Chiriboga CA, et al. Nusinersen versus Sham Control in Later-Onset Spinal Muscular Atrophy. N Engl J Med 2018;378(7):625–35.
49. Mendell JR, Al-Zaidy S, Shell R, et al. Single-Dose Gene-Replacement Therapy for Spinal Muscular Atrophy. N Engl J Med 2017;377(18):1713–22.
50. Writing Group, Edaravone (MCI-186) ALS 19 Study Group. Safety and efficacy of edaravone in well defined patients with amyotrophic lateral sclerosis: a randomised, double-blind, placebo-controlled trial. Lancet Neurol 2017;16(7): 505–12.
51. Aartsma-Rus A, Goemans N. A Sequel to the Eteplirsen Saga: Eteplirsen Is Approved in the United States but Was Not Approved in Europe. Nucleic Acid Ther 2019;29(1):13–5.
52. Finkel RS, Flanigan KM, Wong B, et al. Phase 2a study of ataluren-mediated dystrophin production in patients with nonsense mutation Duchenne muscular dystrophy. PLoS One 2013;8(12):e81302.
53. McDonald C, Reha A, Elfring GL, et al. Timed Function Tests and Other Physical Function Outcomes in Ataluren-Treated Patients with Nonsense Mutation Duchenne Muscular Dystrophy (nmDMD). Neuromuscul Disord 2014;24:861.
54. McDonald CM, Campbell C, Torricelli RE, et al. Ataluren in patients with nonsense mutation Duchenne muscular dystrophy (ACT DMD): a multicentre, randomised, double-blind, placebo-controlled, phase 3 trial. Lancet 2017; 390(10101):1489–98.
55. Available at: https://www.multivu.com/players/English/8420051-ptc-therapeutics-stride-registry-duchenne-muscular-dystrophy-translarna/. Accessed December 1, 2019.
56. Casimersen Shows Promising Phase 3 Results for DMD, May Open Door for FDA New Drug Application. Available at: https://musculardystrophynews.com/

2019/04/05/sareptas-casimersen-shows-promising-results-phase-3-trial/.   Accessed December 19, 2019.

57. Viltolarsen phase 2 data update. Available at: http://www.nspharma.com/pdf/WMS2019_US_P2_Poster_slides_Final.pdf. Accessed December 19, 2019.

58. Biogen to Present New Interim Data from Its Phase 1/2 Clinical Study of Tofersen (BIIB067) for the Potential Treatment of a Subtype of Familial Amyotrophic Lateral Sclerosis (ALS). Available at: http://investors.biogen.com/news-releases/news-release-details/biogen-present-new-interim-data-its-phase-12-clinical-study. Accessed December 19, 2019.

59. Clemens P, Rao V, Connolly A, et al. A Phase II, Dose Finding Study to Assess the Safety, Tolerability, Pharmacokinetics, and Pharmacodynamics of NS-065/NCNP-01 (Viltolarsen) in Boys with Duchenne Muscular Dystrophy (DMD). Neuromuscul Disord 2018;28(Suppl 2):S68. Available at: http://www.nspharma.com/pdf/Poster_slides_WMS_Final.pdf.

60. Komaki H, Nagata T, Saito T, et al. Systemic administration of the antisense oligonucleotide NS-065/NCNP-01 for skipping of exon 53 in patients with Duchenne muscular dystrophy. Sci Transl Med 2018;10(437):eaan0713.

61. Aoki Y, Yokota T, Nagata T, et al. Bodywide skipping of exons 45-55 in dystrophic mdx52 mice by systemic antisense delivery. Proc Natl Acad Sci U S A 2012;109(34):13763–8.

62. Echigoya Y, Aoki Y, Miskew B, et al. Long-term efficacy of systemic multiexon skipping targeting dystrophin exons 45-55 with a cocktail of vivo-morpholinos in mdx52 mice. Mol Ther Nucleic Acids 2015;4:e225.

63. Hwang J, Yokota T. Recent advancements in exon-skipping therapies using antisense oligonucleotides and genome editing for the treatment of various muscular dystrophies. Expert Rev Mol Med 2019;21:e5.

64. Bettica P, Petrini S, D'Oria V, et al. Histological effects of givinostat in boys with Duchenne muscular dystrophy. Neuromuscul Disord 2016;26(10):643–9.

65. Donovan JV, Sweeney K, Tennekoon L, et al. Move DMD Results: Effects of Edasalonexent, an NF-kB Inhibitor, in 4 to 7 Year Old Patients with Duchenne Muscular Dystrophy. AAN annual meeting, Boston, April 22-28, 2017.

66. Taylor M, Jefferies J, Byrne B, et al. Cardiac and skeletal muscle effects in the randomized HOPE-Duchenne trial. Neurology 2019;92(8):E866–78.

67. Nagy S, Hafner P, Schmidt S, et al. Tamoxifen in Duchenne muscular dystrophy (TAMDMD): study protocol for a multicenter, randomized, placebo-controlled, double-blind phase 3 trial. Trials 2019;20(1):637.

68. Raman SV, Hor KN, Mazur W, et al. Stabilization of Early Duchenne Cardiomyopathy With Aldosterone Inhibition: Results of the Multicenter AIDMD Trial. J Am Heart Assoc 2019;8(19):e013501.

69. An Efficacy and Safety Trial of Intravenous Zoledronic Acid Twice Yearly in Osteoporotic Children Treated With Glucocorticoids. Available at: https://clinicaltrials.gov/ct2/show/study/NCT00799266. Accessed December 2, 2019.

70. Strength Training in Duchenne Muscular Dystrophy. Available at: https://clinicaltrials.gov/ct2/show/study/NCT02421523. Accessed December 2, 2019.

71. Flanigan KM. Duchenne and Becker Muscular Dystrophies. Neurol Clin 2014;32(3):671.

72. Wein N, Alfano L, Flanigan KM. Genetics and Emerging Treatments for Duchenne and Becker Muscular Dystrophy. Pediatr Clin North Am 2015;62(3):723–+.

73. Beggs AH, Hoffman EP, Snyder JR, et al. Exploring the Molecular-Basis for Variability among Patients with Becker Muscular-Dystrophy - Dystrophin Gene and Protein Studies. Am J Hum Genet 1991;49(1):54–67.
74. Kaspar RW, Allen HD, Ray WC, et al. Analysis of dystrophin deletion mutations predicts age of cardiomyopathy onset in becker muscular dystrophy. Circ Cardiovasc Genet 2009;2(6):544–51.
75. Mendell JR, Sahenk Z, Malik V, et al. A phase 1/2a follistatin gene therapy trial for becker muscular dystrophy. Mol Ther 2015;23(1):192–201.
76. Available at: https://clinicaltrials.gov/ct2/show/NCT04054375?cond=Becker+Muscular+Dystrophy&draw=5&rank=27. https://clinicaltrials.gov/ct2/show/NCT04054375?cond=Becker+Muscular+Dystrophy&draw=5&rank=27. Accessed December 2, 2019.
77. Chu ML, Moran E. The Limb-Girdle Muscular Dystrophies: Is Treatment on the Horizon? Neurotherapeutics 2018;15(4):849–62.
78. Liewluck T, Milone M. Untangling the Complexity of Limb-Girdle Muscular Dystrophies. Muscle Nerve 2018;58(2):167–77.
79. Wicklund MP, Kissel JT. The Limb-Girdle Muscular Dystrophies. Neurol Clin 2014;32(3):729–+.
80. Lee JJA, Maruyama R, Duddy W, et al. Identification of Novel Antisense-Mediated Exon Skipping Targets in DYSF for Therapeutic Treatment of Dysferlinopathy. Mol Ther Nucleic Acids 2018;13:596–604.
81. Bansal D, Miyake K, Vogel SS, et al. Defective membrane repair in dysferlin-deficient muscular dystrophy. Nature 2003;423(6936):168–72.
82. Sondergaard PC, Griffin DA, Pozsgai ER, et al. AAV.Dysferlin Overlap Vectors Restore Function in Dysferlinopathy Animal Models. Ann Clin Transl Neurol 2015;2(3):256–70.
83. Barthelemy F, Blouin C, Wein N, et al. Exon 32 Skipping of Dysferlin Rescues Membrane Repair in Patients' Cells. J Neuromuscul Dis 2015;2(3):281–90.
84. Mendell JR, Rodino-Klapac LR, Rosales XQ, et al. Sustained alpha-sarcoglycan gene expression after gene transfer in limb-girdle muscular dystrophy, type 2D. Ann Neurol 2010;68(5):629–38.
85. Herson S, Hentati F, Rigolet A, et al. A phase I dose-escalating study of AAV1-gamma-sarcoglycan gene therapy for limb girdle muscular dystrophy type 2C. Mol Ther 2011;19:S20–1.
86. Wyatt EJ, Demonbreun AR, Kim EY, et al. Efficient exon skipping of SGCG mutations mediated by phosphorodiamidate morpholino oligomers. JCI Insight 2018;3(9).
87. Statland J, Tawil R. Facioscapulohumeral muscular dystrophy. Neurol Clin 2014; 32(3):721–8, ix.
88. Miller DG. Gene Therapy for Facioscapulohumeral Muscular Dystrophy (FSHD). In: Duan D, Mendell JR, editors. Muscle gene therapy. Cham, Switzerland: Springer Nature:2019;509-523.
89. Mellion M, Ronco L, Thompson, D. et al. Phase 1 Clinical Trial of Losmapimod in Facioscapulohumeral Muscular Dystrophy (FSHD): Safety, Tolerability and Target Engagement. 2020. Available at: https://mdaconference.org/node/943. Accessed: October 3, 2020.
90. Mercuri E, Bertini E, Iannaccone ST. Childhood spinal muscular atrophy: controversies and challenges. Lancet Neurol 2012;11(5):443–52.
91. Lefebvre S, Burglen L, Reboullet S, et al. Identification and characterization of a spinal muscular atrophy-determining gene. Cell 1995;80(1):155–65.

92. Dubowitz V. Chaos in the classification of SMA: a possible resolution. Neuromuscul Disord 1995;5(1):3–5.

93. Calucho M, Bernal S, Alias L, et al. Correlation between SMA type and SMN2 copy number revisited: An analysis of 625 unrelated Spanish patients and a compilation of 2834 reported cases. Neuromuscul Disord 2018;28(3):208–15.

94. Wirth B, Brichta L, Schrank B, et al. Mildly affected patients with spinal muscular atrophy are partially protected by an increased SMN2 copy number. Hum Genet 2006;119(4):422–8.

95. Messina S. New Directions for SMA Therapy. J Clin Med 2018;7(9):251.

96. A Study for Participants With Spinal Muscular Atrophy (SMA) Who Previously Participated in Nusinersen (ISIS 396443) Investigational Studies. (SHINE). Available at: https://www.clinicaltrials.gov/ct2/show/NCT02594124. Accessed December 4, 2019.

97. De Vivo DC, Bertini E, Swoboda KJ, et al. Nusinersen initiated in infants during the presymptomatic stage of spinal muscular atrophy: Interim efficacy and safety results from the Phase 2 NURTURE study. Neuromuscul Disord 2019; 29(11):842–56.

98. Darras BT, Chiriboga CA, Iannaccone ST, et al. Nusinersen in later-onset spinal-muscular atrophy Long-term results from the phase 1/2 studies. Neurology 2019;92(21):E2492–506.

99. SPINRAZA® (Nusinersen) Approved in the European Union as First Treatment for Spinal Muscular Atrophy. Available at: http://investors.biogen.com/news-releases/news-release-details/spinrazar-nusinersen-approved-european-union-first-treatment. Accessed December 4, 2019.

100. Single-Dose Gene Replacement Therapy Clinical Trial for Patients With Spinal Muscular Atrophy Type 1 (STRIVE-EU). Available at: https://www.clinicaltrials.gov/ct2/show/NCT03461289. Accessed December 4, 2019.

101. Zolgensma FDA approval. Available at: https://www.fda.gov/vaccines-blood-biologics/zolgensma. Accessed December 4, 2019.

102. Ratni H, Ebeling M, Baird J, et al. Discovery of Risdiplam, a Selective Survival of Motor Neuron-2 (SMN2) Gene Splicing Modifier for the Treatment of Spinal Muscular Atrophy (SMA). J Med Chem 2018;61(15):6501–17.

103. A Study to Investigate the Safety, Tolerability, Pharmacokinetics, Pharmacodynamics and Efficacy of Risdiplam (RO7034067) in Type 2 and 3 Spinal Muscular Atrophy (SMA) Participants (SUNFISH). Available at: https://clinicaltrials.gov/ct2/show/NCT02908685. Accessed December 4, 2019.

104. Investigate Safety, Tolerability, PK, PD and Efficacy of Risdiplam (RO7034067) in Infants With Type1 Spinal Muscular Atrophy (FIREFISH). Available at: https://clinicaltrials.gov/ct2/show/NCT02913482. Accessed December 4, 2019.

105. A Study of Risdiplam (RO7034067) in Adult and Pediatric Participants With Spinal Muscular Atrophy (Jewelfish). Available at: https://clinicaltrials.gov/ct2/show/NCT03032172. Accessed December 4, 2019.

106. Risdiplam demonstrates preliminary evidence of clinical benefit in type 1, 2, & 3 spinal muscular atrophy patients [press release]. South Plainfield (NJ), 2018. Available at: https://www.prnewswire.com/news-releases/risdiplam-demonstrates-preliminary-evidence-of-clinical-benefit-in-type-1-2-3-spinal-muscular-atrophy-patients-300723444.html. Accessed October 3, 2020.

107. Bertini E, Dessaud E, Mercuri E, et al. Safety and efficacy of olesoxime in patients with type 2 or non-ambulatory type 3 spinal muscular atrophy: a randomised, double-blind, placebo-controlled phase 2 trial. Lancet Neurol 2017; 16(7):513–22.

108. An Active Treatment Study of SRK-015 in Patients With Type 2 or Type 3 Spinal Muscular Atrophy (TOPAZ). Available at: https://clinicaltrials.gov/ct2/show/NCT03921528?term=SRK-015&rank=1. Accessed December 4, 2019.

109. Reldesemtiv. Available at: https://cytokinetics.com/clinical-trials/. Accessed December 4, 2019.

110. Pasinelli P, Brown RH. Molecular biology of amyotrophic lateral sclerosis: insights from genetics. Nat Rev Neurosci 2006;7(9):710–23.

111. Brown RH, Al-Chalabi A. Amyotrophic Lateral Sclerosis. N Engl J Med 2017; 377(2):162–72.

112. Miller RG, Mitchell JD, Moore DH. Riluzole for amyotrophic lateral sclerosis (ALS)/motor neuron disease (MND). Cochrane Database Syst Rev 2012;(3):CD001447.

113. Shefner J, Heiman-Patterson T, Pioro EP, et al. Long-term edaravone efficacy in amyotrophic lateral sclerosis: Post-hoc analyses of Study 19 (MCI186-19). Muscle Nerve 2019;61(2):218–21.

114. Writing Group On Behalf Of The Edaravone Als 19 Study Group. Open-label 24-week extension study of edaravone (MCI-186) in amyotrophic lateral sclerosis. Amyotroph Lateral Scler Frontotemporal Degener 2017;18(sup1):55–63.

115. D'Amico E, Factor-Litvak P, Santella RM, et al. Clinical perspective on oxidative stress in sporadic amyotrophic lateral sclerosis. Free Radic Biol Med 2013;65:509–27.

116. Mitsumoto H, Santella RM, Liu X, et al. Oxidative stress biomarkers in sporadic ALS. Amyotroph Lateral Scler 2008;9(3):177–83.

117. Writing-Group On Behalf Of The Edaravone ALS 18 Study Group. Exploratory double-blind, parallel-group, placebo-controlled study of edaravone (MCI-186) in amyotrophic lateral sclerosis (Japan ALS severity classification: Grade 3, requiring assistance for eating, excretion or ambulation). Amyotroph Lateral Scler Frontotemporal Degener 2017;18(sup1):40–8.

118. FDA approves drug to treat ALS. Available at: https://www.fda.gov/news-events/press-announcements/fda-approves-drug-treat-als. Accessed Dececmber 9, 2019.

119. Withdrawal of the marketing authorisation application for Radicava (edaravone). Available at: https://www.ema.europa.eu/en/documents/medicine-qa/questions-answers-withdrawal-marketing-authorisation-application-radicava-edaravone_en.pdf. Accessed Dececmber 9, 2019.

120. Renton AE, Chio A, Traynor BJ. State of play in amyotrophic lateral sclerosis genetics. Nat Neurosci 2014;17(1):17–23.

121. Chio A, Logroscino G, Hardiman O, et al. Prognostic factors in ALS: A critical review. Amyotroph Lateral Scler 2009;10(5–6):310–23.

122. Miller TM, Pestronk A, David W. An antisense oligonucleotide against SOD1 delivered intrathecally for patients with SOD1 familial amyotrophic lateral sclerosis: a phase 1, randomised, first-in-man study (vol 12, pg 435, 2013). Lancet Neurol 2013;12(5):423.

123. Cappella M, Ciotti C, Cohen-Tannoudji M, et al. Gene Therapy for ALS-A Perspective. Int J Mol Sci 2019;20(18):4388.

124. Al-Chalabi A, Brown RH Jr. Finding a Treatment for ALS - Will Gene Editing Cut It? N Engl J Med 2018;378(15):1454–6.

125. Gaj T, Ojala DS, Ekman FK, et al. In vivo genome editing improves motor function and extends survival in a mouse model of ALS. Sci Adv 2017;3(12):eaar3952.

126. Staff NP, Madigan NN, Morris J, et al. Safety of intrathecal autologous adipose-derived mesenchymal stromal cells in patients with ALS. Neurology 2016; 87(21):2230–4.

127. Oh KW, Moon C, Kim HY, et al. Phase I trial of repeated intrathecal autologous bone marrow-derived mesenchymal stromal cells in amyotrophic lateral sclerosis. Stem Cells Transl Med 2015;4(6):590–7.

128. Sykova E, Rychmach P, Drahoradova I, et al. Transplantation of Mesenchymal Stromal Cells in Patients With Amyotrophic Lateral Sclerosis: Results of Phase I/IIa Clinical Trial. Cell Transplant 2017;26(4):647–58.

129. Petrou P, Gothelf Y, Argov Z, et al. Safety and Clinical Effects of Mesenchymal Stem Cells Secreting Neurotrophic Factor Transplantation in Patients With Amyotrophic Lateral Sclerosis: Results of Phase 1/2 and 2a Clinical Trials. JAMA Neurol 2016;73(3):337–44.

130. Kaji R, Imai T, Iwasaki Y, et al. Ultra-high-dose methylcobalamin in amyotrophic lateral sclerosis: a long-term phase II/III randomised controlled study. J Neurol Neurosurg Psychiatry 2019;90(4):451–7.

131. Kim HY, Moon C, Kim KS, et al. Recombinant human erythropoietin in amyotrophic lateral sclerosis: a pilot study of safety and feasibility. J Clin Neurol 2014; 10(4):342–7.

132. Urbi B, Broadley S, Bedlack R, et al. Study protocol for a randomised, double-blind, placebo-controlled study evaluating the Efficacy of cannabis-based Medicine Extract in slowing the disease pRogression of Amyotrophic Lateral sclerosis or motor neurone Disease: the EMERALD trial. BMJ Open 2019; 9(11):e029449.

133. Bradley WG, Miller RX, Levine TD, et al. Studies of Environmental Risk Factors in Amyotrophic Lateral Sclerosis (ALS) and a Phase I Clinical Trial of L-Serine. Neurotox Res 2018;33(1):192–8.

134. Elia AE, Lalli S, Monsurro MR, et al. Tauroursodeoxycholic acid in the treatment of patients with amyotrophic lateral sclerosis. Eur J Neurol 2016;23(1):45–52.

135. Al-Chalabi A, Shaw P, Leigh PN, et al. Oral levosimendan in amyotrophic lateral sclerosis: a phase II multicentre, randomised, double-blind, placebo-controlled trial. J Neurol Neurosurg Psychiatry 2019;90(10):1165–70.

136. Benatar M, Wuu J, Andersen PM, et al. Randomized, double-blind, placebo-controlled trial of arimoclomol in rapidly progressive SOD1 ALS. Neurology 2018;90(7):e565–74.

137. Baker M, Griggs R, Byrne B, et al. Maximizing the Benefit of Life-Saving Treatments for Pompe Disease, Spinal Muscular Atrophy, and Duchenne Muscular Dystrophy Through Newborn Screening: Essential Steps. JAMA Neurol 2019. https://doi.org/10.1001/jamaneurol.2019.1206.

138. The UK NSC recommendation on Spinal Muscular Atrophy. Available at: https://legacyscreening.phe.org.uk/sma. Accessed December 10, 2019.

139. Murphy SM, Puwanant A, Griggs RC, et al. Unintended effects of orphan product designation for rare neurological diseases. Ann Neurol 2012;72(4):481–90.

140. Smith GA. The Cost of Drugs for Rare Diseases Is Threatening the U.S. Health Care System. Harv Bus Rev 2017.

141. https://www.fda.gov/news-events/press-announcements/fda-approves-oral-treatment-spinal-muscular-atrophy.

Advances in the Management of Small Fiber Neuropathy

Lawrence A. Zeidman, MD

KEYWORDS

- Small fiber neuropathy • TS-HDS • FGFR-3 • Plexin D1 • IVIg
- Intravenous immunoglobulin • TTR amyloidosis • Sodium channelopathy

KEY POINTS

- Small fiber neuropathy (SFN) is prevalent and sometimes mistaken for other syndromes such as fibromyalgia, cramps, and complex regional pain syndrome.
- Autonomic testing such as quantitative sudomotor axon reflex testing (QSART) and pathologic evaluation by skin punch biopsy are the mainstays of SFN diagnosis, which is negative on nerve conduction studies.
- Sodium channelopathies are an important new potentially treatable SFN etiology, as are other previously known genetic syndromes such as Fabry Disease and TTR amyloidosis.
- Important new inflammatory biomarkers are emerging for SFN, including TS-HDS, FGFR3 Plexin D1, and voltage-gated potassium channel autoantibodies.
- Intravenous Immunoglobulin is showing promise as a form of treatment in immune-mediated SFN syndromes.

BACKGROUND

Small fiber neuropathy (SFN) is a relatively common cause of neurologic morbidity. Currently its minimum estimated worldwide prevalence is 53 per 100,000 population,[1] but that number will likely rise as better testing methods emerge. This probably means that at least 4 million people worldwide have SFN.[2] The prevalence of SFN is higher than other neuromuscular neurologic conditions, including myasthenia gravis (20 per 100,000)[3] and also amyotrophic lateral sclerosis (5 per 100,000).[4] The prevalence of SFN is largely underestimated even since the previous estimated prevalence is based on neurologists' confirmation of the diagnosis, whereas most cases are undiagnosed or misdiagnosed. In fact, recent evidence suggests that 40% of patients with fibromyalgia may have SFN, so the number of people with SFN worldwide may be

Neuromuscular-EMG Division, Department of Neurology, Loyola University Chicago, Loyola University Medical Center, Stritch School of Medicine, 2160 South First Avenue, Maguire Building - Room 2700, Maywood, IL 60153-3328, USA
E-mail addresses: lzeidman@luc.edu; larryzeidman@gmail.com

Neurol Clin 39 (2021) 113–131
https://doi.org/10.1016/j.ncl.2020.09.006
0733-8619/21/© 2020 Elsevier Inc. All rights reserved.
neurologic.theclinics.com

closer to 100 million.[2] SFN has been a burgeoning area of clinical, laboratory, and industry research, especially in the past 20 years with the growing popularity and acceptance of skin punch biopsy as part of the neurologist's armamentarium. This article is not an attempt to rehash what has been discussed in some excellent prior reviews,[5–12] but to provide an overview while providing some updates in this rapidly changing realm and to discuss controversial management and treatment issues regarding SFN.

Small nerve fibers include both the thinly myelinated Aδ fibers that conduct electricity at approximately 20 m/s and are responsible for cold temperature and sharp pain sensation, as well as unmyelinated C fibers (responsible for warm sensation and heat pain) that conduct electricity at approximately 2 m/s and autonomic fibers. The latter include postganglionic sympathetic fibers innervating internal organs along with fibers (sudomotor) innervating sweat glands.[5,13] The extremely slow conduction times of small nerves can be contrasted with large fiber conduction times of 35 to 75 m/s (Aβ) controlling touch sensation, and 80 to 120 m/s for proprioceptive fibers (Aα)[14] (**Fig. 1**). As electromyography/nerve conduction studies (EMG/NCS) typically only test these large myelinated fibers, this test is typically normal in SFN (and patients >75 years old with absent sural sensory responses can still be called isolated SFN).[5,10]

Patients present either with somatic complaints, typically constant or intermittent pain (burning, stabbing, electrical shocks or shooting, tingling, hyperesthesia, allodynia, or dysesthesias such as pebbles or coals on the skin), or autonomic complaints, or an overlap of the two. Patients may not connect the autonomic and somatic complaints. If the autonomic complaints, including postural lightheadedness, syncope, palpitations, dry eyes and mouth, abnormal sweating or skin discoloration, early satiety, constipation, urinary retention, and erectile dysfunction, predominate the syndrome may be called an autonomic neuropathy instead.[6,8,15] But cramps and myalgias can occur as well and can be diffuse over the body, leading to a misdiagnosis of fibromyalgia,[6] and pruritus and restless legs can be seen also.[7] Symptoms can be length-dependent (LD), as in a typical peripheral neuropathy, or non–length-dependent (NLD), with female sex, younger age of onset and SFN diagnosis, and immune-mediated causes more associated with the latter and less association with diabetes. NLD-SFN can be more associated with impaired glucose tolerance (IGT) than LD-SFN, and more association with itchiness and allodynia, along with less responsiveness to pain medications including multiple narcotics (LD-SFN more typically responds to 1 or 2 non-narcotic analgesics). Overall, the ratio of LD to NLD cases is likely 3:1 or 4:1, but NLD cases may be underdiagnosed or misdiagnosed with psychogenic complaints.[7]

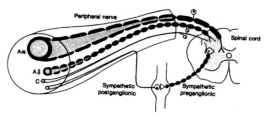

Fig. 1. Some peripheral nerve fibers highlighting the differential fiber size with large myelinated Aβ fibers, small myelinated Aδ fibers, unmyelinated C fibers, and unmyelinated sympathetic fibers. (*From* Vinik AI, Nevoret ML, Casellini C. The New Age of Sudomotor Function Testing: A Sensitive and Specific Biomarker for Diagnosis, Estimation of Severity, Monitoring Progression, and Regression in Response to Intervention. Front Endocrinol (Lausanne). 2015;6:94; with permission.)

Notable also is that SFN can present acutely like a Guillain-Barré syndrome, preceded by an antecedent infection, along with hyporeflexia and albumin-cytologic dissociation. Three such patients either responded to corticosteroid or intravenous immunoglobulin (IVIg) treatment.[16]

On examination, there may be no findings or there may be loss of pin pinprick and thermal sensation in affected regions, or hyperalgesia. Vibration and proprioception sensation, motor strength, coordination, and reflexes are typically normal on examination or vibration may be mildly diminished. Skin and sweating changes may be seen also.[8]

Although up to 50% of SFN cases may be idiopathic,[8] a large differential of causes has been identified in recent years and continues to be updated. Most of these have been well-covered in other reviews but some more novel causes are discussed in further detail in this review (**Box 1**). The cryptogenic incidence may indeed be closer to 25%.[17] Typical causes include diabetes mellitus and IGT, autoimmune (eg, celiac disease, sarcoidosis, Sjögren's syndrome), infectious (eg, human immunodeficiency virus, hepatitis C), alcohol dependence and exposure to toxins, nutritional deficiencies (eg, vitamin B12 deficiency), amyloidosis and paraneoplastic syndromes, and hereditary causes (eg, Fabry's disease, sodium channelopathies).[7] Another consideration regarding the differential diagnosis is whether SFN is one syndrome or multiple

---

Box 1
Some updated causes of small fiber neuropathy

- Diabetes and impaired glucose tolerance
- Rapid glycemic lowering
- Hyperlipidemia, metabolic syndrome
- Chronic kidney disease
- Human immunodeficiency virus, Hepatitis C
- Celiac disease, gluten sensitivity, inflammatory bowel disease (IBD)
- Hypothyroidism, autoimmune thyroiditis
- Vitamin B12 deficiency, Vitamin B1 deficiency, Vitamin B6 toxicity
- Paraproteinemia (MGUS)
- Amyloidosis-familial amyloid polyneuropathy/TTR mutation, primary AL
- Systemic lupus erythematosus, Sjögren syndrome, sarcoidosis, vasculitis, rheumatoid arthritis, Churg-Strauss Disease
- Other immune-mediated – TS-HDS, FGFR-3, Plexin D1, Anti-voltage-gated potassium channel (VGKC) antibody
- Paraneoplastic syndromes (CRMP-5, PCA-2)
- Hereditary- Fabry disease, SCN9A/10A/11A mutations, HSAN, Ehlers-Danlos syndrome
- Pompe disease
- Tangier disease
- Toxic – Alcoholism, chemotherapy (bortezomib), thallium, metronidazole, nitrofurantoin, linezolid, statins, trauma (electrical, cold)
- Pain syndromes-sickle cell disease, fibromyalgia, CRPS Type I (RSD), cramps
- Idiopathic

variants that overlap, and whether SFN is the primary disease or a secondary process from an underlying disease state. A novel way to think about SFN is to categorize it as either small fiber sodium-channel dysfunction, small fiber–mediated painful neuropathy (SFMPN), small fiber–mediated widespread pain (SFMWP, including fibromyalgia and muscle cramps), or small fiber–mediated autonomic dysfunction (SFMAD)[6] (**Fig. 2**).

Now that SFN has been defined and some background including recent updates has been provided, the rest of this review will focus on specific recent developments regarding diagnostic workup, follow-up assessment, specific and overlapping disease states in SFN, as well as disease-modifying treatment. Other reviews contain excellent discussions of symptomatic-only pharmacotherapeutics for neuropathic pain[8,13] and this will not be included here.

SMALL FIBER NEUROPATHY DIAGNOSTICS

Because EMG/NCS is typically normal in SFN, if the diagnosis cannot be made exclusively on the clinical evaluation, the mainstay of diagnostic testing (**Table 1**) is typically autonomic evaluation or skin punch biopsy.[5,7–11] Both can be highly sensitive and specific and have certain advantages and disadvantages, and some ongoing controversies exist. Autonomic testing for SFN includes most commonly quantitative sudomotor axon reflex testing (QSART), quantitative sensory testing (QST), sympathetic skin responses (SSR), or thermoregulatory sweat testing (TST), but newer techniques include laser-evoked potentials, electrochemical skin conductance (ESC; "Sudoscan"), corneal confocal microscopy (CCM),[12] skin wrinkling,[18] and laser-evoked potentials (LEP). Other autonomic testing, such as cardiovagal maneuvers and tilt-table testing may be useful to evaluate cardiovascular symptoms such as orthostatic intolerance, palpitations, and tachycardia.

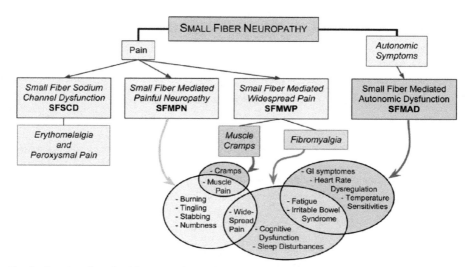

Fig. 2. Overlapping classification scheme for small fiber and autonomic neuropathies, along with sodium channelopathies and pain syndromes based on new evidence. (*From* Levine TD. Small Fiber Neuropathy: Disease Classification Beyond Pain and Burning. J Cent Nerv Syst Dis 2018;10:1–6; with permission.)

Table 1
Primary diagnostic tests for small fiber neuropathy: additive and complementary

Testing qualities	SSR	QSART	QST	TST	IENFD
Sensitivity	10%–41%	80%	60%–85%	72%	88%–90%
Specificity	77.6%	Unknown	Unknown	Unknown	89%–97%
Utility	Fast, simple, reproducible	Sensitive, reproducible, accurate, quantitative, proximal-to-distal topography revealed, dynamic sudomotor function over time	Available, well-tolerated	Sweating tested all over body including head and neck	Highest sensitivity and specificity, gold standard, available anywhere, can see proximal-to-distal gradient
Availability	Widespread – standard EMG machines	Restricted – autonomic labs	Restricted – autonomic labs	Restricted – autonomic labs	Widespread -can order commercial kit to any location
Limitations	Habituates, absent in over 60 yo, qualitative not quantitative	Affected by anticholinergic and other drugs, time-consuming, requires special equipment, not widely available	Requires cooperation of patient, high variability	Cannot distinguish PNS vs CNS	Invasive, high cost relatively
Used to follow?	Unclear	Yes	Unclear	Unclear	Yes

Abbreviations: CNS, central nervous system; EMG, electromyogram; IENFD, intraepidermal nerve fiber density; PNS, peripheral nervous system; QSART, quantitative sudomotor axon reflex testing; QST, quantitative sensory testing; SSR, sympathetic skin response; TST, thermoregulatory sweat testing.

The SSR is perhaps the only autonomic test widely available on routine EMG equipment, making it inexpensive and accessible.[5] Abnormalities in the SSR were shown to be associated with axonal but not demyelinating neuropathies, particularly any neuropathies affecting the small unmyelinated C fibers. The SSR can be triggered by emotional or noxious stimuli, or even more prominently by deep inspiration.[19] The SSR shows abnormalities in a wide variety of neuropathies, especially diabetic neuropathy but also in uremia, alcoholism, and general peripheral neuropathies. One limitation, however, is that the SSR involves more than simply postganglionic sudomotor fibers, and cannot distinguish central from peripheral autonomic failure.[20,21] Other limitations include the fact that the SSR habituates easily, it can be absent physiologically in individuals older than 60, it is only semiquantitative and usually measured as present or absent due to the all-or-nothing conduction along C fibers. But despite the limitations, it is fast, simple, and reproducible,[21] which in addition to the accessibility may make it useful in some cases. A 1988 publication revealed SSR abnormalities in 10% of distal SFN cases.[22] More recently the SSR was shown to have 41% overall sensitivity in diagnosing SFN compared with the clinical data. In this latter series, the SSR was even more sensitive (69.7%) in clinically definite SFN cases.[23] But the latter series notably did not compare SSR or other neurophysiologic tests to skin punch biopsy.

The QSART sensitivity was reported to be 80% for SFN in one report. In the same study, the QSART was more sensitive than TST (72%).[24] The QSART is a quantitative testing method of postganglionic sudomotor function over a restricted zone. Localized sweat production is measured by physiologic response analysis software as a humidity change during and after skin preparation followed by iontophoresis of 10% acetylcholine. Testing sites are the forearm, proximal and distal leg and dorsum of the foot. The sweat response begins after 1 to 2 minutes in healthy controls, increasing until the maximal sweat response is reached at about 5 minutes. Depending on the site mean sweat output in healthy women is 0.25 to 1.2 $\mu L/cm^2$ and in men 2 to 3 $\mu L/cm^2$.[25] QSART may be useful in patients who are anticoagulated and cannot have skin punch biopsies. But limitations include lack of availability of equipment at most centers and time-consuming test administration. Also, because they affect sweating, antihistamines and tricyclic antidepressants must be discontinued 48 hours prior to the study, and caffeine and tobacco should be avoided.[9,10]

The TST, currently a gold standard to measure the pre- and postganglionic sudomotor function of the ventral body surface, is performed in a humidity controlled (35%–40%) and preheated room (to 45–50°C). The supine near-naked patient on a testing table has an indicator dye (that reflects a pH change with a color change) scattered on the complete ventral skin surface (omitting eye, ears, and perioral region). Skin and core temperature are repeatedly checked, with a goal skin temperature of 38.5 to 39.5°C. The maximum heating time is set to 70 minutes to avoid hyperthermia. Digital pictures of the sweating pattern reflecting indicator dye distribution are taken. Any measured anhidrotic skin area is divided by the total skin area and multiplied by 100. A physiologic TST would be symmetric sweating all over the ventral body.[25]

QST is an extension of the physical examination and measures a detection threshold for thermal sensation, thermal pain, and vibration, but cannot distinguish between psychogenic and actual sensory loss. It is widely available, and has been studied not only in SFN diagnosis but longitudinally to determine treatment response in neuropathy clinical trials.[5,8] Whether thermal or cold temperature are better assessed for SFN diagnosis on QST is unclear, and sensitivity has ranged from 60% to 85%.[5] QST has acceptable reproducibility, but high inter-operator, inter-patient, and inter-test variability, especially due to patient cooperation and technical factors, and it cannot differentiate between central and peripheral causes of temperature perception (thus can be affected by impaired cognition or malingering).[5,7] If reasonable standards are applied, QST can assess the patient's somatosensory system functioning, but like the QSART, it is a strong supportive SFN diagnostic tool and cannot be used as a standalone test.[7]

A composite study was performed of autonomic methods in 87 patients with clinically definite or possible SFN from TTR amyloidosis, MGUS, Sjögren's syndrome, Fabry's disease, or idiopathic disease. Clinically definite patients had SFN symptoms and some examination signs of SFN, with no signs of large fiber neuropathy and normal NCS. Clinically possible patients had the preceding symptoms but normal examinations. Five noninvasive tests were used and the SSR sensitivities were reported previously. The following other sensitivities were recorded: QST (Warm [55%] and Cold [32%]), LEP (79%), and ESC (61%).[23] Limitations of this study include a lack of comparison to skin biopsy or QSART, and a "gold standard" was clinical diagnosis alone. Also, the study was not blinded and the relatively uncommon LEP is a specialty of this European neurophysiology laboratory. Notably the premise of ESC has been questioned, with some investigators stating that the "published results violate biologic plausibility." The critics raise the issue of potential bias in that "a single funding source with a vested interest in the study outcomes has supported most of the studies." The critics highlight that ESC values are inconsistent across publications, that large merged data sets do not support the stated high sensitivity and specificity, and that insufficient evidence supports the claim that Sudoscan even tests sudomotor and sensory nerve fiber function.[26]

Skin punch biopsy and the resulting intraepidermal nerve fiber density (IENFD) has been used in clinical practice since original work using double specimens from the thigh and calf stained with a polyclonal antibody to neuron-specific ubiquitin hydrolase (anti-protein gene product 9.5 [PGP 9.5]) demonstrated a high diagnostic efficiency of 88% in diagnosing SFN.[27] PGP 9.5 stains the epidermal somatic nociceptor unmyelinated C fibers.[15] A 2010 joint task force of the European Federation of Neurologic Societies and the Peripheral Nerve Society recommended the skin biopsy as a safe and minimally invasive procedure in SFN diagnosis after its validation in many studies.[28] Sensitivity has been reported as high as 90% and specificity as high as 97%,[29] resulting in some investigators referring to IENFD as the gold standard in SFN diagnosis.[7,9] But others still believe the history and physical is the gold standard. Beside the IENFD, morphologic changes in the skin biopsy may also be useful diagnostically,[8] particularly axonal swelling and nerve fiber branching may predict later development of symptomatic neuropathy. Also the SFN gradient can be determined by sampling multiple sites in the leg, typically the calf and thigh.[13] And some evidence has suggested the utility of using serial skin punches in following treatment response or in clinical trials.[29] Controversial is the utility of the SGNFD because it should be performed at depth of 6 to 8 mm, which is deeper than the typical 3 to 4 mm biopsy done with commercially available testing kits. Also 2010 guidelines recommend against semiquantitative SGNFD analysis being used because of the complex 3-dimensional nature of sweat glands.[28]

Autonomic testing results may be independent and additive to somatic evaluation of SFN. One study comparing autonomic testing to the IENFD in patients with clinical evidence of sensory-only neuropathy and normal NCS showed no significant association. Autonomic tests included autonomic reflex testing (QSART, cardiovagal, and adrenergic testing) and QST. The investigators concluded that autonomic testing and IENFD are independent (complementary) measures of distal SFN, and should be used concurrently in SFN evaluation, if possible.[30] Indeed, an earlier study showed that combining IENFD and autonomic testing (QSART and QST) enhances the likelihood of meeting diagnostic SFN criteria. The investigators of that latter study proposed "pure SFN" criteria with compatible examinatoin, normal EMG, and at least 2 abnormalities of QST, QSART, or IENFD. Adding QSART to the existing criteria (clinical findings, QST, and IENFD) increased the number of patients diagnosed from 38% to 66%.[30]

OBJECTIVE SMALL FIBER NEUROPATHY FOLLOW-UP PARAMETERS

The Utah Early Neuropathy Scale (UENS) provides an examination score, which is specific to early sensory predominant polyneuropathy that prominently involves small-diameter nerve fibers, compared to the Michigan Diabetic Neuropathy Scale (MDNS) and the Neuropathy Impairment Score–Lower Leg (NIS-LL) that focus primarily on large-fiber sensory and motor function. The UENS is out of 42 points, and includes measures of sensation, hypersensitivity to pain, reflexes, and distal strength in both lower extremities (**Fig. 3**). Its sensitivity is 92% as recorded in diabetic or prediabetic subjects, and correlates well with the MDNS and the NIS-LL, both of which were less sensitive (67% and 81%, respectively). But it correlated even more strongly over a 1-year follow-up period with objective testing such as QSART (foot) and IENFD (calf), along with the Visual Analogue Scale (VAS) for pain. Besides its sensitivity the UENS is reproducible, with a high interrater reliability, and may be useful in trials of early neuropathy.[31] Limitations of the UENS are that it was validated on diabetic LD-SFN patients, thus NLD-SFN cases may have artificially low scores on the UENS but have significant symptoms and disease burden. A better scoring system likely will need to be developed for NLD-SFN.

The SFN-SIQ (SFN-Symptom Inventory Questionnaire) is a 13-question, 52-point scale, which along with the 32-question, 64-point SFN-RODS (SFN-Rasch Overall Disability Scale), are aimed at "improving the clinical assessment and care of patients suffering from SFN."[32] The SFN-SIQ asks a number of small fiber neuropathy and autonomic symptoms and a higher number correlates with more severe disease. The SFN-RODS asks a number of daily activity questions regarding functional limitations by neuropathic pain and a lower score correlates with worse disease. The SFN-SL (SFN Screening List), a 21 question (in 2 parts), 84-point scale, was first devised in 2011 in sarcoidosis patients and is a very sensitive and specific way of diagnosing SFN (validated against TST). Higher scores reflect increased disease severity. A score of 11 or more carries 100% sensitivity and 31% specificity for SFN, while a score of greater than 47 is 100% specific and 19% sensitive.[33] The SFN-SL validity has been demonstrated in Pompe disease also.[34] A recent study evaluating IENFD, VAS, and SFN-SIQ and SFN-SL in 55 patients revealed the following: for the SFN-SIQ, using a cutoff value = 5, the sensitivity = 80%, specificity = 81.8%) and for the SFN-SL, using a cut-off value = 8, the sensitivity = 94.1%, specificity = 90.9%.[35]

SMALL FIBER NEUROPATHY MISDIAGNOSED AS OTHER CONDITIONS

A significant, albeit controversial, discovery of the past decade is that SFN may be overlapping or mistakenly diagnosed as fibromyalgia. Fibromyalgia has always likely been a heterogenous group of diseases with myriad symptoms and signs and unsatisfying pathophysiological explanation.[36] Even the 2010 revised criteria did not involve an objective confirmatory diagnostic test.[37] In a 2013 study with 27 patients with fibromyalgia who met American College of Rheumatology (ACR) criteria and 30 matched normal controls, 41% of skin biopsies from fibromyalgia subjects versus 3% of control biopsies were diagnostic for SFN, and Michigan Neuropathy Screening Instrument

Patient Name

Study Number

Visit

Motor Examination	Left	Right
0 normal 2 weak		
Great Toe Extension		
Total both sides (out of 4)		

Pin Sensation:	L	R
0 normal		
1 for each segment with reduced sensation		
2 for each segment with absent sensation		
Total both sides (out of 24)		

Segments for pin sensation reporting

Left Leg Right Leg

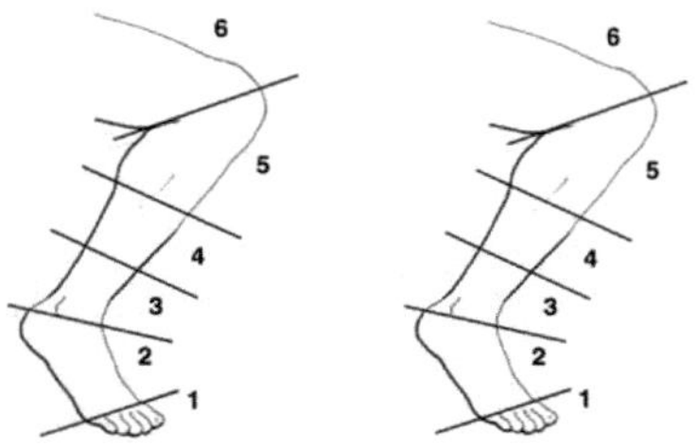

Allodynia/Hyperesthesia	L	R
0 normal		
1 if present in toes or foot		
Total both sides (out of 2)		

Large Fiber Sensation	L	R
0 normal 1 diminished 2 absent		
Great toe vibration		
time	s	s
Great toe joint position		
Total both sides (out of 8)		

Deep Tendon Reflexes	L	R
0 normal 1 diminished 2 absent		
Ankle		
Total both sides (out of 4		

Total Score (out of 42)

Fig. 3. Utah Early Neuropathy Scale. Useful follow-up examination score for distal peripheral neuropathy, including SFN. (*From* Singleton JR, Bixby B, Russell JW, et al. The Utah Early Neuropathy Scale: a sensitive clinical scale for early sensory predominant neuropathy. J Peripher Nerv Syst 2008;13:218–27; with permission.)

(complementary to the preceding MDNS) and UENS scores were higher among patients with fibromyalgia than controls (all $P \leq .001$). Interestingly, all autonomic tests including QSART were equally prevalent in the groups which suggested to the investigators that fibromyalgia-SFN is a somatic-only disorder. Further workup in the newly diagnosed SFN patients revealed etiologies such as dysimmune markers, hepatitis C serologies, or genetic causes.[36] Another study showed that 30% of patients with fibromyalgia had SFN based on abnormal IENFD.[38] And another study of 41 patients with fibromyalgia and 47 controls showed highly statistically significant differences of both thigh and calf IENFD, along with higher interleukin-2R levels in the fibromyalgia group, suggesting LD and NLD-SFN in fibromyalgia and an underlying autoimmune etiology.[39] In another study highlighting the IENFD importance in select patients with fibromyalgia, 34/56 (61%) patients with ACR criteria for fibromyalgia had reduced IENFD on skin biopsy. Of these 34 who actually had SFN and not fibromyalgia, 24 (71%) had laboratory evidence of an underlying potentially treatable and previously unknown etiology for the SFN, including glucose dysmetabolism, Sjögren's syndrome, mixed connective tissue disease, vitamin B6 toxicity, Vitamin B12 deficiency, and Fabry's disease.[37]

Because fibromyalgia may affect 2% to 8% of the population, SFN prevalence could be very high,[36] as noted previously. But questions remain. Is small fiber pathology directly caused by fibromyalgia or is SFN a critical triggering factor in fibromyalgia? Or is it that patients with chronic pain labeled as fibromyalgia have undiagnosed SFN, especially in cases of NLD-SFN.[7] There may be some features of fibromyalgia that help to identify patients who may have SFN and more likely need the punch biopsy. But in one study most symptoms overlapped between fibromyalgia and SFPN, except for dysautonomia and worse paresthesias (trend) that may help predict underlying SFN[40]; the dysautonomia symptom prominence is interesting considering the lack of autonomic testing involvement in the earlier study above.

Questioning the neuropathic pain canon also more recently some investigators have described that complex regional pain syndrome/reflex sympathetic dystrophy (CRPS-I/RSD) may actually be a form of SFN. One of the first studies to show this association contained a significant relationship between QST-mechanical allodynia ($P<.03$) and heat-pain hyperalgesia ($P<.04$) where the CRPS pain was located. And IENFD was diminished at the CRPS-sites of 17 of 18 subjects, by 29% ($P<.001$) on average. The IENFD was highly correlated on both sides in patients with CRPS, including the asymptomatic side.[41] In another more recent study IENFD was obtained in symptomatic and contralateral limbs of 8 patients with CRPS-I and from equivalent sites in controls. IENFD was significantly lower in both the affected and contralateral limbs of patients with CRPS-I, and similarly to the prior study, the IENFD did not differ between symptomatic and contralateral limbs in the patients with CRPS-I. On QST the thermal pain threshold was significantly lower in the affected limb in patients with CRPS-I compared with controls but the other thresholds were not, likely reflecting the higher sensitivity of IENFD. The investigators concluded that CRPS-I may be actually a form of SFN given the bilateral involvement, which could be from a systemic injury response that increases the risk of developing RSD after trauma.[42] It has been noted that small nerve fibers have critical vasomotor and trophic efferent functions that may lead to CRPS symptoms by antidromic release of vasoactive neuropeptides such as calcitonin gene-related peptide and substance P. Additionally it has been shown that after traumatic sciatic neuropathy in rats the cell bodies of small-diameter axons in the dorsal root ganglion and their central axons preferentially degenerate, thus explaining why trauma can lead to SFN and CRPS without obvious large-fiber injury.[43] Another study only showed that 20% of patients with CRPS-I had a low IENFD, and QST and IENFD did not correlate. The investigators questioned whether commercial skin biopsy testing caused false-negative testing because of skipped patches of low IENFD, as well as the fact that commercial skin biopsy laboratories may not use stereological techniques to quantitate the IENFD.[44]

Cramp symptoms are also associated with SFN. Patients with and without neuropathic complaints had skin biopsies performed in one study in which 12 patients were biopsied; 8 of these had normal small-fiber sensation. Of the 12, 7 patients (58%) had reduced IENFD and 2 of these had NLD-SFN. A cause for neuropathy was found in 1 patient who previously had a diagnosis of cramp-fasciculation syndrome. The creatine kinase was even elevated in 8 patients and half of those had decreased IENFD. Muscle biopsy was also performed in 8 patients, but was diagnostic in only 1 patient who had McArdle disease. The investigators concluded that nearly 60% of muscle cramp patients without neuropathic complaints have SFN, and that cramps may in these cases be caused by local inflammatory mediators released from damaged small nerve fibers that excite intramuscular nerves.[45] One questions whether one uniform inflammatory syndrome may cause the overlapping syndromes of cramps, fibromyalgia, and CRPS, the so-called SFMWP as mentioned previously.

SMALL FIBER NEUROPATHY CAUSED BY INHERITED CONDITIONS

Exciting developments in the past decade also have included elucidation of novel and potentially treatable genetic causes of SFN. Hereditary causes of SFN should be suspected in younger patients presenting with SFN, patients with a family history,[9] or patients with phenotypic findings typical of hereditary neuropathies or of specific syndromes.

Previously known were autosomal recessive sensory autonomic neuropathy (HSAN) types II, III, and IV that have small fiber involvement, occurring predominantly in patients of Eastern European Jewish descent.[7] The X-linked rare disorder of glycosphingolipid metabolism, Fabry disease, has a prominently associated SFN syndrome.[46] Besides acroparesthesias and anhidrosis, it features disseminated angiokeratomas, which may clue in the astute examiner to investigate for Fabry.[47] Fabry may be seen in 21% of otherwise idiopathic SFN cases, per one study (5/24 patients),[48] and can even be seen in female carriers, which makes testing for alpha-galactosidase mutations a strong consideration because enzyme replacement therapy may work quite well for this condition.[47] However, more recent evidence suggests that the association between Fabry and idiopathic SFN is low and that only patients with clinical features of Fabry should be genetically tested.[9] Also on the hereditary front, late-onset Pompe disease was shown to be associated with SFN in 2 cases, which then led to a study in which 50% of 44 cases had positive SFN-SL scores of $\geq$11.[34] And patients with Ehlers-Danlos syndrome (EDS) all had abnormal IENFD and 19 of 20 had neuropathic pain in one series, suggesting that SFN is common in EDS.[49]

Transthyretin (TTR) amyloidosis has emerged in the quest for etiologic identification of SFN because novel treatments have emerged to sequester, or silence the production of, insoluble, misfolded amyloid fibrils that can deposit in multiple organs, especially the heart and large and small nerves. TTR can present as a wild-type or hereditary mutation (ATTRwt and ATTRm, respectively). The neuropathy in ATTRm had been referred to as familial amyloid polyneuropathy in the past. But the neuropathy and autonomic features, along with other organ involvement may be delayed and carpal tunnel syndrome can be the initial symptom in 33%, preceding other symptoms by 4 to 6 years. The most common mutation is the V30M and this is endemic in Portugal, Japan, and Sweden. It presents with painful LD-SFN pattern that progresses to a large fiber sensorimotor neuropathy. Up to 75% of patients with ATTRm develop an autonomic neuropathy, which can severely affect the cardiac, gastrointestinal, and genitourinary systems. Cardiac involvement is more common in late-onset ATTRm, and additionally, amyloid patients typically lose 10% of body weight. Two disease-modifying ATTRm treatments therapies work by stabilizing the TTR tetramer (Diflunisal and Tafamidis), and orthotopic liver transplant was a good gene silencing option. But in 2018, anti-sense oligonucleotide treatments which halt ATTRm or ATTRwt production in the liver were released, under the names Patirisan and Inotersen. These 2 agents reduce serum amyloid by 81% and 79%, respectively, and result in significantly improved neuropathy impairment and quality of life scores compared with placebo.[50]

Primarily 3 voltage-gated sodium channels, NaV 1.7 (SCN9A gene), Nav1.8 (SCN10A gene), and Nav1.9 (SCN11A gene) have been found on dorsal root ganglion (DRG), peripheral small fiber, trigeminal, and sympathetic neurons and are responsible for normal and pathologic pain sensation. Mutations in these genes have been demonstrated in SFN syndromes, either as loss or gain-of-function.[51,52] Nav 1.7 mutations cause inherited erythromelalgia and paroxysmal extreme pain disorder as well as SFN (gain-of-function) or loss of function (congenital insensitivity to pain) (**Fig. 4**). Nav1.8 mutations cause SFN, and Nav 1.9 mutations cause loss of pain perception and familial episodic pain.[51] Gain-of-function Nav1.7 mutations were seen in 28% of patients in a series of 28 subjects with biopsy-proven idiopathic SFN.[51] In another paper Nav 1.8 mutations were found in 8.7% (9/104) of patients with panful SFN who were negative for Nav 1.7 mutations. And in a larger cohort negative for Nav 1.7 and 1.8 mutations, 12/345 patients (3.5%) had Nav 1.9 mutations and painful SFN.[52] Despite knowledge of the sodium channelopathy pathophysiology in these novel hereditary SFN cases, not many trials have yet occurred to study the effect of sodium-channel blocker medications, though carbamazepine has been mentioned to be "protective" of DRG neurons.[51] Lacosamide was recently shown to be safe and well-tolerated, and to significantly improve pain, general well-being, and sleep quality in Nav1.7-related SFN.[53]

NOVEL IMMUNE BIOMARKERS IN SMALL FIBER NEUROPATHY

A larger recent study revealed that up to 48% of otherwise cryptogenic SFN cases may have novel autoantibodies to trisulfated heparan disaccharide IdoA2S-GlcNS-

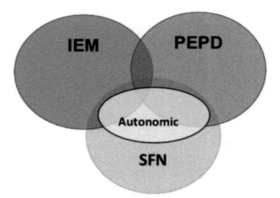

Fig. 4. Varied pain disorders due to gain-of-function Nav1.7 mutations. The overlapping scope of human pain syndromes associated with Nav 1.7 mutations is illustrated. IEM, inherited erythromelalgia; PEPD, paroxysmal extreme pain disorder. (*From* Brouwer BA, Bakkers M, Hoeijmakers JGJ, et al. Improving assessment in small fiber neuropathy. Journal of the Peripheral Nervous System 2015;20:333–40; with permission.)

6S (TS-HDS)[a] or fibroblast growth factor receptor 3 (FGFR3). This was the first published paper specifically describing these new antibodies in cryptogenic SFN, and involved a relatively large multicenter cohort of 155 patients.[17] Previously TS-HDS had only been described in combined cohorts of axonal mixed large and small fiber neuropathies. In these latter cases it was demonstrated that prominent anti-TS-HDS-C5b-9 complement deposits formed on endoneurial capillaries,[54] as well as TS-HDS-IgM and kappa light chains deposited around the rim of intermediate-sized perimysial and epineurial veins.[55] Notably, however, some of the patients, including one "representative" patient in one of these 2 original papers on anti-TS-HDS neuropathy had severe neuropathic pain and normal nerve conduction studies,[54] thus presumably had SFN. And anti-FGFR3, an antibody against the receptor's intracellular domain, had only been shown previously to have a high positive predictive value (94.1%) in detecting NLD immune sensory neuronopathy. Anti-FGFR-3 IgG likely impairs neural repair following injury at the DRG level and at the Schwann cell–axon level.[56]

The preceding recent SFN paper regarding these novel antibodies also showed the following: 37% of the patients had TS-HDS-IgM and 15% had FGFR3-IgG. TS-HDS antibodies were more frequent in SFN patients than in controls ($P = .0012$); but this was not the case for FGFR3 antibodies. Both antibodies were more common in women, and NLD pathology was more common (but not a clinical NLD pattern, a disconnect). Acute onset was seen in 12 of 155 patients, and 92% of these had TS-HDS antibodies.[17] Other recent studies have also addressed TS-HDS and FGFR3 antibodies. Evaluating patients with fibromyalgia in St. Louis, 19 (86%) of 22 had abnormal IENFD (looking at the raw data table), and of these 19, 9 (47%) had either TS-HDS or FGFR3 antibodies (similarly to the previous study), and 5 (56%) of 9 with antibodies had NLD-SFN. Of the TS-HDS positive patients, there was a significant association with NLD-SFN pathologically, and a trend toward all the patients with fibromyalgia having NLD-SFN. As in the previous study there was a disconnect between clinical and pathologic evidence of NLD-SFN. And there was no significant difference comparing signs and symptoms to presence or absence of TS-HDS antibodies.[57] Yet there are cautionary words from other centers in interpretation of these novel antibodies. At Stanford, 7 neuropathy patients were tested for FGFR3 antibodies and 4 were positive, 3 had SFN, and 4 had large fiber neuropathy on EMG, and repeat testing of FGFR3-positive cases revealed normalized titers in 2 and significant titer reduction in another without any treatment.[58]

Another novel antibody was identified in a targeted search for human autoantibodies from 110 patients with neuropathic pain from various inflammatory neurologic diseases or neuropathies whose sera would selectively bind to mouse unmyelinated C-fiber type DRG neurons (compared with 50 controls without neuropathic pain). Anti-DRG neuron antibodies were more frequent in patients with neuropathic pain than non-neuropathic pain subjects (10% vs 0%; $P<.05$). These autoantibodies

---

[a] Sulfated oligosaccharide domains in heparin and heparan sulfate bind extracellular proteins such as growth factors and affect a variety of functions. TS-HDS oligosaccharides strongly bind to fibroblast growth factor (FGF)-1, and they modulate oligomerization of FGF-2 and binding of FGF-2 to FGFR-1. Also, heparan sulfate–dependent pathways moderate actions of vascular endothelial growth factor (VEGF), and angiogenesis is stimulated in several tissues by the interplay between FGF, VEGF, and heparan sulfate oligosaccharides. All of these proteins exist in peripheral nerves and likely play roles in maintenance and repair. Because TS-HDS oligosaccharides play such a vital role in these extracellular matrix pathways, this could explain why impairment of their function through an immune attack could lead to peripheral, and especially small fiber, neuropathy. See Pestrock and colleagues, 2003.[55]

were identified to be anti–Plexin D1 antibodies. Main comorbidities were atopy and collagen-vascular disease. Reverse-application of anti–Plexin D1 antibody-positive patient sera to DRG neurons increased membrane permeability, leading to cellular swelling. Neuropathic pain patients with anti–Plexin D1 antibodies developed burning pain and QST threshold abnormalities for C fibers. In 7 neuropathic pain cases with Plexin-D1 antibodies unlisted immunotherapies reduced their pain. The investigators concluded that Plexin D1 antibodies are a novel biomarker for immunotherapy-responsive neuropathic pain.[59]

Paraneoplastic antibodies may also be associated with SFN, but there is a paucity of cases in the literature. One report showed paraneoplastic SFN followed by chorea in a patient with small cell lung cancer found to have antibodies to Purkinje cell cytoplasmic autoantibody type 2 (PCA-2) and collapsin response-mediator protein-5 (CRMP-5) autoantibodies. The EMG was normal but the patient had NLD-SFN by IENFD.[60] In a larger retrospective series of 159 patients with voltage-gated potassium channel (VGKC)-complex-IgG antibodies from the Mayo Clinic who presented with chronic idiopathic or subacute pain, 6.3% of patients had only SFN and 64% of patients had normal EMGs. Most had other complaints such as autonomic or cognitive issues, hyperexcitability such as cramps, fasciculations, or myokymia, besides having typical neuropathic pain. It was shown that the CASPR2-IgG subtype significantly associates with pain, and that impairment of repolarization with resultant channel hyperexcitability of nociceptive pathways is the pathophysiologic mechanism for VGKC-complex autoimmune pain. As evidence of the hyperexcitability the patients had documented hyperhidrosis on TST, EMG-hyperexcitability, and abnormal heat-pain hyperalgesia on QST. Only 12% had cancers found, suggesting this is largely an autoimmune and not a paraneoplastic syndrome. Supporting the latter, 14 (88%) of 16 who received immunotherapy (IVIg, plasmapheresis, steroids, steroid-sparing agents) had pain reductions, as well as improvements in other neurologic complaints.[61]

TREATMENT WITH INTRAVENOUS IMMUNOGLOBULIN

Already discussed previously were specific treatments in TTR amyloidosis sodium channelopathies. Here the treatment of some specific inflammatory SFN syndromes is discussed. SFN from sarcoidosis is more effectively treated with IVIg than with other immunomodulatory treatments. In a retrospective series 47 (76%) of 62 patients treated with IVIg improved, but only 4 (15%) of 27 untreated patients improved. By contrast, 8 patients (67%) of 12 who received anti-TNF (tumor necrosis factor) therapy and 10 (71%) of 14 patients who received combination IVIg and anti-TNF therapy improved.[62] With celiac neuropathy, 3 patients with biopsy-proven celiac disease had cerebellar ataxia and neuropathic pain despite a strict gluten-free diet, and had reduced IENFD on skin biopsy. All symptoms responded to IVIG treatment, and ataxia worsened when IVIG was discontinued, supporting its efficacy and the immune pathophysiology. Symptoms improved when IVIg was resumed.[63] Besides these cases, 6 patients with Sjögren's SFN in 2 papers responded to IVIg.[2] And 62% of patients in a smaller series of 8 juvenile patients with "early-onset SFN" improved clinically with improved skin biopsies and autonomic testing, and a multicenter, double-blind trial of IVIg in 23 patients with eosinophilic granulomatosis with polyangiitis (Churg-Strauss) reported improved secondary outcome of pain reduction.[2]

But given the high cost of IVIg of more than $100,000 annually, drug shortages, and administration issues and requirements of nursing support, many insurers do not approve it as therapy even for SFN with clear evidence of autoimmunity. That was the rationale for a Class IV retrospective study of IVIg treatment in immune SFN. A total

---

Box 2
SFN syndromes possibly responsive to intravenous immunoglobulin

- TS-HDS (trisulfated heparan disaccharide IdoA2S-GlcNS-6S) and FGFR3 (fibroblast growth factor receptor 3) antibody-mediated
- Plexin D1 antibody-mediated
- Sarcoidosis SFN
- Sjögren's SFN
- Celiac SFN
- IBD SFN
- Sensory Chronic Inflammatory Demyelinating Polyneuropathy (CIDP)/Guillain-Barre Syndrome (GBS)
- Voltage-gated potassium channel-antibody-mediated

---

of 55 patients with immune SFN confirmed by biopsies and autonomic testing, as well as evidence of autoimmunity by history (27% had systemic autoimmune diseases) or ≥1/5 unexplained nonspecific inflammatory markers such as Anti-Nuclear Antibody (≥1:160 dilution), elevated erythrocyte sedimentation rate (≥15 mm/h), low complement component 4 (C4; <20 mg/dL), low complement component 3 (C3; <85 mg/dL) and Sjögren autoantibodies (SSA/Ro, SSA/La). The proportion of abnormal autonomic tests indicating SFN dropped from 89% to 55% (P<.001) and QSARTs improved significantly with 69% abnormal before treatment and 49% abnormal afterward (P = .039). Among patients with pain ≥3/10 before IVIg (average 6.3 ± 1.7) their scores dropped significantly after treatment (5.2 ± 2.1; P = .007). Overall, 74% rated themselves 'improved' and neurologists labeled 77% of patients as 'IVIg responders' (especially male patients). The "IVIg responders" were treated on average for 38 ± 23 months and 16% of patients entered sustained remissions even after IVIg discontinuation. All adverse events were expected; most were typical infusion reactions, but 2 had deep venous thromboses and one had hemolytic anemia.[2]

As with the abovementioned response of immune-mediated SFN to PlexinD1 or VGKC antibodies to immunotherapy, SFN related to TS-HDS or FGFR-3 antibodies has been shown to respond in small series to IVIg (**Box 2**), and is the topic of 2 current ongoing Phase II clinical trials.[64] Given the potential prevalence of SFN and that 48% of cryptogenic SFN cases may have these novel antibodies, proven efficacy of IVIg in this syndrome has the potential to impact thousands of patients. In one presented series of 3 cases IVIg was demonstrated to cause normalization of skin biopsies and 54% pain reduction in patients with TS-HDS or FGFR-3 antibodies. The cases in this series were treated with monthly high dose (2 g/kg) infusions for 6 months.[65] In another presented and ongoing series in which 62% of 34 cryptogenic SFN cases had TS-HDS or FGFR3 antibodies, 9 cases had treatment with IVIg; 7 improved (78%) as measured by pain reduction, improved UENS, and/or improved IENFD, including 1 patient who went into remission, but 2 patients had to stop due to aseptic meningitis (and patient refusal to try again even with mitigating measures) or hemolytic anemia. Notably the latter adverse events were after the initial 2 g/kg IVIg loading dose.[66]

SUMMARY

The field of SFN is has had exciting developments in recent years, and shows promise for future burgeoning findings regarding diagnostics and management to improve symptoms and quality of life in this patient population. Improved autonomic and pathologic diagnostics have allowed discovery of SFN in a much more definitive fashion. More and more cases of so-called fibromyalgia or nonspecific cramps and even CRPS are now being diagnosed as SFN. And etiologic investigation and treatment have been more elucidated by advances in knowledge about sodium channelopathy neuropathies, familial TTR amyloid neuropathy, and novel biomarkers for immune-mediated SFN such as TS-HDS, FGFR-3, and Plexin D1. Clinical trials for therapies in these novel etiologies, with objective endpoints and using the new biomarkers, will hopefully continue to emerge, such as IVIg for inflammatory SFN.

CLINICS CARE POINTS

- Small fiber neuropathy can present as a diffuse pain syndrome and be non-length dependent, unlike typical neuropathies.
- Skin biopsy and autonomic testing such as QSART are the mainstays of SFN diagnosis, with EMG typically being normal in isolated SFN cases.
- Diabetes and alcohol abuse are important SFN causes, but testing for vitamin deficiencies, channelopathies, TTR mutation, and autoimmune causes are paramount.
- Immunotherapy such as IVIG may be effective and is being studied.

ACKNOWLEDGMENTS

Special thanks to my former neurology residents Ali Zandieh, Fang Bai, and Anjali Garg, along with fellow Martha Cruz. Also special thanks to Dr Tibor Valyi-Nagy (UIC neuropathology) and Dr Charles Abrams (UIC Neurology) for advice and mentorship, and the same to Dr Todd Levine (Phoenix Neurologic Associates), Dr Alan Pestronk (Washington University), and Dr Christopher Gibbons (Harvard-Beth Israel). Special thanks to my former nurse Linda Querry, current nurse Donna Starsiak, former EMG techs Jessie Alverio and Erica Chapman, and to Pam Markham (Therapath, Inc).

DISCLOSURE

Dr L.A. Zeidman has participated on a scientific advisory board for Akcea Therapeutics.

REFERENCES

1. Peters MJ, Bakkers M, Merkies IS, et al. Incidence and prevalence of small-fiber neuropathy: a survey in the Netherlands. Neurology 2013;81(15):1356-60.
2. Liu X, Treister R, Lang M, et al. IVIg for apparently autoimmune small-fiber polyneuropathy: first analysis of efficacy and safety. Ther Adv Neurol Disord 2018;11. 1756285617744484.
3. Phillips LH 2nd. The epidemiology of myasthenia gravis. Ann N Y Acad Sci 2003; 998:407-12.
4. Mehta P, Kaye W, Raymond J, et al. Prevalence of amyotrophic lateral sclerosis — United States, 2015. MMWR Morb Mortal Wkly Rep 2018;67:1285-9.
5. Lacomis D. Small-fiber neuropathy. Muscle Nerve 2002;26(2):173-88.
6. Levine TD. Small fiber neuropathy: disease classification beyond pain and burning. J Cent Nerv Syst Dis 2018;10:1-6.
7. Chan ACY, Wilder-Smith EP. Small fiber neuropathy: getting bigger! Muscle Nerve 2016;53:671-82.

8. Hovaguimian A, Gibbons CH. Diagnosis and treatment of pain in small-fiber neuropathy. Curr Pain Headache Rep 2011;15(3):193–200.

9. Zhou L. Small fiber neuropathy. Semin Neurol 2019;39(5):570–7.

10. Tavee JO. Office approach to small fiber neuropathy. Cleve Clin J Med 2018; 85(10):801–12.

11. Lauria G, Merkies IS, Faber CG. Small fibre neuropathy. Curr Opin Neurol 2012; 25(5):542–9.

12. Farhad K. Current diagnosis and treatment of painful small fiber neuropathy. Curr Neurol Neurosci Rep 2019;19(12):103.

13. Freeman RL. Painful peripheral neuropathy: diagnosis and assessment. Chronic Inflammatory Demyelinating Polyneuropathy/Guillain-Barre Syndrome 2009; 15(5):13–29. Miller AE, ed. Neuropathic pain.

14. Somatosensory system. In: Siegel A, Sapru H, editors. Essential neuroscience. Baltimore (MD): Lippincott Williams & Wilkins; 2005. p. 255–67.

15. Devigili G, Tugnoli V, Penza P, et al. The diagnostic criteria for small fibre neuropathy: from symptoms to neuropathology. Brain 2008;131:1912–25.

16. Yuki N, Chan AC, Wong AHY, et al. Acute painful autoimmune neuropathy: a variant of Guillain-Barré syndrome. Muscle Nerve 2018;57(2):320–4.

17. Levine TD, Kafaie J, Zeidman LA, et al. Cryptogenic small-fiber neuropathies: serum autoantibody binding to trisulfated heparan disaccharide and fibroblast growth factor receptor-3. Muscle Nerve 2020;61(4):512–5.

18. Teoh HL, Chow A, Wilder-Smith EP. Skin wrinkling for diagnosing small fibre neuropathy: comparison with epidermal nerve density and sympathetic skin response. J Neurol Neurosurg Psychiatry 2008;79:835–7.

19. Shahani BT, Halperin JJ, Boulu P, et al. Sympathetic skin response-a method of assessing unmyelinated axon dysfunction in peripheral neuropathies. J Neurol Neurosurg Psychiatry 1984;47:536–42.

20. Navarro X, Espadeler JM, Miralles R. The value of the absence of the sympathetic skin response in Sjogren's syndrome. Muscle Nerve 1990;13(5):460.

21. Ravits JM. AAEM minimonograph #48: autonomic nervous system testing. Muscle Nerve 1997;20:919–37.

22. Evans BA, Lussky D, Knezevic W. The peripheral autonomic surface potential in suspected small fiber peripheral neuropathy [abstract]. Muscle Nerve 1988; 11:982.

23. Lefaucheura JP, Wahabh A, Planté-Bordeneuveb V, et al. Diagnosis of small fiber neuropathy: a comparative study of five neurophysiological tests. Clin Neurophysiol 2015;45:445–55.

24. Stewart JD, Low PA, Fealey RD. Distal small fiber neuropathy: results of tests of sweating and autonomic cardiovascular reflexes. Muscle Nerve 1992;15(6): 661–5.

25. Buchmann SJ, Penzlin AI, Kubasch ML, et al. Assessment of sudomotor function. Clin Auton Res 2019;29(1):41–53.

26. Rajan S, Campagnolo M, Callaghan B, et al. Sudomotor function testing by electrochemical skin conductance: does it really measure sudomotor function? Clin Auton Res 2019;29(1):31–9.

27. McArthur JC, Stocks EA, Hauer P, et al. Epidermal nerve fiber density: normative reference range and diagnostic efficiency. Arch Neurol 1998;55(12):1513–20.

28. Lauria G, Hsieh ST, Johansson O, et al. European Federation of Neurological Societies/Peripheral Nerve Society Guideline on the use of skin biopsy in the diagnosis of small fiber neuropathy. Report of a joint task force of the European

Federation of Neurological Societies and the Peripheral Nerve Society. Eur J Neurol 2010;17:903–12.

29. Hays AP. Utility of skin biopsy to evaluate peripheral neuropathy. Curr Neurol Neurosci Rep 2010;10:101–7.

30. Thaisetthawatkul P, Fernandes Filho JA, Herrmann DN. Autonomic evaluation is independent of somatic evaluation for small fiber neuropathy. J Neurol Sci 2014;344:51–4.

31. Singleton JR, Bixby B, Russell JW, et al. The Utah Early Neuropathy Scale: a sensitive clinical scale for early sensory predominant neuropathy. J Peripher Nerv Syst 2008;13:218–27.

32. Brouwer BA, Bakkers M, Hoeijmakers JGJ, et al. Improving assessment in small fiber neuropathy. J Peripher Nerv Syst 2015;20:333–40.

33. Hoitsma E, De Vries J, Drent M. The small fiber neuropathy screening list: construction and cross-validation in sarcoidosis. Respir Med 2011;105(1):95–100.

34. Hobson-Webb LD, Austin SL, Jain S, et al. Small-fiber neuropathy in Pompe disease: first reported cases and prospective screening of a clinic cohort. Am J Case Rep 2015;16:196–201.

35. Sun B, Li Y, Liu L, et al. SFN-SIQ, SFNSL and skin biopsy of 55 cases with small fibre involvement. Int J Neurosci 2018;128(5):442–8.

36. Oaklander AL, Herzog ZD, Downs HM, et al. Objective evidence that small-fiber polyneuropathy underlies some illnesses currently labeled as fibromyalgia. Pain 2013;154:2310–6.

37. Levine TD, Saperstein DS. Routine use of punch biopsy to diagnose small fiber neuropathy in fibromyalgia patients. Clin Rheumatol 2015;34(3):413–7.

38. Giannoccaro MP, Donadio V, Incensi A, et al. Small nerve fiber involvement in patients referred for fibromyalgia. Muscle Nerve 2014;49(5):757–9.

39. Caro XJ, Winter EF. Evidence of abnormal epidermal nerve fiber density in fibromyalgia: clinical and immunologic implications. Arthritis Rheumatol 2014;66(7):1945–54.

40. Lodahl M, Treister R, Oaklander AL. Specific symptoms may discriminate between fibromyalgia patients with vs without objective test evidence of small-fiber polyneuropathy. Pain Rep 2017;3(1):e633.

41. Oaklander AL, Rissmiller JG, Gelman LB, et al. Evidence of focal small-fiber axonal degeneration in complex regional pain syndrome-I (reflex sympathetic dystrophy). Pain 2006;120(3):235–43.

42. Rasmussen VF, Karlsson P, Drummond PD, et al. Bilaterally reduced intraepidermal nerve fiber density in unilateral CRPS-I. Pain Med 2018;19(10):2021–30.

43. Oaklander AL, Fields HL. Is reflex sympathetic dystrophy/complex regional pain syndrome type I a small-fiber neuropathy? Ann Neurol 2009;65(6):629–38.

44. Kharkar S, Venkatesh YS, Grothusen JR, et al. Skin biopsy in complex regional pain syndrome: case series and literature review. Pain Physician 2012;15(3):255–66.

45. Lopate G, Streif E, Harms M, et al. Cramps and small-fiber neuropathy. Muscle Nerve 2013;48(2):252–5.

46. Dütsch M, Marthol H, Stemper B, et al. Small fiber dysfunction predominates in Fabry neuropathy. J Clin Neurophysiol 2002;19(6):575–86.

47. El-Abassi R, Singhal D, England JD. Fabry's disease. J Neurol Sci 2014;344:5–19.

48. Tanislav C, Kaps M, Rolfs A, et al. Frequency of Fabry disease in patients with small-fibre neuropathy of unknown aetiology: a pilot study. Eur J Neurol 2011;18:631–6.

49. Cazzato D, Castori M, Lombardi R, et al. Small fiber neuropathy is a common feature of Ehlers-Danlos syndromes. Neurology 2016;87(2):155–9.
50. Kapoor M, Rossor AM, Laura M, et al. Clinical presentation, diagnosis and treatment of TTR amyloidosis. J Neuromuscul Dis 2019;6(2):189–99.
51. Brouwer BA, Merkies IS, Gerrits MM, et al. Painful neuropathies: the emerging role of sodium channelopathies. J Peripher Nerv Syst 2014;19(2):53–65.
52. Hoeijmakers JG, Faber CG, Merkies IS, et al. Painful peripheral neuropathy and sodium channel mutations. Neurosci Lett 2015;596:51–9.
53. de Greef BTA, Hoeijmakers JGJ, Geerts M, et al. Lacosamide in patients with Nav1.7 mutations-related small fibre neuropathy: a randomized controlled trial. Brain 2019;142(2):263–75.
54. Pestronk A, Schmidt RE, Choksi RM, et al. Clinical and laboratory features of neuropathies with serum IgM binding to TS-HDS. Muscle Nerve 2012;45(6):866–72.
55. Pestronk A, Choksi R, Logigian E, et al. Sensory neuropathy with monoclonal Igm binding to a trisulfated heparin disaccharide. Muscle Nerve 2003;27:188–95.
56. Antoine JC, Boutahar N, Lassablière F, et al. Antifibroblast growth factor receptor 3 antibodies identify a subgroup of patients with sensory neuropathy. J Neurol Neurosurg Psychiatry 2015;86:1347–55.
57. Malik A, Lopate G, Hayat G. Prevalence of axonal sensory neuropathy with IgM binding to trisulfated heparin disaccharide in patients with fibromyalgia. J Clin Neuromuscul Dis 2019;20:103–10.
58. Samara V, Sampson J, Muppidi S. FGFR3 antibodies in neuropathy: what to do with them? J Clin Neuromuscul Dis 2018;20(1):35–40.
59. Fujii T, Yamasaki R, Iinuma K, et al. A novel autoantibody against Plexin D1 in patients with neuropathic pain. Ann Neurol 2018;84(2):208–24.
60. Waheed W, Boyd J, Khan F, et al. Double trouble: para-neoplastic anti-PCA-2 and CRMP-5-mediated small fibre neuropathy followed by chorea associated with small cell lung cancer and evolving radiological features. BMJ Case Rep 2016; 2016. bcr2016215158.
61. Klein CJ, Lennon VA, Aston PA, et al. Chronic pain as a manifestation of potassium channel-complex autoimmunity. Neurology 2012;79(11):1136–44.
62. Tavee JO, Karwa K, Ahmed Z, et al. Sarcoidosis-associated small fiber neuropathy in a large cohort: clinical aspects and response to IVIG and anti-TNF alpha treatment. Respir Med 2017;126:135–8.
63. Souayah N, Chin RL, Brannagan TH, et al. Effect of intravenous immunoglobulin on cerebellar ataxia and neuropathic pain associated with celiac disease. Eur J Neurol 2008;15(12):1300–3.
64. https://clinicaltrials.gov/ct2/show/NCT03401073 Gamunex-C (Grifols, Inc) in SFN with TS-HDS or FGFR3 antibodies – Beth Israel Hospital (Boston) and Phoenix Neurological Associates.
65. Levine T, Saperstein D, Pestronk A, et al. Identification of a novel immune mediated cause for small fiber neuropathy (P4.137). Neurology 2017;88 (16 Supplement).
66. Zeidman LA. Clinical Features in Immune-Mediated Small Fiber Neuropathy with TS-HDS or FGFR-3 Antibodies. Poster 227, AANEM Annual Meeting in Austin, Texas, October 16th-19th 2019. Muscle and Nerve 2019;60 (S1):S1-S140. Also included is unpublished or unpresented data on 3 extra patients not presented at the meeting.

Update in the Management of Myasthenia Gravis and Lambert-Eaton Myasthenic Syndrome

Cynthia Bodkin, MD[a],[1],*, Robert M. Pascuzzi, MD[b],[1]

KEYWORDS

- Lambert Eaton myasthenic syndrome • Myasthenia gravis • Weakness
- Complement inhibitor • Thymectomy

KEY POINTS

- History, acuity of presentation, family history, medication and physical exam are very important when evaluating a patient with muscle weakness.
- Disorders of the NMJ often have fatigable weakness. MG usually present with ocular and/or bulbar symptoms, while LEMS have more arm and leg weakness.
- Choice of medication needs to be taken in contexts of severity of disease, co-morbid diagnosis, and antibody status.

MYASTHENIA GRAVIS
Clinical Features

Fatigable or variable weakness is a hallmark of myasthenia gravis (MG). Ocular symptoms such as diplopia and ptosis are seen in approximately 50% of patients at onset of illness. Within 1 month of onset of symptoms, 80% of patients will have some degree of ocular involvement. Presenting symptom of generalized weakness, leg weakness, or bulbar symptoms each account for about 10% of the patients. Patients lack sensory symptoms and prominent muscle pain. On examination patients may demonstrate variable extraocular movement with normal pupillary reflexes, ptosis, nasal speech, flaccid dysarthria, and/or variable weakness with manual muscle strength testing. However, at times the patient's examination maybe completely normal at the time of their clinic visit.

[a] Clinical Neurology, Physical Medical Rehabilitation, Indiana University School of Medicine, Indiana University Health, Indianapolis, IN, USA; [b] Neurology Department, Indiana University School of Medicine, Indiana University Health, Indianapolis, Indiana, USA
[1] Present address: 335 W16th Street, Suite 4700, Indianapolis, IN 46202.
* Corresponding author.
E-mail address: cbodkin@iu.edu

Neurol Clin 39 (2021) 133–146
https://doi.org/10.1016/j.ncl.2020.09.007
0733-8619/21/© 2020 Elsevier Inc. All rights reserved.

Diagnosis

Acetylcholine receptor

MG is an autoimmune disorder caused by the production of antibodies directed against the nicotinic acetylcholine receptor (AChR). Roughly 80% to 90% of patients with MG will have measurable antibodies to the AChR in their serum. Overall antibody testing for AChR is fairly specific, with false-positive antibodies being extremely rare from a reliable laboratory. Thymoma is present in about 10% of patients with AChR-positive MG (and most of them have thymic hyperplasia). Therefore, patients positive for AChR antibodies must be screened with a computed tomography (CT) or MRI of the chest for thymoma.

In patients without AChR antibodies, muscle-specific receptor tyrosine kinase (MuSK) or low-density lipoprotein receptor-related protein 4 (LRP4) antibodies maybe found.

Muscle-specific receptor tyrosine kinase

The second most common antibody found is MuSK antibody. Series vary in the percentage found to be positive for MuSK but in general about one-fourth of all patients negative for AChR will be found positive for MuSK (roughly 25% of all patients negative for the AChR Ab or 5% of all patients with autoimmune MG). MuSK patients often have distinctive clinical characteristics. Such patients tend to be younger women (younger than 40 years) with disproportionate bulbar, neck extensor, shoulder, and respiratory symptoms with increased likelihood of "fixed weakness" and have a lower likelihood of abnormal repetitive stimulation and edrophonium test results. MuSK patients have no associated thymus abnormalities (and are not candidates for thymectomy) and are more likely to be refractory to a variety of therapies (such as cholinesterase inhibitors and many immune therapies). Conversely the MuSK patients tend to respond very favorably to rituximab and plasmapheresis.

Low-density lipoprotein receptor-related protein 4

A less common MG antibody seen in patients without AChR and MuSK (often referred to as the "double-negative" patients) is the LRP4. The LRP4 antibody is found in about 1% to 2% of all patients with autoimmune MG. The LRP4-positive patients do not have association with thymic pathology, and thymectomy is not indicated in their management. Patients with LRP4 MG were noted to have a younger age of onset and was more common in women compared with other "double-negative" patients who do not have LRP4. LRP4 patients tend to have relatively mild severity and often have pure ocular manifestations, and LRP4 patients are observed to generally respond favorable to pyridostigmine or prednisone.[1] Studies looking at patterns of clinical characteristics and distinctive responses to the various MG treatment options are ongoing. Regarding specificity, LRP4 antibodies have also been found in occasional patients with amyotrophic lateral sclerosis and thus positive results should be interpreted in the proper clinical context.[2]

Anti-agrin

Occasional patients without AChR, MuSK, and LRP4 ("triple-negative" patients) are found to have anti-agrin antibodies.[3] However, most cases of anti-agrin antibodies are also found along with MuSK, LRP4, or AChR antibodies.[4] Agrin is a protein of the basal lamina with 2 isoforms. Neural agrin seems to bind to LRP4, which activates MuSK, leading to clustering of AChR.

Electrophysiological testing

When antibody testing is negative (10%–15% of patients with MG), Electromyography (EMG) can aid in the diagnosis. An EMG can confirm a disorder of the NMJ as well as evaluate for other possible causes of weakness including myopathy or motor neuron disease. Repetitive stimulation of a motor nerve at a slow frequency (2–3 Hz) can demonstrate decrement greater than 10% in patients with dysfunction of the NMJ. Decrement is more prominent in patients with postsynaptic disorders than presynaptic. Overall sensitivity is about 50% but higher in clinically weak muscles and lower with ocular MG. Single-fiber EMG is more sensitive (about 90%) than repetitive stimulation.

Treatment

First part of management is patient education. The Muscular Dystrophy Association and Myasthenia Gravis Foundation are the 2 organizations that offer educational material and pamphlets for patients. Another crucial part of management is recognizing when to hospitalize a patient with MG. Patients with rapidly worsening symptoms, moderate-to-severe dysphagia, or dyspnea should be evaluated and admitted urgently. Signs of respiratory failure should be monitored closely. Evaluation of MG crisis triggers, such as surgery, medication, infection, hyper- or hypothyroidism, or medication change, should be performed and addressed promptly.

Cholinesterase inhibitors

Pharmacologic treatment should be individualized and based on patient's symptoms and comorbid diagnosis. First-line treatment in MG is reversible cholinesterase inhibitors (CEI) such as pyridostigmine or neostigmine. CEI are generally safe without significant long-term complications. However, too much of CEI can lead to skeletal muscle weakness (cholinergic weakness), uncommon in patients on oral CEI.

Immunotherapy

Corticosteroids

Corticosteroids are commonly used for moderate to severe MG, although prospective controlled trials documenting benefits are lacking. Expert opinion and patient compliance despite complications support its use in patients with moderate to severe symptoms. There is no consensus on dosing of corticosteroids but typically aim for a higher dose (60–80 mg/d of prednisone) initially. Most of the patients (approximately 80%) will show marked improvement or remission, and only 5% have no response. A lack of response should raise the question of the diagnosis. Typical improvement begins around the 1 to 2 weeks and gradually continues over the next 3 to 9 months. Approximately half of the patients will experience temporary worsening of weakness starting 1 to 2 days after initiating steroids and lasting 3 to 4 days. The weakness can be severe enough in 10% of patients to require ventilation or a feeding tube. Therefore, many patients with moderate to severe disease should be hospitalized for initiation of steroids. An alternating dose (AD) schedule is often used to avoid early exacerbations (prednisone, 25 mg, AD with increasing 12.5 mg every third dose to a maximum dose of 100 mg AD or until optimal improvement occurs). Improvement typically takes longer, with improvement starting around 1 month. Low-AD prednisone with gradual titration was beneficial in ocular MG compared with placebo, although recruitment was much lower than planned.[5] To avoid myasthenia crisis or flare-up of disease, steroids should be slowly tapered at about 10 mg every 1 to 2 months when greater than 20 mg/d and slower taper less than 20 mg/d. If symptoms recur while tapering steroids, a steroid-sparing medication is initiated to aid in the steroid taper and minimize long-term complications with prednisone.

Alternative Immunosuppressive Drug Therapy

Steroid-sparing immunosuppressive medication is often needed in patients who suffer relapse in symptoms with tapering of steroids, whose steroids are contraindicated, and are intolerant or continue to have symptoms. Azathioprine, mycophenolate mofetil, and cyclosporine have historically been used as steroid-sparing agents. Double-blind controlled studies with cyclosporine demonstrated improvement in strength and symptoms.[6] Mycophenolate mofetil failed to show improvement in 3 months in a controlled double-blind trial.[7] In a second trial mycophenolate was no more effective than placebo in reducing prednisone dose over 9 months in patients who were steroid dependent. However, retrospective studies of mycophenolate mofetil suggest that time to improvement takes longer than 6 to 12 months, and therefore 3 months in the controlled trial may have been too short in duration to demonstrate a statistical improvement.[8] Tacrolimus is used in some centers for refractory MG although studies have failed to demonstrate a major benefit.[9,10] Methotrexate is also used although a recent prospective study failed to demonstrate steroid-sparing benefit in 12 months.[11]

Complement inhibitors

Given that the pathogenesis of MG involves AChR-binding antibodies at the postsynaptic membrane attracting complement and leading to complement-mediated lysis, there is a logical interest in using a monoclonal antibody to block C5 complement and ostensibly reduce complement-mediated lysis and reduce malfunction at the neuromuscular junction. Eculizumab blocks C5 complement and was originally Food and Drug Administration (FDA)-approved for treatment of paroxysmal nocturnal hemoglobinuria. This drug binds to human terminal complement protein C5 and inhibits enzymatic cleavage of C5 to C5a and C5b, thus preventing C5a-induced attraction of proinflammatory cells and related lysis of the postsynaptic membrane. Recent studies (REGAIN) have demonstrated clinical benefit in the treatment of MG.[12] In a 6-month randomized, double-blind, placebo-controlled REGAIN study of eculizumab in 125 patients with refractory generalized, AChR + MG, the primary analysis showed no significant difference between eculizumab and placebo. However, MG exacerbations were seen in 6 (10%) of the patients in the eculizumab group compared with 15 (24%) in the placebo group. A requirement for rescue therapy was seen in only 6 (10%) of the patients in the eculizumab group compared with 12 (19%) in the placebo group. Eculizumab was well tolerated and associated with improvement in activities of daily living, muscle power, functional, and quality of life. Given the mechanism of action of eculizumab, patients are recommended to receive meningococcal vaccination before the first infusion to limit the risk of meningococcal meningitis. Complement is not thought to play a major role in MuSK MG pathophysiology, and therefore complement inhibitors would not be indicated in MuSK + patients.

A subsequent analysis of an open-label extension reported on eculizumab's long-term safety and efficacy (1200 mg every 2 weeks for a median duration of 22.7 month in 117 patients), indicating a favorable safety profile including no cases of meningococcal meningitis. The MG exacerbation rate was 75% less than what patient experienced in the year before beginning eculizumab, and statistically significant improvement in activities of daily living, muscle power, functional, and quality of life were maintained. During this time 56% of patients improved to a clinical state of minimal manifestations or pharmacologic remission. And those patients initially on placebo in the initial study demonstrated rapid and sustained improvement on open-label eculizumab.[13]

Rituximab

Rituximab is a monoclonal antibody directed against the CD20 antigen on B cells, which has over the last decade become widely used in the treatment of patients with AChR-positive MG and MuSK MG. Major benefit is well established for most of the MuSK-positive patients. Hehir and colleagues[14] reported results of a prospective controlled double-blind trial in MuSK-positive patients with MG. The primary clinical endpoint was the "Myasthenia Gravis Status and Treatment Intensity" (MGSTI), a measure reflecting Myasthenia Gravis Foundation of America (MGFA) postintervention status as well as requirements for additional immunotherapy. With median follow-up of 3.5 years 58% (14/24) of the rituximab-treated patients achieved the primary outcome target compared with 16% (5/31) of controls. In addition, at the time of last visit, 29% of rituximab-treated patients were taking prednisone (mean dose 4.5 mg/d) compared with 74% of controls (mean dose 13 mg/d). This study provides class IV evidence for benefit of rituximab in MuSK patients with MG.

For patients with AChR-positive myasthenia there is abundant anecdotal and retrospective evidence for benefit but overall a more limited success rate in such patients compared with MuSK-positive patients with MG.[15–17] A large retrospective national study in patients with MG from Austria included 56 patients, 70% of which were AChR positive and 25% with MuSK-positive MG (5% seronegative). Three months after rituximab, 14 of 53 (26.4%) patients were in remission. At last follow-up after a median of 20 (10; 53) months, remission was present in 42.9% of patients and another 25% had minimal manifestations. Remission was observed in 71% of the MuSK patients with MG compared with 36% of those with AChR MG. Rituximab usage was without major side effects in this retrospective study.[16]

Plasmapheresis

Plasma exchange (plasmapheresis or PLEX) removes antibodies (including AChR antibodies) from the plasma. Improvement is typically seen within 1 to 2 weeks but only lasting 1 to 2 months. Because of the rapid improvement with PLEX, it is commonly used in MG crises. A typical exchange removes 5 L of plasma every other day for about 5 exchanges. Complications included bradycardia, hypotension, electrolyte imbalance, hemolysis, infection, and access problems. Maintenance PLEX (one exchange every 1–8 weeks) has been used in patients with refractory myasthenia, especially MuSK patients.[18,19]

Intravenous immunoglobulin

High-dose intravenous immunoglobulin (IVIg) and subcutaneous Ig have been associated with clinical improvement in MG symptoms similar to the time-frame of PLEX.[20,21] Improvement can be seen within the first week and last 4 to 8 weeks. The usual dose for IVIg is 2 g/kg spread out over 5 days. Common practice in the management of patients with moderate to severe MG, especially those refractory or intolerant of multiple immune therapies, is to use IVIg not only for acute crisis and exacerbations (for which there are prospective controlled double-blind trial data to support such use) but also for maintenance therapy.[22] Many experienced neuromuscular clinicians use maintenance IVIg in selected cases and provide anecdotal attestation as to its effectiveness in a significant proportion of patients. The lack of published prospective controlled double-blind evidence for IVIg benefit as a maintenance therapy is an understandable barrier to access for IVIg in many patients, particularly given the substantial cost of the drug. Although prospective double-blind trials are in progress, there is substantial published anecdotal and retrospective literature providing support for this form of maintenance therapy.

A report of 52 patients with MG from one center who had not responded to pyridostigmine, prednisone, azathioprine, or combination were given IVIg as maintenance treatment. Sustained improvement was seen in 37 of these patients, and treatment was continued for an average of 6 years. The improvement was generally mild to moderate in degree without full remission. Favorable response was associated with AChR seropositivity including higher titers, older age-group, and those with bulbar onset. Use of maintenance IVIg was associated with reduced needs for other treatments including CEI, prednisone, and azathioprine.[23]

Complications with IVIg include flulike symptoms, fever, chills, and headache. Decreasing the rate of the infusion and pretreatment with diphenhydramine may improve the side effects. Rare cases of stroke, nephritic syndrome, and renal failure have been reported. Screening for selective IgA deficiency is recommended to avoid anaphylaxis reaction. Compared with PLEX, IVIg is considerate and equally efficacious for severe generalized MG.[22] However, IVIg seems to be superior for pretreatment before thymectomy.[24]

Exercise

Historically patients with MG have often been advised to be cautious about prolonged physical exertion. To learn if progressive resistance training or aerobic training are possible and effective in patients with MG 15 patients with generalized MG were randomly assigned to 20 sessions over an 8-week period. Overall only 1 patient dropped out of the training session, and adverse events were seen in both groups, including 2 with increased bulbar symptoms and 3 with increased fatigue. The progressive resistance-training group showed increases in maximal strength and functional capacity. This study would suggest that most of the patients with MG can tolerate exercise therapy and some demonstrate improved strength and function.[25]

Thymectomy

Association of the thymus gland with MG was first noted around the1900s, and thymectomy for treatment of myasthenia was initially reported in the 1930s. Around the 1940s this procedure had been considered a standard of care, especially for younger patients and those with moderate to severe disease. Debate over the effectiveness of thymectomy persisted for decades[26] until recently when results of a large randomized international multicenter controlled trial indicatec clear benefit in patients having AChR-positive generalized nonthymoma MG.[27]

The MGTX randomized 126 patients to thymectomy plus prednisone or prednisone alone. Patients in this study had been symptomatic for less than 5 years, were seropositive for AChR antibodies, and had MGFA class II to IV clinical involvement. Follow-up was 3 years. Patients in both groups received oral prednisone titrated up to 100 mg alternate day until acquiring a clinical status of minimal manifestations. Extended transsternal thymectomy was performed. Primary outcome measures included clinical status and total prednisone requirement. Secondary outcome measures included serious adverse events, total hospitalization over the 3 years, and surveys for quality of life. Patients randomized to thymectomy had significant improvement in MG symptoms, including an average Quantitative Myasthenia Gravis (QMG) scale (6.15 vs 8.99). Lower dose of prednisone was needed to maintain optimal clinical status (44 mg vs 60 mg alternate day). Complications were similar in both groups. Additional favorable measures the time-weighted average score on the Myasthenia Gravis Activities of Daily Living scale (2.24 vs 3.41), requirement for azathioprine use (17% vs 48%), and the percent of patients with minimal-manifestation status at month 36 (67% vs 47%). Hospitalizations were lower in the thymectomy group (9% vs 37%).[27]

A subsequent rater-blinded 2-year extension study for patients who completed the initial 3-year MGTX further supported the benefit of thymectomy. Endpoints in the extension study included time-weighted means of the QMG score and the alternate-day prednisone dose from month 0 to month 60. Sixty-eight (61%) of the 111 patients who completed the initial 3-year MGTX entered the extension study and 50 patients completed the 60-month study. At 5 years, patients in the thymectomy plus prednisone group had significantly lower QMG scores and mean alternate-day prednisone doses (24 mg vs 48 mg) than did those in the prednisone group. There is now clear evidence supporting the benefit of thymectomy in the treatment of MG.[28]

In a recent American Academy of Neurology Practice Advisory: Thymectomy for Myasthenia Gravis (Practice Parameter Update) the guidelines listed 2 level B recommendations:

1. "Clinicians should discuss thymectomy with patients who have AChR antibody + generalized MG and are 18 to 65 years of age. The discussion should clearly indicate the anticipated benefits and risks of the procedures and uncertainties surrounding the magnitude of these benefits and risks."
2. Clinicians should counsel patients with AChR antibody + generalized MG considering minimally invasive thymectomy techniques that it is uncertain whether the benefit attained by extended transsternal thymectomy will also be attained by minimally invasive approaches.

Because extended transsternal thymectomy is a big procedure with multiple days of hospitalization, there is an increasing practice to consider the less invasive approach to thymectomy.[29] The International consensus guidance for management of myasthenia gravis states, *"Endoscopic and robotic approaches to thymectomy are increasingly performed and have a good track record for safety in experienced centers. Data from randomized, controlled comparison studies are not available. Based on comparisons across studies, less invasive thymectomy approaches appear to yield similar results to more aggressive approaches."*[22]

Regarding presurgical treatment with IVIg or plasma exchange a randomized clinical trial of 24 patients with MG (IVIg group) received IVIg 1 g/kg/d for 2 consecutive days was compared with plasma exchange 5 L every other day, 10 to 30 days before thymectomy. Intubation period and duration of surgery differed between the plasma exchange and IVIg groups, suggesting that IVIG may be a more effective preoperative option.[24]

Historically there has been limited acceptance of thymectomy for treatment of ocular MG. A recent meta-analysis of studies assessing the outcome of thymectomy in patients with nonthymomatous ocular MG was favorable.[30]

The International consensus guidance for management of MG also provides consensus opinion regarding other clinically relevant question with respect to thymectomy.

"Thymectomy may be considered in patients with generalized MG without detectable AChR antibodies if they fail to respond adequately to IS therapy, or to avoid/minimize intolerable adverse effects from IS therapy." And, *"Current evidence does not support an indication for thymectomy in patients with MuSK, LRP4, or agrin antibodies."*[22]

Neonatal Fc receptor–targeted therapy for myasthenia gravis
Of the many new strategies being considered as novel treatment of MG, there is particular interest in the role of the neonatal Fc receptor. The neonatal Fc receptor

(FcRn) plays an important role in the regulation of IgG levels. The FcRn "saves" IgG from degradation by rescuing and recycling, leading to a longer half-life and greater blood levels than other immunoglobulins. FcRn is present in myeloid cells and in endothelial cells throughout the lifespan. With monoclonal antibody inhibition of FcRn there is an overall reduction in the levels of pathogenic IgG and in preliminary studies in MG biomarker and clinical evidence to suggest a meaningful therapeutic role for treatment of patients with MG. Current ongoing clinical trial results should be anticipated to clarify the role of such strategy in patient management.[31,32]

Medications to avoid

There is an extensive list of medications that have been observed to interfere with neuromuscular transmission and aggravate symptoms in patients with MG. Those drugs most commonly observed to increase symptoms and thus wise to avoid if possible in patients with known MG include chloroquine, quinine, quinidine, procainamide, and botulinum toxin. Aminoglycoside antibiotics should be avoided unless needed for a life-threatening infection. Fluoroquinolones (ciprofloxacin) and erythromycin have significant neuromuscular blocking effects, and some patients will experience worsening of their symptoms on exposure. Telithromycin has been reported to cause life-threatening weakness in patients with MG and should not be used. Neuromuscular blocking drugs such as pancuronium and D-tubocurarine can produce marked and prolonged paralysis in patients with MG. Depolarizing drugs such as succinylcholine can also have a prolonged effect and should be used by a skilled anesthesiologist who is well aware of the patient's MG. Debate continues over the likelihood of current-day iodinated contrast agents to aggravate MG, but the overall risk seems to be low.[33]

A distinctive drug concern is that several therapeutic agents have been found to "induce" autoimmune MG (cause the disease as opposed to aggravating preexisting MG). The most widely studied and reported historically is D-penicillamine, in which about 5% of patients seem to develop MG symptoms and the presence of AChR antibodies. When penicillamine is stopped most patients clinically improve and serology reverts to normal. More recently α-interferon has been observed to induce autoimmune MG. Patients having received a bone marrow transplant may develop MG as part of a chronic graft versus host syndrome.

Of greater recent concern is the observation for immune checkpoint inhibitors (ICI) to induce or aggravate MG and be associated with a relatively severe and at times refractory clinical presentation. The ICI are increasingly and widely used as standard care in the treatment of a variety of malignancies. They include ipilimumab, nivolumab, pembrolizumab, atezolizumab, durvalumab, and avelumab. Checkpoint inhibitor complications include the induction of a variety of immune-mediated conditions that can in some cases be severe and require discontinuation of the ICI and the addition of aggressive immune therapy. Checkpoint inhibitor use in patients with known preexisting autoimmune disease seems to be associated with exacerbation of the preexisting autoimmune disorder in half of such patients and the induction of new autoimmune disease in 30%.[34] Although most patients improved, 17% required a permanent discontinuation of checkpoint inhibitor treatment.[34]

Specific neurologic complications from checkpoint inhibitors are less common, but the risk of MG is of sufficient frequency and severity to warrant attention from the practicing neurologist. Patients can have new onset MG induced by checkpoint inhibitors or a flare-up of preexisting MG. A retrospective review of a large cohort of 65 patients with MG with checkpoint inhibitor exposure emphasized the severity and the rapidly progressive course of MG in such patients and indicated potential benefit with early use of plasma exchange and IVIg.[35]

Congenital myasthenia encompasses a group of rare hereditary disorders of the neuromuscular junction. The patients tend to have life-long relatively stable symptoms of generalized fatigable weakness. These disorders are not immune-mediated and do not respond to immune therapy (steroids, thymectomy, and plasma exchange). Most patients improve on CEI. Although there are many established subtypes of congenital myasthenia, several are noteworthy for their therapeutic options. The *fast-channel congenital myasthenic syndrome* tends to be static or slowly progressive but usually very responsive to combination therapy with amifampridine and pyridostigmine. In *congenital slow-channel myasthenic syndrome* the disease typically worsens over years as the endplate myopathy progresses. Cholinesterase inhibitors typically worsen symptoms, but quinidine and fluoxetine, which reduce the duration of AChR channel openings, are both effective treatments for *slow-channel syndrome*. The *congenital myasthenic syndrome associated with AChR deficiency* tends to be nonprogressive and may even improve slightly as the patient ages. Treatment includes pyridostigmine and/or amifampridine, and ephedrine produces benefit in some. Patients with *endplate acetylcholinesterase deficiency* usually present in infancy or early childhood with generalized weakness, muscle underdevelopment, slow pupillary responses to light, and either no response or worsening with CEI therapy. Albuterol is reported effective in treating patients with *endplate acetylcholinesterase deficiency*. A homozygous mutation of *Dok-7* is responsible for a form of congenital myasthenia characterized by weakness in limbs and trunk but largely sparing the face, eyes, and oropharyngeal muscles. The formation of neuromuscular synapses requires the MuSK. Dok-7 is necessary for the activation of MuSK. Albuterol is reported effective in treating patients with *Dok-7* congenital myasthenia.[36]

LAMBERT-EATON MYASTHENIC SYNDROME
Clinical Features

Lambert-Eaton myasthenic syndrome (LEMS) (also commonly referred to as Lambert-Eaton syndrome and Lambert-Eaton myasthenia) is a presynaptic disease characterized by chronic fluctuating weakness of proximal limb muscles. Symptoms (**Table 1**) include difficulty walking, climbing stairs, or rising from a chair. In LEMS there may be some improvement in power with sustained or repeated exercise. Although the predominant symptoms are those of symmetric proximal weakness particularly involving the lower extremities, up to half of patients have some degree of bulbar involvement[37] and half may complain of ptosis or diplopia,[38] although ocular and bulbar symptoms are typically less pronounced than in patients with MG. In contrast with the MG severe respiratory failure is less common. In addition, patients with LEMS often complain of myalgia, muscle stiffness of the legs and back, limb paresthesia, metallic taste, severe

Table 1 Symptoms and signs of Lambert-Eaton myasthenic syndrome	
Symptoms	**Signs on Examination**
Proximal limb weakness (legs > arms)	Proximal weakness
Cranial weakness (20%)	Mild cranial weakness
Fluctuating symptoms	Objective weakness is less than predicted based on
Dry mouth	symptoms
Other anticholinergic autonomic	Absent/reduced muscle stretch reflexes
symptoms	Lambert sign (2–3 s of maximal grip produces
Metallic taste	increase strength)

dry mouth, impotence, and other autonomic symptoms from muscarinic cholinergic insufficiency. The examination typically shows proximal lower extremity weakness, although the objective bedside assessment may suggest relatively mild weakness relative to the patient's history. The muscle stretch reflexes are absent. On testing sustained maximal grip there is a gradual increase in power over the initial 2 to 3 seconds (Lambert sign).

Overall LEMS is rare compared with MG, which is about 100 times more common. About half of patients with LME have an underlying malignancy that is usually small cell carcinoma of the lung. Occasional patients will have a small cell carcinoma originating elsewhere in the body.[39] Patients with LEMS should be evaluated with CT scan and fluorodeoxyglucose PET to evaluate for underlying tumor. If no tumor is found, evaluation and screen should be repeated at regular intervals (ie, every 6 months for about 2–4 years). In patients without malignancy, LEMS is an autoimmune disease and is often associated with other autoimmune diseases. In general, patients older than 40 years are more likely to be men and have an associated malignancy, whereas younger patients are more likely to be women and have no neoplasm. LEMS symptoms can precede detection of the malignancy by 1 to 2 years. Another serologic indicator of associated small cell lung cancer is the SOX1 antibody, an immunogenic tumor antigen in SCLC. SOX1 antibodies were detected in 64% of patients with LEMS with SCLC but in none of 50 patients with nonparaneoplastic LEMS.[40]

Diagnosis

The pathogenesis involves autoantibodies directed against presynaptic P/Q-type voltage-gated calcium channels at cholinergic nerve terminals, resulting in reduced presynaptic calcium concentration and reduced quanta release of acetylcholine These IgG antibodies also inhibit cholinergic synapses of the autonomic nervous system. More than 90% of patients with LEMS are seropositive, and thus serologic testing is essential in screening and confirming the diagnosis. The diagnosis is confirmed with EMG studies, which typically show low amplitude of the compound muscle action potentials and a decrement to slow rates or repetitive stimulation in more than 95% of patients. Following brief exercise, there is marked facilitation of the CMAP amplitude (greater than 100% increase) in 90% of patients. At high rates of repetitive stimulation, there may be an incremental response. Single-fiber EMG is markedly abnormal in virtually all patients with LEMS.

Treatment of Lambert-Eaton Myasthenic syndrome

Treatment options include treating of the underlying small cell lung cancer when present, use of cholinesterase inhibitors such as pyridostigmine, use of voltage-gated potassium channel blocker 3,4-diaminopyridine/amifampridine, and for severe and refractory patients, treatment with immunotherapy.[41]

Cancer treatment: successful treatment of small cell lung cancer can in some patients be "curative" for LEMS. Evaluation of the impact of concurrent LEMS on the survival of patient with small cell lung cancer suggests that the presence of LEMS with small cell lung cancer conferred a significant survival advantage independently of the other prognostic variables.[42]

3,4-diaminopyridine/amifampridine

First-line medical therapy involves the use of 3,4-diaminopyridine/amifampridine. Both names refer to the same drug. There are currently 2 slightly different preparations of this drug made by different manufacturers, both of which have received FDA approval for the treatment of LEMS. Amifampridine/3,4-diaminopyridine is a quaternary ammonium drug that exerts its effect by blocking the presynaptic voltage-gated potassium channels and in doing so keeps the motor nerve terminal depolarized longer, thus allowing more time for calcium channels to remain open, leading to increased calcium concentration at the motor nerve terminal, thus enhancing the presynaptic release of ACh. Ever since the initial prospective double-blind placebo-controlled studies showing benefit of 3,4-diaminopyridine in the 1989,[43] patients have been required to receive such medication through approved research centers until the recent FDA approval of 2 forms of amifampridine resulting in the drug being commercially available. Amifampridine phosphate is the active ingredient of FDA-approved form named *Firdapse*.[44] In 2018 the FDA approved *Firdapse* amifampridine for treatment of adults aged 17 years and older with LEMS. The second form of amifampridine, historically referred to as 3,4 diaminopyridine, has also demonstrated clear benefit in patients with LEMS,[45] and in 2019 this base form of amifampridine called *Ruzurgi* became FDA approved for treatment of juvenile LEMS (age 6 years to <17 years). Accordingly, the potential access to these drugs with FDA approval has markedly improved. Both agents have proved efficacy. Although there are now 2 FDA-approved drugs for treatment of LEMS, a new challenge involves cost of the drug and insurance coverage. Before FDA approval patient would acquire the drug through neuromuscular centers having an investigation new drug program to allow access at no or minimal financial cost. As of 2020 the established charge for *Ruzurgi*-Jacobus is $80/10 mg pill. *Firdapse*-Catalyst established charge in 2020 is $180/10 mg pill. Programs exist although both manufacturers provide cost assistance for patients with limited resources. One difference in the 2 products is that *Ruzurgi* requires refrigeration and *Firdapse*, being more stable, does not. Concerns over the processes and policies of the FDA in approval for 2 competing manufacturers of similar drugs and potential negative consequences have been expressed by the neuromuscular physician community.[46] Side effects include transient paresthesia (10%) and rarely seizures, especially in high doses. A comparison of dosing recommendations for these agents is found in **Table 2**.

Table 2 Amifampridine[47,48]		
	Firdapse®	**Ruzurgi®**
FDA approval	>17 y/o with LES	617 y/o with LES
Starting Dose	15mg-30 mg PO divided 3–4 times a day[a]	Wt. ≥45 kg start 15–30 mg (wt. <45 kg start 7.5–15 mg) daily PO divided 2–3 times a day
Dose titration	5 mg daily every 3–4 d	Wt. ≥45 kg increase 5–10 mg divided (wt. <45 kg increase 2.5 mg to 5 mg) in up to 5 doses daily
Maximum dose	20 mg single dose and 80 mg daily	Wt. ≥45 kg 30 mg single dose and 100 mg daily Wt. <45 kg 15 mg single dose and 50 mg daily dose
Refrigeration	Not needed	Needed
Contraindications	Seizures	Seizures

[a] Starting dosage is 15 mg daily for patients with renal impairment, hepatic impairment and in known N-acetyltransferase 2 (NAT2) poor metabolizers.

Data from Jacobus Ruzergi prescribing information. (https://www.accessdata.fda.gov/drugsatfda_docs/label/2019/209321s000lbl.pdf); and Catalyst Firdapse prescribing information. (https://www.accessdata.fda.gov/drugsatfda_docs/label/2018/208078s000lbl.pdf).

Although pyridostigmine offer limited benefit in patients with LEMS, it is safe and in many patients significantly effective. This drug is also widely available and relatively inexpensive.

Lambert-Eaton myasthenic syndrome

Immune therapy Prednisone, azathioprine, rituximab, IVIg, and plasma exchange are all used in patients having limited benefit from amifampridine.[41]

CLINICS CARE POINTS

- Patients with a disorder of the NMJ and rapid deterioration or moderate to severe dysphagia or dyspnea should be hospitalized.
- Patients with MG may temporarily deteriorate after starting steroids before they improve, therefore patients should be monitored closely and may need to be hospitalized when initiating steroids.
- Tapering immunotherapy very slowly in patients with MG to prevent MG crisis.
- Patient's should receive meningococcal vaccination at least 2 weeks prior to starting a complement inhibitor.
- Providers should discuss thymectomy with patients who have AChR antibody with generalized MG and are 18 to 65 years of age.

DISCLOSURE

The authors have nothing to disclose.

REFERENCES

1. Bacchi S, Kramer P, Chalk C. Autoantibodies to Low-Density Lipoprotein Receptor-Related Protein 4 in Double Seronegative Myasthenia Gravis: A Systematic Review. Can J Neurol Sci 2018;45:62–7.
2. Lazaridis K, Tzartos SJ. Autoantibody Specificities in Myasthenia Gravis; Implications for Improved Diagnostics and Therapeut cs. Front Immunol 2020;11:212.
3. Zhang B, Shen C, Bealmear B, et al. Autoantibodies to agrin in myasthenia gravis patients. PLoS One 2014;9:e91816.
4. Gasperi C, Melms A, Schoser B, et al. Anti-agrin autoantibodies in myasthenia gravis. Neurology 2014;82:1976–83.
5. Benatar M, McDermott MP, Sanders DB, et al. Efficacy of prednisone for the treatment of ocular myasthenia (EPITOME): a randomized, controlled trial. Muscle Nerve 2016;53:363–9.
6. Tindall RS, Phillips JT, Rollins JA, et al. A clinical therapeutic trial of cyclosporine in myasthenia gravis. Ann N Y Acad Sci 1993;681:539–51.
7. Sanders DB, Hart IK, Mantegazza R, et al. An international, phase III, randomized trial of mycophenolate mofetil in myasthenia gravis. Neurology 2008;71:400–6.
8. Cahoon WD Jr, Kockler DR. Mycophenolate mofetil treatment of myasthenia gravis. Ann Pharmacother 2006;40:295–8.
9. Wang L, Zhang S, Xi J, et al. Efficacy and safety of tacrolimus for myasthenia gravis: a systematic review and meta-analysis. J Neurol 2017;264:2191–200.
10. Yoshikawa H, Kiuchi T, Saida T, et al. Randomised, double-blind, placebo-controlled study of tacrolimus in myasthenia gravis. J Neurol Neurosurg Psychiatry 2011;82:970–7.
11. Pasnoor M, He J, Herbelin L, et al. A randomized controlled trial of methotrexate for patients with generalized myasthenia gravis. Neurology 2016;87:57–64.

12. Howard JF Jr, Utsugisawa K, Benatar M, et al. Safety and efficacy of eculizumab in anti-acetylcholine receptor antibody-positive refractory generalised myasthenia gravis (REGAIN): a phase 3, randomised, double-blind, placebo-controlled, multicentre study. Lancet Neurol 2017;16:976–86.

13. Muppidi S, Utsugisawa K, Benatar M, et al. Long-term safety and efficacy of eculizumab in generalized myasthenia gravis. Muscle Nerve 2019;60:14–24.

14. Hehir MK, Hobson-Webb LD, Benatar M, et al. Rituximab as treatment for anti-MuSK myasthenia gravis: Multicenter blinded prospective review. Neurology 2017;89:1069–77.

15. Tandan R, Hehir MK 2nd, Waheed W, Howard DB. Rituximab treatment of myasthenia gravis: A systematic review. Muscle Nerve 2017;56:185–96.

16. Topakian R, Zimprich F, Iglseder S, et al. High efficacy of rituximab for myasthenia gravis: a comprehensive nationwide study in Austria. J Neurol 2019;266:699–706.

17. Di Stefano V, Lupica A, Rispoli MG, et al. Rituximab in AChR subtype of myasthenia gravis: systematic review. J Neurol Neurosurg Psychiatry 2020;91:392–5.

18. Yamada C, Teener JW, Davenport RD, et al. Maintenance plasma exchange treatment for muscle specific kinase antibody positive myasthenia gravis patients. J Clin Apher 2015;30:314–9.

19. Usmani A, Kwan L, Wahib-Khalil D, et al. Excellent response to therapeutic plasma exchange in myasthenia gravis patients irrespective of antibody status. J Clin Apher 2019;34:416–22.

20. Adiao KJB, Espiritu AI, Roque VLA, et al. Efficacy and tolerability of subcutaneously administered immunoglobulin in myasthenia gravis: A systematic review. J Clin Neurosci 2020;72:316–21.

21. Ortiz-Salas P, Velez-Van-Meerbeke A, Galvis-Gomez CA, et al. Human immunoglobulin versus plasmapheresis in Guillain-Barre syndrome and myasthenia gravis: a meta-analysis. J Clin Neuromuscul Dis 2016;18:1–11.

22. Sanders DB, Wolfe GI, Benatar M, et al. International consensus guidance for management of myasthenia gravis: Executive summary. Neurology 2016;87:419–25.

23. Hellmann MA, Mosberg-Galili R, Lotan I, et al. Maintenance IVIg therapy in myasthenia gravis does not affect disease activity. J Neurol Sci 2014;338:39–42.

24. Alipour-Faz A, Shojaei M, Peyvandi H, et al. A comparison between IVIG and plasma exchange as preparations before thymectomy in myasthenia gravis patients. Acta Neurol Belg 2017;117:245–9.

25. Rahbek MA, Mikkelsen EE, Overgaard K, et al. Exercise in myasthenia gravis: A feasibility study of aerobic and resistance training. Muscle Nerve 2017;56:700–9.

26. McQuillen MP, Leone MG. A treatment carol: thymectomy revisited. Neurology 1977;27:1103–6.

27. Wolfe GI, Kaminski HJ, Aban IB, et al. Randomized Trial of Thymectomy in Myasthenia Gravis. N Engl J Med 2016;375:511–22.

28. Wolfe GI, Kaminski HJ, Aban IB, et al. Long-term effect of thymectomy plus prednisone versus prednisone alone in patients with non-thymomatous myasthenia gravis: 2-year extension of the MGTX randomised trial. Lancet Neurol 2019;18:259–68.

29. Gronseth GS, Barohn R, Narayanaswami P. Practice advisory: thymectomy for myasthenia gravis (practice parameter update): report of the guideline development, dissemination, and implementation subcommittee of the American Academy of Neurology. Neurology 2020;94:705–9.

30. Zhu K, Li J, Huang X, et al. Thymectomy is a beneficial therapy for patients with non-thymomatous ocular myasthenia gravis: a systematic review and meta-analysis. Neurol Sci 2017;38:1753–60.

31. Howard JF Jr, Bril V, Burns TM, et al. Randomized phase 2 study of FcRn antagonist efgartigimod in generalized myasthenia gravis. Neurology 2019;92: e2661–73.

32. Gable KL, Guptill JT. Antagonism of the neonatal Fc receptor as an emerging treatment for myasthenia gravis. Front Immunol 2019;10:3052.

33. Mehrizi M, Pascuzzi RM. Complications of radiologic contrast in patients with myasthenia gravis. Muscle Nerve 2014;50:443–4.

34. Abdel-Wahab N, Shah M, Lopez-Olivo MA, et al. Use of Immune Checkpoint Inhibitors in the Treatment of Patients With Cancer and Preexisting Autoimmune Disease: A Systematic Review. Ann Intern Mec 2018;168:121–30.

35. Safa H, Johnson DH, Trinh VA, et al. Immune checkpoint inhibitor related myasthenia gravis: single center experience and systematic review of the literature. J Immunother Cancer 2019;7:319.

36. Vanhaesebrouck AE, Beeson D. The congenital myasthenic syndromes: expanding genetic and phenotypic spectrums and refining treatment strategies. Curr Opin Neurol 2019;32:696–703.

37. Burns TM, Russell JA, LaChance DH, et al. Oculobulbar involvement is typical with Lambert-Eaton myasthenic syndrome. Ann Neurol 2003;53:270–3.

38. Young JD, Leavitt JA. Lambert-Eaton Myasthenic syndrome: ocular signs and symptoms. J Neuroophthalmol 2016;36:20–2.

39. Kennelly KD, Dodick DW, Pascuzzi RM, et al. Neuronal autoantibodies and paraneoplastic neurological syndromes associated with extrapulmonary small cell carsinoma. Neurology 1997;48:A31–2.

40. Sabater L, Titulaer M, Saiz A, et al. SOX1 antibodies are markers of paraneoplastic Lambert-Eaton myasthenic syndrome. Neurology 2008;70:924–8.

41. Kesner VG, Oh SJ, Dimachkie MM, et al. Lambert-Eaton Myasthenic Syndrome. Neurol Clin 2018;36:379–94.

42. Maddison P, Gozzard P, Grainge MJ, et al. Long-term survival in paraneoplastic Lambert-Eaton myasthenic syndrome. Neurology 2017;88:1334–9.

43. McEvoy KM, Windebank AJ, Daube JR, et al. 3,4-Diaminopyridine in the treatment of Lambert-Eaton myasthenic syndrome. N Engl J Med 1989;321:1567–71.

44. Oh SJ, Shcherbakova N, Kostera-Pruszczyk A, et al. Amifampridine phosphate (Firdapse((R))) is effective and safe in a phase 3 clinical trial in LEMS. Muscle Nerve 2016;53:717–25.

45. Sanders DB, Juel VC, Harati Y, et al. 3,4-diaminopyridine base effectively treats the weakness of Lambert-Eaton myasthenia. Muscle Nerve 2018;57:561–8.

46. Burns TM, Smith GA, Allen JA, et al. Editorial by concerned physicians: Unintended effect of the orphan drug act on the potential cost of 3,4-diaminopyridine. Muscle Nerve 2016;53:165–8.

47. Jacobus Ruzergi prescribing information. Available at: https://www.accessdata. fda.gov/drugsatfda_docs/label/2019/209321s000lbl.pdf. Accessed September 30, 2020.

48. Catalyst Firdapse prescribing information. Available at: https://www.accessdata. fda.gov/drugsatfda_docs/label/2018/208078s000lbl.pdf. Accessed September 30, 2020.

Update in the Management of Idiopathic Intracranial Hypertension

Matthew J. Thurtell, MD[a,b], Aki Kawasaki, MD, PhD[c],*

KEYWORDS

- Idiopathic intracranial hypertension • Pseudotumor cerebri • Papilledema
- CSF shunting • Optic nerve sheath fenestration • Venous sinus stenting

KEY POINTS

- Idiopathic intracranial hypertension is a syndrome of increased intracranial pressure of unknown cause that most often occurs in overweight/obese women of childbearing age.
- Papilledema is the hallmark clinical sign of idiopathic intracranial hypertension and can result in severe, irreversible vision loss if left untreated.
- For patients with papilledema and minimal-to-mild visual loss, sustained weight loss and medical therapy are usually effective treatments.
- For patients with papilledema and moderate visual loss, more aggressive medical therapy is often required.
- Surgical therapy is usually reserved for patients with a fulminant presentation who have rapidly declining vision or severe vision loss at presentation, although can also be considered in patients who fail to improve or worsen despite maximally tolerated medical therapy.

INTRODUCTION

Idiopathic intracranial hypertension (IIH) is a syndrome of increased intracranial pressure of unknown cause.[1] The term "idiopathic" implies that history, examination, and investigations (ie, neuroimaging and cerebrospinal fluid analysis) have ruled out other etiologies of increased intracranial pressure (**Table 1**).[1,2]

The only known risk factor for this syndrome is weight gain.[3] More than 90% of patients with IIH have a high body mass index (BMI), being either overweight (BMI >25) or obese (BMI >30). Even weight gain of 5% to 15% has been demonstrated to increase the risk of developing IIH.[3,4]

[a] Department of Ophthalmology and Visual Sciences, University of Iowa, Iowa City, IA 52242, USA; [b] Department of Neurology, University of Iowa, Iowa City, IA 52242, USA; [c] University of Lausanne, Hôpital Ophtalmique Jules Gonin, Avenue de France 15, Lausanne 1004, Switzerland
* Corresponding author.
E-mail address: aki.kawasaki@fa2.ch

Neurol Clin 39 (2021) 147–161
https://doi.org/10.1016/j.ncl.2020.09.008
0733-8619/21/© 2020 Elsevier Inc. All rights reserved.

Table 1
Conditions and medications that have been reported to cause or be associated with increased intracranial pressure

Hematological	Anemia Polycythemia vera
Obstruction to venous drainage	Cerebral venous sinus thrombosis Jugular vein thrombosis Superior vena cava syndrome Jugular vein ligation following bilateral radical Neck dissection Increased right heart pressure Arteriovenous fistulas Previous infection or subarachnoid hemorrhage Causing decreased cerebrospinal fluid absorption
Medications	Fluoroquinolones Tetracycline class antibiotics Corticosteroid withdrawal Danazol Vitamin A derivatives (including isotretinoin and all transretinoic acid) Levothyroxine Nalidixic acid Tamoxifen Ciclosporin Levonorgestrel implant Lithium Growth hormone Indomethacin Cimetidine
Systemic disorders	Chronic kidney disease/renal failure Obstructive sleep apnoea syndrome Chronic obstructive pulmonary disease Systemic lupus erythematosus Psittacosis
Endocrine	Addison disease Adrenal insufficiency Cushing syndrome Hypoparathyroidism Hypothyroidism Hyperthyroidism
Syndromic	Down syndrome Craniosynostosis Turner syndrome

From Mollan SP, Davies B, Silver NC, et al. Idiopathic intracranial hypertension: consensus guidelines on management. J Neuro Neurosurg Psychiatry 2018;89:1088-1100; with permission.

The etiology of IIH remains unclear. In pre-pubertal children, IIH is relatively rare and there is no gender predilection.[5] After puberty, the prevalence of IIH in women is 9 times the prevalence in men, and most affected women are 20 to 50 years old. The preponderance of IIH in women of childbearing age suggests a hormonal influence in the disease pathophysiology, but the exact mechanism has not yet been established.[6–8]

Common symptoms, reported by more than 50% of patients with IIH, include headache, transient visual obscurations, back pain, pulsatile tinnitus, and dizziness. **Fig. 1** shows the frequency of all symptoms reported by 165 patients enrolled in the Idiopathic Intracranial Hypertension Treatment Trial (IIHTT).[9] Headache was the most common symptom (in 84% of patients), but had no defining feature. In 51% of patients, it was a constant head pain and mean pain intensity was 6 out of 10. Approximately 40% of patients had a preexisting history of migraine.[9]

The primary cause of symptoms is increased intracranial pressure (ICP). Although documentation of increased ICP is necessary for confirming the diagnosis, successful management of IIH does not require a lumbar puncture to confirm that there has been reduction in ICP. Clinical measures are considered sufficient to guide management and include the following:

- Preservation of vision
- Resolution of papilledema
- Alleviation of symptoms
- Control of risk factors (weight)
- Management of psychosocial issues

The remainder of this article is focused on the management of IIH in adults. Patients with IIH often struggle to lose weight and can have coexisting psychosocial issues, such as depression. Consequently, a multidisciplinary approach to management is beneficial. Regular surveillance of the patient's ophthalmic status, weight, and psychosocial state is necessary to optimize outcome of therapy; each of these will be discussed in further detail.

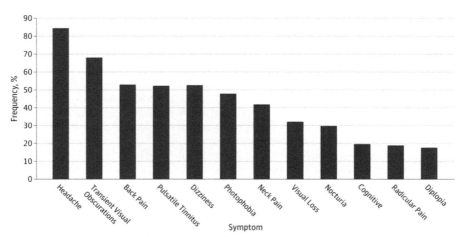

Fig. 1. Bar graph showing the frequency of symptoms in patients with IIH at the time of enrollment into the IIHTT. (*From* Wall M, Kupersmith MJ, Kieburtz KD, et al. The idiopathic intracranial hypertension treatment trial: clinical profile at baseline. JAMA Neurol 2014;71:693-701; with permission.)

ASSESSMENT AND MONITORING OF THE PATIENT WITH IDIOPATHIC INTRACRANIAL HYPERTENSION
Ophthalmologic Surveillance

The major morbidity of IIH is permanent visual loss and, thus, ophthalmic surveillance is crucial for the assessment and monitoring of IIH. At each visit, the following ophthalmic tests are recommended:

- Visual acuity
- Pupil examination
- Color vision testing
- Formal visual field assessment
- Funduscopy

Visual acuity is the most common measure of central vision and is assessed one eye at a time with the patient wearing their glasses. When possible, acuity is tested at distance (20 feet or 6 m) and at near (15.5 inches or 400 mm). Papilledema rarely causes an acute loss of visual acuity, although it can be mildly decreased due to globe flattening, presence of chorioretinal folds, or presence of subretinal fluid caused by the increased ICP.[10] Visual acuity is usually spared unless papilledema is chronically untreated or inadequately treated. In contrast, most patients with IIH have at least mild visual field loss in one or both eyes at presentation.[9,11]

The pupils are evaluated for the presence of a relative afferent pupillary defect. This sign appears if there is optic nerve dysfunction that is asymmetric between the 2 eyes.

Dyschromatopsia is an early sign of optic nerve dysfunction and can be detected by checking color vision with a booklet, such as the Ishihara color plates for evaluating color blindness. This and other standardized color vision tests are available as online tests.

Changes in the visual fields are likely the result of axoplasmic flow stasis leading to intraneuronal ischemia. In addition to an enlarged physiologic blind spot, early visual field changes of papilledema include localized nerve fiber bundle defects, in particular nasal defects and arcuate defects in the inferior and superior hemifield. These early visual field changes are usually not evident to the patient and not detectable with confrontation visual field testing, yet they are important markers to guide therapy. Although visual loss can occur in the periphery of the visual field in patients with IIH, it is current practice to test and monitor the central 24 or 30° of visual field.[11] Automated static threshold perimetry is favored over kinetic perimetry because of its high sensitivity, repeatability, and quantitative analysis of the visual field. **Fig. 2** shows automated static perimetry from patients with IIH who have an enlarged physiologic blind spot, nasal arcuate visual field defects, and severe generalized visual field constriction. One quantitative parameter derived from automated static threshold perimetry is the mean deviation (MD), which is a measure (in dB) of the average deviation of all test locations compared with age-matched controls. In general, a normal visual field will have an MD less than -2 dB. The IIHTT defined mild visual loss as an MD between -2 and -7 dB.[12]

Papilledema is the hallmark sign of increased ICP. It is important to describe the fundus appearance at every visit, paying attention to the following features: degree of disc elevation, opacification of the peripapillary nerve fibers and vessels, disc hyperemia, hemorrhages, venous dilation and tortuosity, and any associated changes in the macula. Papilledema can also be graded from 0 (no papilledema) to 5 (severe papilledema) using the modified Frisén scale.[13] When available, fundus photography is an objective means to document the optic disc appearance. More recently, optical

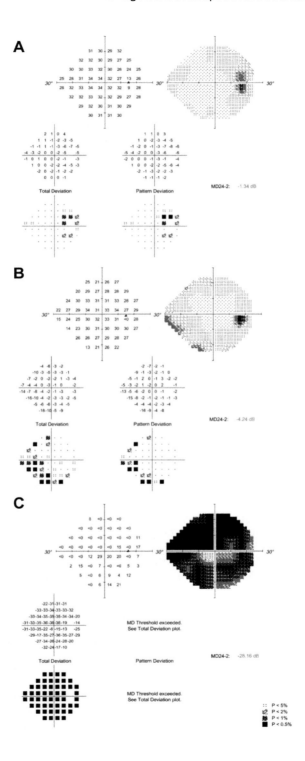

coherence tomography (OCT) parameters, including optic disc volume, peripapillary retinal nerve fiber layer thickness, and macular retinal ganglion cell layer thickness, have been used to monitor papilledema in IIH.[13–15] In addition, OCT can detect other pathology, such as macular subretinal fluid, chorioretinal folds, or peripapillary choroidal neovascularization, which can occasionally develop in patients with IIH.[10,16]

Weight Surveillance

Weight plays an important role in patients with IIH. Approximately 90% of patients with IIH are overweight or obese and weight gain of 5% to 15% can pose a risk for developing IIH.[3] In addition, weight is associated with visual outcome; one study reported a poorer visual prognosis with increasing BMI, particularly if BMI was greater than 40 kg/m^2.[17] Thus, weight surveillance is an integral component of the monitoring of patients with IIH. Ideally, weight should be checked at every visit, although many offices and clinics do not have easily accessible scales. Self-reported weight tends to be an underestimate of the patient's actual weight, but periodic weight measurement can be used for validation.[18]

Psychosocial Surveillance

Patients with IIH have more problems with hearing, fatigue, and sleep compared with overweight and obese persons without IIH.[19] Headache, present in 90% of patients, is often multifactorial and can become refractory to treatment despite normalization of ICP.[20] Neck, back, and shoulder pain, as well as other fibromyalgialike complaints are common.[21] Depression is an important comorbidity and was present in up to 37% of patients in one study.[22] Overall, patients with IIH tend to have more pain, poorer physical function, and less ability to meet daily demands. Independent of obesity, quality of life is decreased in patients with IIH; quality of life is correlated with decreased visual function and severity of pain symptoms.[23] Assessment of any psychosocial issues is tailored to the individual patient; there is no consensus regarding the use of standardized questionnaires to evaluate anxiety, depression, sleep quality, and quality of life in routine practice.

TREATMENT OF THE PATIENT WITH IDIOPATHIC INTRACRANIAL HYPERTENSION
Weight Loss

It is recommended to weigh the patient at the initial consultation and to discuss weight loss goals for overweight patients. As little as 6% to 15% weight loss can be effective to reduce or even to resolve papilledema.[24,25] Although patients are initially motivated to lose weight, in our experience, they often struggle to maintain their weight loss. Weight regain and weight fluctuations are associated with recurrence of the symptoms and signs of IIH.[4]

Weight loss can be attained with either lifestyle changes (eg, exercise, dietary) or bariatric surgery. In general, "lose weight fast" dietary programs are difficult to maintain long-term. We prefer to work with a nutritionist or dietician, who can, for example,

---

Fig. 2. Automated static perimetry (Humphrey 24–2 SITA-standard protocol) results from the right eye in 3 patients with IIH. (*A*) Enlarged physiologic blind spot with MD of −1.34 dB in a patient with mild papilledema. (*B*) Inferonasal arcuate defect and subtle superonasal arcuate defect with MD of −4.24 dB in a patient with moderately severe papilledema. (*C*) Severe generalized (superior more than inferior) visual field constriction with MD of −28.16 dB in a patient with severe papilledema.

set a goal of 1% weight reduction per month until the desired weight is achieved. Thereafter, follow-up consultation with a nutritionist or dietician is recommended to help maintain the desired weight and ensure a balanced dietary intake.

Bariatric surgery is superior to any lifestyle or dietary weight loss program for inducing a greater amount of weight loss and for sustaining significant weight loss. In one study of obese patients, mean weight loss was 17% of baseline weight at 10 years postoperatively.[26] Bariatric surgery is generally safe and complication rates are less than 5%. A meta-analysis of the existing literature examined the outcomes of 65 patients with IIH who had bariatric surgery and 277 who had nonsurgical management.[27] Although the 2 groups had differences in baseline characteristics (the bariatric surgery group had mean baseline BMI of 48.3 kg/m² compared with the nonsurgical group with BMI of 37.7 kg/m²), weight loss, improvement in clinical symptoms, and resolution of papilledema were found to be superior in patients who underwent bariatric surgery.[27] Of note, mean BMI reduction was 17.5 kg/m² for the surgical group compared with 4.2 kg/m² for the nonsurgical group.

Because weight control has a central role in the management of patients with IIH, the upcoming multicenter, open-label, randomized controlled clinical trial comparing bariatric surgery with a dietary weight loss program over 5 years will help to answer unresolved questions, such as when should bariatric surgery be considered; what are the short-term and long-term risks; and how effective is bariatric surgery in the management of IIH.

Medical Therapy

Medical therapy of IIH mostly involves the use of acetazolamide, a carbonic anhydrase inhibitor. The IIHTT reported that acetazolamide plus weight loss was superior to weight loss alone after 6 months for improving visual field loss (MD), papilledema, symptoms, and quality of life.[28,29] Although acetazolamide doses up to 4 g per day were reportedly well-tolerated in the IIHTT, doses of more than 2 g per day are often not needed.

For patients with no or mild visual loss (eg, with MD better than −7 dB), we recommend acetazolamide 500 mg twice daily and a 1% weight reduction in the first month. Patients are informed of common, reversible side effects, including paresthesias in extremities and around the mouth, dysgeusia, nausea, and less commonly diarrhea. Use of acetazolamide should be avoided in pregnant women, especially during the first trimester. Monitoring of serum electrolytes and renal function with acetazolamide use is not usually necessary.[2] After 1 month, if vision is stable or improved, but the papilledema has not changed, the acetazolamide dose should be increased and another 1% weight reduction recommended. Many patients with mild vision loss respond well to acetazolamide doses of 500 to 1000 mg twice a day, especially if concomitant weight reduction can be achieved, and the papilledema usually resolves over 6 months. Once the papilledema has resolved and the vision has stabilized, we decrease the acetazolamide dose by 500 mg per month while continuing to monitor weight. Although some patients experience reduction of their headaches with acetazolamide, headache in patients with IIH is often multifactorial and may persist despite improvement of other parameters.[30] Consequently, headache often needs to be managed separately of visual symptoms and signs; headache prophylactic agents and other nonpharmacologic approaches can be effective.[20]

For patients with moderate visual loss (eg, with MD between −7 and −15 dB) or high-grade papilledema at presentation, the starting dose of acetazolamide is higher at 1000 mg twice a day and should be titrated upward more rapidly. Treatment of these patients has 2 acute objectives: preservation of vision and reduction of papilledema (**Fig. 3**). Weight loss is neither essential nor effective for these acute objectives and, as such, may be deferred until the situation has stabilized. Such patients should be monitored closely. If there is failure to improve or worsening despite maximally tolerated medical therapy, more aggressive (surgical) treatment is required.

Furosemide (in low-moderate dose) can be added to acetazolamide for added diuretic effect. With this combination therapy, regular monitoring of electrolytes and potassium supplementation is required. However, furosemide is not recommended as monotherapy for IIH due to lack of clinical evidence of efficacy.

Topiramate is a weak carbonic anhydrase inhibitor and is commonly used for treating primary headache disorders. It also appears to be effective in treatment of IIH.[31] Thus, topiramate is a reasonable alternative medical treatment for patients who are unable tolerate acetazolamide (eg, due to side effects or an allergic reaction) or when headache is a prominent symptom (**Fig. 4**). The starting dose for topiramate is low at 25 to 50 mg daily and can be titrated up to 100 mg twice daily for improved

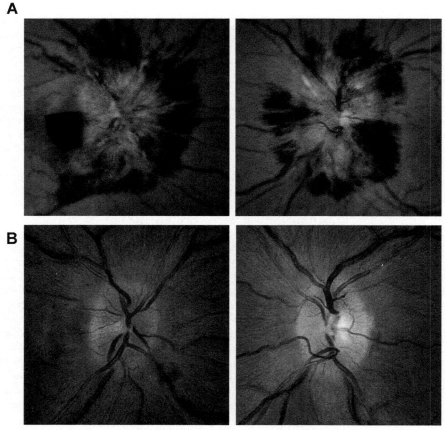

Fig. 3. (*A*) Fundus photographs showing moderately severe papilledema with marked peripapillary hemorrhages in both eyes in a patient with IIH at presentation. (*B*) Fundus photographs showing almost complete resolution of papilledema and peripapillary hemorrhages in both eyes following 6 weeks of high-dose acetazolamide treatment.

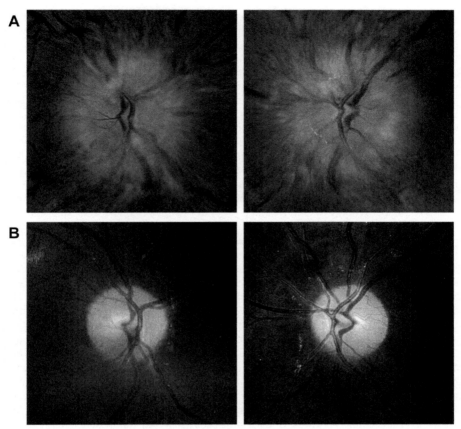

Fig. 4. (*A*) Fundus photographs showing moderately severe papilledema in both eyes in a patient with IIH at presentation. The patient developed an urticarial rash following the first dose of acetazolamide. (*B*) Fundus photographs showing complete resolution of papilledema in both eyes following 4 months of topiramate treatment. Note peripapillary discoloration ("high water" marks) from prior papilledema.

symptom control. Common side effects of topiramate include mental slowing, lethargy, paresthesias, and loss of appetite. Other important, but less common, side effects include renal stones and acute angle-closure glaucoma.

Corticosteroids are not used in the management of patients with IIH. Even its exceptional use in patients who have a fulminant presentation and are awaiting surgical intervention is controversial.[32] In the scenario of a fulminant presentation with rapidly declining vision, a lumbar drain may be offered as a temporizing measure while awaiting surgical intervention.[32] However, repeat lumbar punctures are not recommended for the long-term management of patients with IIH.

Surgical Therapy

Surgical therapy options for patients with IIH include cerebrospinal fluid (CSF) shunting, optic nerve sheath fenestration (ONSF), and cerebral venous sinus stenting.[33] The selection and timing of surgical therapy remains controversial, because there have been no prospective randomized controlled trials evaluating or comparing these therapies. In general, surgical therapy is reserved for patients who fail to improve or worsen despite maximally tolerated medical therapy. In addition, it is often indicated for patients with a fulminant presentation of IIH who have rapidly declining vision or severe vision loss at presentation (eg, with MD worse than −15 dB). Surgical therapy also can be considered in patients with IIH who are unable to tolerate medical therapy, yet have persistent or worsening symptoms, signs, and vision loss. The choice of surgical therapy often depends on local resources and practices. When more than 1 option is available, the severity of symptoms, signs, and visual loss should be considered when deciding between therapies. For example, a patient with vision loss from papilledema who has no other symptoms or signs of increased ICP might be best treated with ONSF, whereas a patient with vision loss from papilledema who has other symptoms of increased ICP (eg, headache, diplopia, and pulsatile tinnitus) might be best treated with CSF shunting or venous sinus stenting.

CSF shunting rapidly reduces the ICP and, therefore, results in a rapid improvement in papilledema. A variety of CSF shunting procedures have been used for treatment of IIH; the most commonly used shunting procedures are lumbo-peritoneal (LP) and ventriculo-peritoneal (VP) shunting, although ventriculo-atrial and ventriculo-jugular shunting are also options when there is a contraindication to peritoneal drainage (eg, in patients with intra-abdominal adhesions). Stereotactic VP shunting is preferred to LP shunting due to its lower failure and complication rate.[34] In addition, an adjustable valve can be incorporated into the VP shunt apparatus so that the CSF flow rate can be adjusted according to the patient's symptoms and signs. Although most case series have reported improvement in symptoms and signs of IIH with shunting, there is a significant complication rate; potential complications include infection, obstruction, and migration of the shunt tubing, as well as intracranial hypotension.[33] Thus, shunt revisions are often required. Given the potential for significant complications and need for shunt revision, CSF shunting is not recommended for management of patients with IIH with mild or moderate vision loss at presentation. It is also not recommended for the management of isolated headache in patients with IIH unless the headache is documented to respond to decreases in ICP (eg, following a lumbar puncture) and nonsurgical management options have been exhausted. Although headache initially improves in most patients with IIH following CSF shunting, almost 50% had recurrent headaches at 36 months following shunting in one study.[35]

ONSF is a surgical therapy to consider when the main issue is vision loss from papilledema.[33] ONSF consists of either fashioning a window or making a series of slits in the retrobulbar optic nerve sheath, thereby creating a fistula between the subarachnoid space and orbital cavity. The decompression of the optic nerve results in improvement of papilledema with stabilization of or improvement in visual function. ICP may also be modestly decreased after ONSF. Consequently, in some patients, unilateral ONSF improves the papilledema and visual function in the contralateral eye.[36] Up to 50% of patients also have postoperative improvement in their headaches.[37] However, the magnitude and duration of any decrease in ICP with ONSF has not been established, and may be influenced by local anatomic factors, such as the density of trabeculations in the retrobulbar subarachnoid space.[38] Consequently, many patients require bilateral sequential ONSF as well as ongoing medical therapy for IIH. Potential complications of ONSF include transient or persistent worsening of visual function (eg, due to optic nerve trauma or central retinal artery occlusion), tonic pupil (eg, from damage to the ciliary ganglion or post-ganglionic parasympathetic fibers), and diplopia.

Imaging of the cerebral venous system often shows smoothly tapered stenoses in the transverse venous sinuses of patients with IIH.[39] It is thought that the stenoses occur because of mechanical compression and collapse of the venous sinuses in the setting of increased ICP.[40] Catheter manometry often shows a pressure gradient across the stenoses, with increased venous pressures in the superior sagittal sinus and transverse venous sinus proximal to the stenoses.[41] It has been proposed that the stenoses might play a role in the pathogenesis of IIH or perhaps exacerbate it, because the increased venous pressures likely impede CSF absorption. Consequently, venous sinus stenting may reduce cerebral venous hypertension resulting in increased CSF absorption, reduced ICP, and, thus, improved symptoms and signs of IIH. Indeed, several retrospective and prospective studies have reported an improvement in symptoms, signs, visual function, and ICP following venous sinus stenting.[42–44] There is no consensus regarding the indications for venous sinus stenting, although it should be considered only in patients who have a pressure gradient of more than 8 mm Hg across the stenosis and increased venous pressures in the venous sinuses proximal to the stenosis (**Fig. 5**). Potential complications of venous sinus stenting include in-stent thrombosis, subdural hemorrhage, and development of recurrent stenosis immediately proximal to the stent.

Psychosocial Therapy

Patients with IIH frequently have coexisting psychosocial problems, including depression, and report a poor quality of life.[22,23] Successful treatment of IIH with weight loss, medical therapies, and surgical therapies can lead to improvement in quality of life due to improvement in symptoms and visual function. However, we encourage a multidisciplinary approach, especially for patients with psychosocial issues; consultation with a psychologist or psychiatrist is recommended. Because headache is often multifactorial and can persist despite normalization of ICP, consultation with a neurologist or chronic pain specialist who has expertise in headache management is recommended for patients with refractory headache.[20]

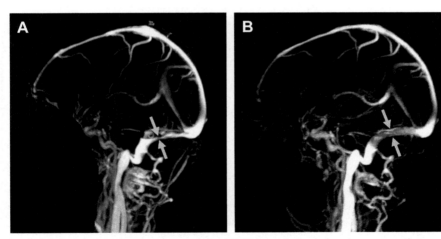

Fig. 5. (*A*) Magnetic resonance venography (MRV, lateral view) showing a smooth-tapered stenosis (*arrows*) in the right transverse sinus of a patient with IIH. There was a pressure gradient (10 mm Hg) across the stenosis and the left transverse sinus was hypoplastic. The patient was unable to tolerate medical therapy and elected to undergo right transverse venous sinus stenting. (*B*) MRV (lateral view) after right transverse venous sinus stenting, showing resolution of the stenosis. The patient's symptoms and signs had resolved 3 months following the procedure.

SUMMARY

The management approach for IIH depends on the severity of visual loss on the basis of automated static perimetry, severity of papilledema, severity of symptoms, response to medical therapy, and ability to tolerate medical therapy. Patients with no visual loss (eg, with MD better than −2 dB) can be managed with weight loss alone, although medical therapy may be needed depending on the severity of symptoms and response to weight loss attempts. Patients with mild vision loss (eg, with MD of −2 to −7 dB) can usually be successfully managed with weight loss plus medical therapy. Patients with moderate vision loss (eg, with MD −7 dB to −15 dB) can often be managed with weight loss plus more aggressive medical therapy, although surgical therapy may be needed depending on the response to weight loss and medical therapy. Patients with severe vision loss (eg, with MD worse than −15 dB) often require aggressive medical therapy and consideration for early surgical therapy (eg, CSF shunting, ONSF, or venous sinus stenting), although the selection and timing of surgical therapy remains controversial.

Patients with IIH require long-term monitoring, because this is a chronic disease that is prone to relapses in association with weight gain. Because the severity of vision loss, papilledema, and symptoms influences treatment decisions, ophthalmic surveillance is crucial; the timing of follow-up is tailored according to the severity of symptoms and signs at presentation, response to treatment, and subsequent clinical course. A multidisciplinary approach is recommended to optimize management of weight loss, refractory headaches, and coexisting psychosocial issues.

CLINICS CARE POINTS

- For patients with no or mild visual loss, we recommend acetazolamide 500 mg twice daily and a 1%weight reduction, if the patient is overweight, with re-examination of the patient in one month.
- For patients with moderate visual loss or high-grade papilledema at presentation, we suggest starting acetazolamide at 1000 mg twice a day with 1% weight loss and re-examination in one month.
- Steady weight reduction by 6-15% over 6 months or more can be effective to reduce or even to resolve papilledema.

DISCLOSURE

Dr M.J. Thurtell has nothing to disclose. Dr A. Kawasaki has nothing to disclose.

REFERENCES

1. Friedman DI, Liu GT, Digre KB. Revised diagnostic criteria for the pseudotumor cerebri syndrome in adults and children. Neurology 2013;81:1159–65.
2. Mollan SP, Davies B, Silver NC, et al. Idiopathic intracranial hypertension: consensus guidelines on management. J Neuro Neurosurg Psychiatry 2018;89:1088–100.
3. Daniels AB, Liu GT, Volpe NJ, et al. Profiles of obesity, weight gain, and quality of life in idiopathic intracranial hypertension (pseudotumor cerebri). Am J Ophthalmol 2007;143:635–41.
4. Ko MW, Chang SC, Ridha MA, et al. Weight gain and recurrence in idiopathic intracranial hypertension: a case-control study. Neurology 2011;76:1564–7.
5. Balcer LJ, Liu GT, Forman S, et al. Idiopathic intracranial hypertension: relation of age and obesity in children. Neurology 1999;52:870–2.

6. Markey KA, Uldall M, Botfield H, et al. Idiopathic intracranial hypertension, hormones, and 11β-hydroxysteroid dehydrogenases. J Pain Res 2016;19:223–32.
7. McGeeney BE, Friedman DI. Pseudotumor cerebri pathophysiology. Headache 2014;54:445–58.
8. Hornby C, Mollan SP, Botfield H, et al. Metabolic concepts in idiopathic intracranial hypertension and their potential for therapeutic intervention. J Neuroophthalmol 2018;38:522–30.
9. Wall M, Kupersmith MJ, Kieburtz KD, et al. The idiopathic intracranial hypertension treatment trial: clinical profile at baseline. JAMA Neurol 2014;71:693–701.
10. Chen JJ, Thurtell MJ, Longmuir RA, et al. Causes and prognosis of visual acuity loss at the time of initial presentation in idiopathic intracranial hypertension. Invest Ophthalmol Vis Sci 2015;56:3850–9.
11. Wall M, Subramani A, Chong LX, et al. Threshold static automated perimetry of the full visual field in idiopathic intracranial hypertension. Invest Ophthalmol Vis Sci 2019;60:1898–905.
12. Keltner JL, Johnson CA, Cello KE, et al. Baseline visual field findings in the Idiopathic Intracranial Hypertension Treatment Trial (IIHTT). Invest Ophthalmol Vis Sci 2014;55:3200–7.
13. Scott CJ, Kardon RH, Lee AG, et al. Diagnosis and grading of papilledema in patients with raised intracranial pressure using optical coherence tomography vs clinical expert assessment using a clinical staging scale. Arch Ophthalmol 2010;128:705–11.
14. Kardon R. Optical coherence tomography in papilledema: what am I missing? J Neuroophthalmol 2014;34:S10–7.
15. Auinger P, Durbin M, Feldon S, et al. Baseline OCT measurements in the idiopathic intracranial hypertension treatment trial, part II: correlations and relationship to clinical features. Invest Ophthalmol Vis Sci 2014;55:8173–9.
16. Sibony PA, Kupersmith MJ, Feldon SE, et al. Retinal and choroidal folds in papilledema. Invest Ophthalmol Vis Sci 2015;56:5670–80.
17. Szewka AJ, Bruce BB, Newman NJ, et al. Idiopathic intracranial hypertension: relation between obesity and visual outcomes. J Neuroophthalmol 2013;33:4–8.
18. Parish DC, Bidot S, Bruce BB, et al. Self-reported weight and height among idiopathic intracranial hypertension patients. J Neuroophthalmol 2019. https://doi.org/10.1097/WNO.0000000000000861.
19. Kleinschmidt JJ, Digre KB, Hanover R. Idiopathic intracranial hypertension: relationship to depression, anxiety, and quality of life. Neurology 2000;54:319–24.
20. Friedman DI. Headaches in idiopathic intracranial hypertension. J Neuroophthalmol 2019;39:82–93.
21. Hulens M, Rasschaert R, Vansant G, et al. The link between idiopathic intracranial hypertension, fibromyalgia, and chronic fatigue syndrome: exploration of a shared pathophysiology. J Pain Res 2018;11:3129–40.
22. Puustinen T, Tervonen J, Avellan C, et al. Psychiatric disorders are a common prognostic marker for worse outcome in patients with idiopathic intracranial hypertension. Clin Neurol Neurosurg 2019;186:105527.
23. Digre KB, Bruce BB, McDermott MP, et al. Quality of life in idiopathic intracranial hypertension at diagnosis: IIH treatment trial results. Neurology 2015;84:2449–56.
24. Subramaniam S, Fletcher WA. Obesity and weight loss in idiopathic intracranial hypertension. J Neuroophthalmol 2017;37:197–205.

25. Sinclair AJ, Burdon MA, Nightingale PG, et al. Low energy diet and intracranial pressure in women with idiopathic intracranial hypertension: prospective cohort study. BMJ 2010;341:c2701.

26. Sjöström L. Review of the key results from the Swedish Obese Subjects (SOS) trial - a prospective controlled intervention study of bariatric surgery. J Intern Med 2013;273:219–34.

27. Manfield JH, Yu KK, Efthimiou E, et al. Bariatric surgery or non-surgical weight loss for idiopathic intracranial hypertension? A systematic review and comparison of meta-analyses. Obes Surg 2017;27:513–21.

28. Wall M, McDermott MP, Kieburtz KD, et al. Effect of acetazolamide on visual function in patients with idiopathic intracranial hypertension and mild visual loss: the idiopathic intracranial hypertension treatment trial. JAMA 2014;311: 1641–51.

29. Bruce BB, Digre KB, McDermott MP, et al. Quality of life at 6 months in the idiopathic intracranial hypertension treatment trial. Neurology 2016;87:1871–7.

30. Friedman DI, Quiros PA, Subramanian PS, et al. Headache in idiopathic intracranial hypertension: findings from the idiopathic intracranial hypertension treatment trial. Headache 2017;57:1195–205.

31. Celebisoy N, Gokcay F, Sirin H, et al. Treatment of idiopathic intracranial hypertension: topiramate vs acetazolamide, an oper-label study. Acta Neurol Scand 2007;116:322–7.

32. Thambisetty M, Lavin PJ, Newman NJ, et al. Fulminant idiopathic intracranial hypertension. Neurology 2007;68:229–32.

33. Kalyvas AV, Hughes M, Koutsarnakis C, et al. Efficacy, complications and cost of surgical interventions for idiopathic intracranial hypertension: a systematic review of the literature. Acta Neurochir (Wien) 2017;159:33–49.

34. Menger RP, Connor DE Jr, Thakur JD, et al. A comparison of lumboperitoneal and ventriculoperitoneal shunting for idiopathic intracranial hypertension: an analysis of economic impact and complications using the Nationwide Inpatient Sample. Neurosurg Focus 2014;37:E4.

35. McGirt MJ, Woodworth G, Thomas G, et al. Cerebrospinal fluid shunt placement for pseudotumor cerebri-associated intractable headache: predictors of treatment response and an analysis of long-term outcomes. J Neurosurg 2004;101: 627–32.

36. Keltner JL, Albert DM, Lubow M, et al. Optic nerve decompression. A clinical pathologic study. Arch Ophthalmol 1977;95:97–104.

37. Corbett JJ, Nerad JA, Tse DT, et al. Results of optic nerve sheath fenestration for pseudotumor cerebri. The lateral orbitotomy approach. Arch Ophthalmol 1988; 106:1391–7.

38. Killer HE, Jaggi GP, Flammer J, et al. Cerebrospinal fluid dynamics between the intracranial and the subarachnoid space of the optic nerve. Is it always bidirectional? Brain 2007;130:514–20.

39. Farb RI, Vanek I, Scott JN, et al. Idiopathic intracranial hypertension: the prevalence and morphology of sinovenous stenosis. Neurology 2003;60: 1418–24.

40. King JO, Mitchell PJ, Thomson KR, et al. Manometry combined with cervical puncture in idiopathic intracranial hypertension. Neurology 2002;58:26–30.

41. King JO, Mitchell PJ, Thomson KR, et al. Cerebral venography and manometry in idiopathic intracranial hypertension. Neurology 1995;45:2224–8.

42. Ahmed RM, Wilkinson M, Parker GD, et al. Transverse sinus stenting for idiopathic intracranial hypertension: a review of 52 patients and of model predictions. Am J Neuroradiol 2011;32:1408–14.
43. Dinkin MJ, Patsalides A. Venous sinus stenting in idiopathic intracranial hypertension: results of a prospective trial. J Neuroophthalmol 2017;37:113–21.
44. Patsalides A, Oliveira C, Wilcox J, et al. Venous sinus stenting lowers the intracranial pressure in patients with idiopathic intracranial hypertension. J Neurointerv Surg 2018;11:175–8.

What is New in Neuro-oncology?

Jigisha P. Thakkar, MD[a],*, Vikram C. Prabhu, MD[b], Katherine B. Peters, MD, PhD[c], Rimas V. Lukas, MD[d,e]

KEYWORDS

- Neuro-oncology update • Immune therapy • Targeted therapy
- Brain tumor classification

KEY POINTS

- Discuss update on brain tumor classification.
- Discuss updates in molecular neuro-oncology.
- Discuss update on management of primary brain tumors and future directions.

INTRODUCTION

Neuro-oncology, the study of primary and secondary cancers of the nervous system, is advancing forward because of an improved understanding of the basic mechanisms of carcinogenesis and development of targeted therapies. Because the scope of the subspecialty is broad, the authors narrow the focus of this review on primary central nervous system (CNS) tumors. Because the number of parallel investigations is enormous, the discussion is limited to certain key themes.

UPDATE ON BRAIN TUMOR CLASSIFICATION

Before the updated 2016 World Health Organization classification of brain tumors, microscopic histopathology evaluation defined how brain tumors were classified. This system changed in 2016 with the incorporation of molecular characterization leading to a layered diagnostic approach with each component (histology, molecular pathology) being complementary to the other.[1] In this molecular era there is now a

[a] Department of Neurology, Division of Neuro-oncology, Loyola University Chicago, Stritch School of Medicine, 2160 South 1st Avenue, Building 105, Room 2716, Maywood, IL 60153, USA; [b] Department of Neurological Surgery, Duke University School of Medicine, 40 Duke Medicine Circle, Durham, NC 27711, USA; [c] Department of Neurology, Duke University School of Medicine, 40 Duke Medicine Circle, Durham, NC 27711, USA; [d] Department of Neurology, Northwestern University, 303 East Chicago Avenue, Chicago, IL 60611, USA; [e] Lou & Jean Malnati Brain Tumor Institute of the Robert H. Lurie Comprehensive Cancer Center
* Corresponding author.
E-mail address: jigisha.thakkar@lumc.edu

Neurol Clin 39 (2021) 163–179
https://doi.org/10.1016/j.ncl.2020.09.009
0733-8619/21/© 2020 Elsevier Inc. All rights reserved.

restructured classification of several CNS tumors. One aspect of the restructuring that has had substantial clinical and research impact is the categorization of infiltrating gliomas. For example, descriptions are now used as glioblastoma (GBM) lacking isocitrate dehydrogenase (IDH) mutation (GBM IDH wild-type), infiltrating astrocytomas (grade 2–4) harboring IDH mutations, oligodendrogliomas (defined by IDH mutation and 1p19q co-deletion), infiltrating astrocytomas with histone mutations (most frequently H3 K27M), and other infiltrating glial neoplasms. Specific highlights are detailed in **Table 1**. It is anticipated that as the understanding broadens the classification system will continue to develop.

These advances are being actively codified within the context of the Consortium to Inform Molecular and Practical Approaches to CNS Tumor Taxonomy (cIMPACT-NOW) series of manuscripts (see **Table 1**).

UPDATE ON DIAGNOSTICS

In light of the advances detailed earlier, molecular testing has become essential for the optimal workup of CNS tumors.[9] Application of molecular analysis including next-generation sequencing (NGS) in combination with copy number array analyses and even whole genome methylation profiling has become more widely used. However, substantial variability across institutions remains regarding the utilization of molecular neuropathology. Because of benefit and drawbacks of specific techniques and their respective platforms for conducting tumor tissue interrogation there is not a standardized approach established. There is, however, consensus in the neuro-oncology community that molecular neuropathology has clinical value for diagnosis, prognostication, and guidance of therapeutic management (**Table 2**).[10,11]

UPDATE ON BRAIN TUMOR THERAPEUTICS

Several therapeutic strategies are being investigated in CNS tumors. The clinical trial designs used are tailored to the specific questions asked. Patient populations being studied can be broadly classified into 2 groups: those that are defined by their histological-molecular classification and those that are defined purely by their molecular characteristics. Traditional neuro-oncologic clinical trial design relied on histologic classification. The contemporary layered classification system has allowed for a narrowing of the study population leading to more homogeneity among subjects' tumors. As an example, moving from evaluating a therapeutic modality in high-grade gliomas to glioblastoma *IDH wild-type* or infiltrating astrocytoma *IDH* mutated. This approach is being used across a range of study types from early phase to late-phase trials. The other approach occurring in parallel is the inclusion of subjects based solely on a specific molecular characteristic, agnostic to tissue histology. Such basket trials allow for the evaluation of promising targets. They have led to tissue agnostic regulatory approval of therapeutic agents for patients with tumors harboring neurotrophic tropomyosin receptor kinase (*NTRK*) fusions, as an example.

Recent advances can be broadly grouped into thematic categories. In this article the authors discuss refinement of existing efficacious therapeutic modalities, targeted therapeutics (both for narrow molecularly defined subpopulations and more broad indications), immunotherapeutic approaches, oncolytic viral therapies, and other novel approaches.

Refinement of Existing Therapeutic Approaches: What is Old is New

For patients with malignant gliomas there have been multiple clinical trials aiming to refine existing therapeutic approaches to help reduce treatment toxicities and improve

Table 1 **Consortium to inform molecular and practical approaches to CNS tumor taxonomy series**	
Update 1[2]	Clarified NOS and NEC entities: *NOS*: necessary diagnostic information (histologic or molecular) to assign a specific WHO diagnosis is not available. *NEC*: available diagnostic information (typically molecular) is not yet sufficient for making a specific WHO diagnosis. NEC diagnoses must be accompanied by full histologic and molecular data in the report.
Update 2[3]	Clarified diagnostic criteria for the following entities: Diffuse midline glioma: H3K27M-mutant This term should be reserved for tumors that are diffuse (ie, infiltrating). Midline (eg, thalamus, brain stem, spinal cord, etc.) gliomas and H3K27M mutant; should not be applied to other tumors that are H3 K27M mutant. *Diffuse astrocytic tumors that are WHO grade II or grade III with IDH mutation.* There is no need for 1p19q testing for diffuse astrocytoma, IDH-mutant, or anaplastic astrocytoma(respectively) if there is definite loss of ATRX nuclear expression and/or strong, diffuse p53 immunopositivity. 1p19q testing should be reserved for only oligodendrogliomas and mixed oligodendroglioma–astrocytoma.
Update 3[4]	Clarified diagnosis of IDH-wt diffuse astrocytic gliomas WHO grade II or III: Presence of EGFR amplification, +7/−10, or TERT promoter mutation in these tumors is associated with significantly shorter patient survival compared with patients with other WHO grade II or III gliomas, and patients have outcomes similar to patients with IDH-wt glioblastoma. This entity is now called diffuse astrocytic glioma, IDH-wt with molecular features of glioblastoma, WHO grade IV. Subsets of IDH-wt diffuse astrocytic gliomas associated with better clinical outcomes include gliomas with MYB/MYBL or BRAF alterations as individual drivers. IDH-wt diffuse gliomas that occur predominantly in childhood and adolescence: H3 K27M mutant diffuse midline glioma with aggressive clinical behavior corresponding to WHO grade IV. H3 G34 mutant with high-grade biology with only modestly longer survivals than other IDH-wt glioblastomas.
Update 4[5]	Clarified approach to the diagnosis of pediatric diffuse gliomas IDH-wt/H3-wt. Recommend integration of diagnosis to combine their histologic and genetic features. • Diffuse glioma, MYB-altered • Diffuse glioma, MYBL1-altered • Diffuse glioma, FGFR1 TKD-duplicated • Diffuse glioma, FGFR1-mutant • Diffuse glioma, BRAF V600E mutant • Diffuse glioma, other MAPK pathway alteration WHO grade II diffuse gliomas from children and adolescents IDH-wt/H3-wt with a mutation in either BRAFV600E, FGFR alteration, or an MYB or MYBL1 rearrangement describe an indolent clinical behavior and rare anaplastic progression. Diffuse glioma and other MAPK pathway alterations could be used for those rare tumors in which another genetic alteration (mutations of KRAS and fusions of FGFR2 or BRAF) capable of activating the MAPK pathway is detected.

(continued on next page)

Table 1 (continued)	

Update 5[6]	Risk stratification of IDH-mutant diffuse astrocytoma based on histologic features and molecular markers.
	Grading criteria for IDH-mutant astrocytomas:
	Astrocytoma, IDH-mutant, grade 2
	    A diffusely infiltrative astrocytic glioma with an IDH1 or IDH2 mutation that is well differentiated and lacks histologic features of anaplasia. Mitotic activity is not detected or low. Microvascular proliferation, necrosis, and CDKN2A/B homozygous deletions are absent.
	Astrocytoma, IDH-mutant, grade 3
	    A diffusely infiltrative astrocytic glioma with an IDH1 or IDH2 mutation that exhibits focal or dispersed anaplasia and displays significant mitotic activity. Microvascular proliferation, necrosis, and CDKN2A/B homozygous deletions are absent.
	Astrocytoma, IDH-mutant, grade 4
	    A diffusely infiltrative astrocytic glioma with an IDH1 or IDH2 mutation that exhibits microvascular proliferation or necrosis or CDKN2A/B homozygous deletion or any combination of these features.
	CDKN2A/B is associated with shorter survival in patients with IDH-mutant astrocytomas, and its presence corresponds to WHO grade IV clinical behavior.
	Other markers associated with poor prognosis that need further validation include CDK4 amplification, RB1 mutation/homozygous deletion, PDGFRA amplification, mutations in PIK3R1 and PIK3CA, amplifications in MYCN, and G-CIMP-low DNA methylation pattern.

Update 6[7]	Arabic numeral grades were assigned
	Cataloged newly recognized or changed types/subtypes/criteria/families
	• Diagnostic criteria for glioblastoma, IDH-wt, WHO grade 4
	    Microvascular proliferation or necrosis or 1 (or more) of the 3 genetic alterations (TERT promoter mutation, EGFR gene amplification, +7/−10 chromosome copy number changes).
	    Simplified nomenclature by eliminating the term "diffuse astrocytic glioma, IDH-wt, with molecular features of glioblastoma, WHO grade IV".
	• Diffuse glioma, H3.3 G34 mutant will be included in future classification as diffuse glial tumor, WHO grade IV, novel tumor type distinct from the established types of IDH-mutant and IDH-wt gliomas, as well as from the H3 K27M-mutant diffuse midline gliomas.
	    Overall survival with standard of care is slightly longer compared with patients with glioblastoma, IDH-wt, but considerably shorter compared with patients with WHO grade IV IDH-mutant astrocytomas.
	• Astroblastoma, MN1-altered should be classified as "other gliomas."
	• Astroblastomas with lack of MN1 alterations should be classified as "Astroblastoma, NEC."
	• Neuronal and mixed neuronal-glial tumors should include the following entities:
	    Diffuse leptomeningeal glioneuronal tumor (DLGNT)
	    Myxoid glioneuronal tumor
	    Polymorphous low-grade neuroepithelial tumor of the young (PLNTY)
	    Multinodular and vacuolating neuronal tumor
	• CNS neuroblastoma, FOXR2-activated should be classified as embryonal tumor
	• CNS neuroblastomas with MYC amplification could be designated as CNS neuroblastoma, NEC
	• CIC sarcoma should be classified under tumors of Soft Tissue and Bone

(continued on next page)

Table 1 (*continued*)	
Update 7[8]	Updated classification of ependymoma based on anatomic site and genetic and epigenetic alterations found in these tumors. Meaningful data related to the outcome of patients on clinical trials are not yet available for a WHO grade to be assigned to types of ependymoma defined by molecular alterations. Supratentorial ependymoma C11orf95-RELA fusion-positive (grade 2–3) YAP1-MAMLD1 fusion-positive Posterior fossa ependymoma (2 subgroups distinguished by histone H3 K27 trimethylation) Group PF-A (seen in children) Group PF-B (seen in adults) Spinal ependymoma Subependymoma grade 1 Myxopapillary ependymoma grade 2 Classic spinal ependymoma grade 2/3 (elimination of morphologic subsets due to lack of clinical utility) Spinal ependymoma MYCN-amplified (aggressive)

Abbreviations: ATRX, alpha thalassemia/mental retardation syndrome X-linked; CDK, cyclin-dependent kinase inhibitor; EGFR, epidermal growth factor receptor; *FGFR*, fibroblast growth factor receptors; G-CIMP, cytosine-phosphate-guanine (CpG) island methylator phenotype; IDH, isocitrate dehydrogenase enzyme; *MAPK*, mitogen-activated protein kinase; NEC, not elsewhere classified; NOS, not otherwise specified; PA posterior fossa; PDGFRA, platelet derived growth factor receptor alpha; TERT, *telomerase reverse transcriptase*; WHO, World Health Organization; wt, wild type.

survival. The larger trials discussed later were designed and initiated before the widespread incorporation of the molecular characterization previously discussed. In turn, unplanned subgroup analyses are being conducted. The interpretability of these analyses is limited, as the trials were not powered to answer questions for these molecularly defined subgroups definitively.

Anaplastic astrocytoma

The phase III CATNON trial (EORTC [European Organization for Research and Treatment of Cancer] 26053/22054; NCT00626990) is evaluating optimal treatment of grade 3 astrocytoma. Interim analysis of the trial reported superiority in overall survival (OS) with 12 months adjuvant temozolomide compared with radiotherapy alone.[16] Molecular analysis of the study revealed benefit of using concurrent temozolomide only in *IDH* mutant tumors.[17] This finding is at odds with the results of the pivotal EORTC/NCIC (National Cancer Institute of Canada Clinical Trials Group) phase III trial for newly diagnosed GBM, which demonstrated improved survival with the addition of temozolomide (TMZ) to a population that was presumably IDH wild-type.[18]

Glioblastoma

TMZ has been a part of standard-of-care therapy for GBM since 2005.[18] Despite the standard of care being 6 adjuvant cycles, the practice of prescribing 12 cycles is common and used in many clinical trials, including key phase III studies such as RTOG 0525.[19] A meta-analysis revealed no additional survival benefit of more than 6 cycles of TMZ.[20] However, a progression-free survival benefit was noted. This must be weighed against an increased toxicity in patients receiving more than 6 cycles as well as a decreased benefit from salvage treatment.[20] Combination of TMZ with

Table 2
Overview of important molecular alterations in glioma and their significance

IDH mutation	Prognostic value, potential therapeutic target
MGMT methylation status	Prognostic value, predictive value for response to temozolomide
EGFR amplification	Diagnostic maker for glioblastoma, potential therapeutic target
TERT promoter mutation	Diagnostic maker for glioblastoma, seen in oligodendroglioma
Gain for 7p and loss of 10q	Diagnostic maker for glioblastoma
ATRX loss	Diagnostic maker for low-grade astrocytoma
TP53 mutation	Diagnostic maker for low-grade astrocytoma
CDKN2A/B homozygous deletion	Poor prognostc marker in IDH mutant glioma
CDK4	Poor prognostic marker in glioma
MYCN	Poor prognostic marker in glioma
PDGFRA	Poor prognostic marker in glioma
PIK3CA and PIK3R1	Poor prognostic marker in glioma
BRAF fusion	Diagnostic marker for pilocytic astrocytoma, therapeutic target
BRAF V600E mutations	Diagnostic marker for pleomorphic xanthoastrocytomas, pilocytic astrocytoma and gangliogliomas, therapeutic target
1p/19q codeletion	Diagnostic marker for oligodendroglioma
H3F3A	Diagnostic marker for a subset of gliomas (H3 K27M-mutant and H3 G34 mutant), therapeutic target
FGFR fusions	Therapeutic target
NTRK fusions	Therapeutic target
Tumor mutational burden	Therapeutic implication for immune therapy, predictive marker for response to oncolytic virus therapy, prognostic factor for patients with IDH-mutant glioma

Abbreviations: ATRX, alpha thalassemia/mental retardation syndrome X-linked; CDK, cyclin-dependent kinase inhibitor; EGFR, epidermal growth factor receptor; *FGFR*, fibroblast growth factor receptors; IDH, isocitrate dehydrogenase enzyme; *MAPK*, mitogen-activated protein kinase; MGMT, O^6-methylguanine-DNA methyltransferase; NTRK, neurotrophic tropomyosin receptor kinase; PDGFRA, platelet derived growth factor receptor alpha; TERT, *telomerase reverse transcriptase.*
Data from Refs.[6,10,12–15]

radiation and CCNU for newly diagnosed MGMT promoter-methylated GBM demonstrated encouraging results in the moderately sized randomized phase III CeTeG/NOA-09 trial.[21,22] There are plans to further investigate this within the context of another cooperative group trial.

Tumor-treating fields (TTFields) are another approved treatment of newly diagnosed and recurrent GBM.[23–25] It is an antimitotic treatment that delivers low-intensity alternating electric fields to the tumor via a wearable scalp device. Although in standard practice it is initiated approximately 1 month after the completion of radiation, there is interest to move up the initiation of TTFields during radiation therapy (RT) and in the post-RT period where patients are not receiving any treatment before initiating adjuvant TMZ. Phase I results have been presented, and plans are moving forward for a larger multicenter trial (EF-32 trial).

Standard of care RT for GBM consists of 60 Gy via 3-dimensional conformal RT over 6 weeks.[18] Use of more directive radiation therapies, in particular dose-escalated photon intensity-modulated RT (IMRT) or proton beam technology, is now being explored. In the NRG cooperative randomized phase II clinical trial, researchers will compare standard of care RT with dose-escalated photon IMRT or photon beam RT in patients with newly diagnosed GBM (NCT02179086). Accrual is currently active for this study.

Targeted Therapies

The therapeutic success of targeting specific molecular pathway aberrancies in a variety of non-CNS cancers has stimulated similar interest for CNS tumors. Thus far, under most circumstances, this approach has been unsuccessful. This approach is broadly divided into targeting a single pathway versus targeting multiple (possibly complimentary) pathways.

One area of particular interest is the large population of infiltrating gliomas (both astrocytomas and oligodendrogliomas) harboring *IDH* mutations. Success in this realm has the potential to positively affect a wide swath of patients, many of them younger than the typical neuro-oncology patient population. One approach to targeting IDH is via small molecule inhibitors. Vorasidenib (VOR; AG-881), an oral, potent, reversible, brain-penetrant pan inhibitor of mutant IDH1/2 enzymes in a phase I perioperative trial demonstrated decrease in 2-hydroxyglutarate levels on advanced imaging studies and in resected tumor samples.[26,27] This drug is currently being investigated in a phase III trial in subjects with residual or recurrent grade 2 glioma (oligodendroglioma or astrocytoma) with an IDH1 or IDH2 mutation (NCT04164901). Similar small compounds are being studied, which include olutasidenib, an oral brain penetrant IDH1 inhibitor, in a phase Ib/II study of relapsed IDH1 mutant gliomas.[28]

BRAF–MAPK (mitogen-activated protein kinase) pathway is mutated in select glial tumors and offers potential as a therapeutic target. Targeting of the V600E BRAF mutation has proved successful in melanoma with CNS responses observed.[29–31] Several glioma subtypes harbor *BRAF* V600E mutations and include pleomorphic xanthoastrocytomas (PXA), pilocytic astrocytomas, and gangliogliomas.[32] Successful use of BRAF inhibitors in patients with BRAFV600E-mutant gliomas has been demonstrated.[33,34] The VE-BASKET phase I trial is the largest published study of this approach in glial tumors.[35] In this study efficacy was shown to vary with histology with genetically more complex tumors demonstrating less robust responses. PXA often demonstrated marked responses while glioblastoma most often demonstrating stable disease when efficacious. In clinical practice, the combination of a BRAF inhibitor with an MEK inhibitor,[36] mimicking what is typically used in melanoma, is often used in glial tumors as well, although this approach has not been consistently successful.[37,38]

Activating fusions are known cancer drivers and are actionable therapeutic mutations. Two, which are highlighted later, are fusions involving fibroblast growth factors receptor (FGFR) and NTRK. FGFR aberrations are implicated in tumor development and progression. Fusions between *FGFR* and *TACC* (transforming acidic coiled-coil containing proteins) genes are oncogenic in GBM. These fusions occur in only about 3% of patients with GBM[39,40] and are a potential therapeutic target (NCT04439240, NCT01948297).

NTRK fusion alterations also have oncogenic potential. These occur in pediatric gliomas and adult GBMs. Targeting NTRK with entrectinib or larotrectinib has demonstrated marked radiographic responses in CNS tumors.[41–43] A current phase I/II trial is evaluating repotrectinib in pediatric and young adult subjects harboring ALK, ROS1, or NTRK1-3 alterations (NCT04094610).

Because targeted therapies have proved effective for treating some brain metastases, there is considerable interest in further refining this approach. Because brain metastases demonstrate branched evolution differentiating their genetic profile from their original primary tumor,[44] there is potential benefit in interrogating the molecular characterization of the brain metastasis when embarking on a targeted therapy approach. NGS may help tailor treatment of each mutation. An ongoing phase II trial cooperative group trial, Alliance A071701 (NCT03994796), for brain metastases from solid tumors is analyzing targeted therapies for genes found to be altered or mutated in the brain metastases (NTRK, ROS1, CDK, or PI3K targeted by abemaciclib, GDC-0084, and entrectinib).

Other Therapeutics

Another approach is to target pathways essential to tumor cells survival. A more broad ranging approach entails targeting a range of pathways frequently aberrant in tumors, including gliomas.

Proteasome inhibition with marizomib sensitizes glioma cells to TMZ and RT, providing a novel therapeutic strategy for GBM.[45] It is currently undergoing a phase III evaluation in newly diagnosed GBM (NCT03345095).

Regorafenib is a pan-tyrosine kinase inhibitor. It is an oral agent that targets angiogenic, stromal (VEGFR1/3, platelet-derived growth factor receptor-β and fibroblast growth factor receptor 1) and oncogenic (KIT, RET, and B-RAF) receptor tyrosine kinases.[46] The phase II REGOMA trial in recurrent GBM demonstrated improved survival when compared with lomustine.[47] GBM Adaptive, Global, Innovative Learning Environment (AGILE) is an international, seamless phase II/III response adaptive randomization platform trial designed to evaluate multiple therapies in newly diagnosed and recurrent GBM. Goal is to identify effective therapies for glioblastoma and match effective therapies with patient subtypes. Protocol allows multiple drugs and drug combinations to be evaluated simultaneously with addition of new experimental therapies and remove therapies as they complete their evaluation (NCT03970447). Regorafenib is undergoing further investigation currently in the debut arm for the ongoing GBM AGILE trial. A post hoc analysis suggests that a specific gene transcript and miRNA pattern may be predictive of benefit from regorafenib,[48] which requires further validation.

Immune Therapies

Immunotherapeutic approaches have revolutionized the treatment of many cancers. Immune therapies being investigated in patients with malignant gliomas include vaccine therapies, immune checkpoint inhibitors (ICI), modulators of immunosuppression, chimeric antigen receptor (CAR) T cells, and gene therapy based approaches.

Vaccines

Vaccine therapies are designed to induce immune response against tumor. Tumor antigen vaccines target specific tumor antigens (eg, EGFRvIII, survivin). Conjugated EGFRvIII-specific peptide failed to show improvement in survival in a phase III study.[49,50] One interesting vaccine-based approach generating interest combines a multivalent vaccine with a DNA plasmid for expression of the proinflammatory cytokine IL-12 and the programmed cell death protein 1 (PD-1) antibody cemiplimab. Preliminary results have demonstrated favorable OS in recurrent GBM.[51]

Patient-derived vaccines require a minimum volume of resectable tumor to generate a vaccine. This has been most extensively investigated in studies of DC-Vax-L and HSPPC-96 vaccines. DC-Vax-L uses whole tumor lysate to generate a personalized vaccine that activates patient's dendritic cells (antigen presenting cells) by exposure to tumor lysate. Phase III study of DC-Vax-L in newly diagnosed GBM resulted in a mOS of 23.1 months for all participants (90% of whom received the DC-Vax-L treatment due to crossover design). Mature study results are awaited. HSPPC-96 (Prophage) demonstrated improved survival in patients with low PD-1 expression in a phase II study.[52] However, the randomized phase II cooperative group trial was unable to demonstrate superiority to bevacizumab.[53] It is currently being studied in combination with check point blockade (NCT03018288).

Immune checkpoint inhibitors

ICI block inhibitory signals for T cells allowing the adaptive immune system to target tumor cells without being converted to an exhausted phenotype. This class of drugs includes antibodies that target PD-1 (nivolumab, pembrolizumab, cemiplimab), programmed death ligand 1 (atezolizumab, avelumab, durvalumab), or cytotoxic T-lymphocyte–associated protein 4 (ipilimumab). They are approved for a variety of cancers, including melanoma, lung cancer, renal cancer, bladder cancer, and lymphomas. Their potential role in treatment of primary brain tumors is undergoing investigation.[54,55] Glioblastomas are resistant to immune therapies due to a frequently low tumor mutational burden (TMB) and a highly immunosuppressive microenvironment. Responses to checkpoint inhibition have been reported in a small population of malignant gliomas with germline mutations, DNA mismatch repair deficiencies, high microsatellite instability, and high de-novo tumor mutational burden.[56,57] It has recently been demonstrated that the chemotherapy-induced tumoral hypermutation in gliomas may not be responsive to PD-1 blockade.[56]

Although the large phase III trials in recurrent GBM and newly diagnosed GBM did not achieve their primary endpoints,[58,59] glimmers of hope remain for checkpoint inhibition in gliomas. One observation was the lack of efficacy in patients treated with steroids with trends toward better outcomes when patients were off steroids.[60] The area of ICIs is moving forward combinatorial approaches with other immunotherapies (including vaccines as mentioned above), cytotoxic chemotherapies, antiangiogenics, and oncolytic viruses. Other immune checkpoints including lymphocyte activation gene 3, T-cell immunoglobulin mucin 3, and glucocorticoid-induced tumor necrosis factor receptor are often upregulated in GBM and are under active investigation in this disease.[56]

Modulators of immunosuppression

Several approaches have been investigated to help modulate the tumor microenvironment with a goal of making it less immunosuppressive. Targeting of indoleamine 2, 3-dioxygenase 1 (IDO; IDO1; INDO) is one such approach. IDO is a rate-limiting enzyme that metabolizes the essential amino acid, tryptophan, into downstream kynurenines. IDO inhibits immune cell effector functions and/or facilitates T-cell death by accumulation of kynurenine. IDO also suppresses immunity through nonenzymic effects. Preclinical work combining radiation with anti-PD1 mAb and IDO inhibition showed durable survival benefit.[61] This combination is currently being evaluated in a phase I study (NCT04047706). IDO inhibitor monotherapy has demonstrated favorable control of disease in recurrent GBM within the context of a phase I trial.[62]

Table 3
Viral therapy–based approaches for glioma

Disease	Trial	ClinicalTrials.gov Identifier
Oncolytic Viruses		
Recurrent	Phase I trial of carcinoembryonic antigen-expressing measles virus (MV-CEA) in patients with recurrent GBM	NCT00390299
Recurrent	Phase II study of M032 (NSC 733972), a genetically engineered HSV-1 expressing IL-12, in patients with recurrent/progressive GBM, anaplastic astrocytoma, or gliosarcoma	NCT02062827
Recurrent	Phase I trial of IRS-1 HSV C134 administered intratumorally in patients with recurrent malignant glioma	NCT03657576
Recurrent	Phase Ib, randomized, multicenter, open-label study of a conditionally replicative adenovirus (DNX-2401) and interferon gamma (IFN-γ) for recurrent GBM or gliosarcoma (TARGET-I)	NCT02197169
Recurrent	Phase I study of intratumoral/peritumoral HSV-1 mutant HSV1716 in patients with refractory or recurrent HGG	NCT02031965
Recurrent	Phase I clinical trial of allogeneic bone marrow human mesenchymal stem cells loaded with a tumor selective oncolytic adenovirus, DNX-2401, administered via intraarterial injection in patients with recurrent HGG	NCT03896568
Recurrent	Phase I dose-finding and safety study of an oncolytic polio/rhinovirus recombinant against recurrent WHO grade IV malignant glioma	NCT01491893
Recurrent	Phase Ib study of oncolytic polio/rhinovirus recombinant against recurrent malignant glioma in children	NCT03043391
Newly diagnosed	Phase I neural stem cell oncolytic adenoviral virotherapy of newly diagnosed malignant glioma	NCT03072134
Recurrent	Phase, multicenter, open-label study of a conditionally replicative adenovirus (DNX-2401) with pembrolizumab for recurrent glioblastoma or gliosarcoma	NCT02798406
Viral Vector Gene therapies		
Recurrent	Phase I protocol ATI001-102 expansion substudy: evaluation of Ad-RTS-hIL-12 + veledimex in subjects with recurrent or progressive glioblastoma	NCT03679754
Recurrent	Phase I protocol ATI001-102 substudy: evaluation of Ad-RTS-hIL-12 + veledimex in combination with nivolumab in subjects with recurrent or progressive glioblastoma	NCT03636477
Recurrent	Phase I study of Ad-RTS-hIL-12, an inducible adenoviral vector engineered to express hIL-12 in the presence of the activator ligand veledimex in subjects with recurrent or progressive glioblastoma or grade III malignant glioma	NCT02026271

(continued on next page)

Table 3 *(continued)*		
Disease	Trial	ClinicalTrials.gov Identifier
Recurrent	Phase II study of Ad-RTS-hIL-12 + veledimex in combination with cemiplimab-rwlc in subjects with recurrent or progressive glioblastoma	NCT04006119
Recurrent	Phase I/II study of Ad-RTS-hIL-12, an inducible adenoviral vector engineered to express hIL-12 in the presence of the activator ligand veledimex in pediatric brain tumor	NCT03330197
Recurrent	Phase Ib study of Toca 511, a retroviral replicating vector, combined With Toca FC in patients with solid tumors or lymphoma	NCT02576665
Recurrent	Continuation protocol for patients previously enrolled in a study of Toca 511	NCT04327011
Recurrent	A Phase I ascending dose trial of the safety and tolerability of Toca 511 in patients with recurrent HGG	NCT01156584
Recurrent	Phase I ascending dose trial of the safety and tolerability of Toca 511, a retroviral replicating vector, administered intravenously before, and intracranially at the time of, subsequent resection for recurrent HGG followed by treatment with extended-release 5-FC	NCT01985256
Recurrent	Phase I ascending dose trial of the safety and tolerability of Toca 511, a retroviral replicating vector administered intracranially at the time of resection for recurrent HGG followed by treatment with extended-release 5-FC	NCT01470794

Abbreviations: HGG, high-grade gliomas; HSV, herpes simplex virus.

Chimeric antigen receptor T cells

CAR T cells are T cells that have been engineered to express receptors, which allow the cells to target specific proteins expressed on the surface of tumor cells. CAR T cells are currently approved for specific hematologic malignancies and are being explored in a variety of solid tumors including primary CNS tumors.[63] For CNS tumors CAR-T target is being studied in intratumoral, intraventricular, and dual delivery systems. Tumor antigens investigated for CAR targets in GBM to date are IL-13 receptor alpha 2, EGFRvIII, and human epidermal growth factor receptor 2.[64–66] Current studies suggest encouraging results regarding safety, feasibility, and penetrance of CAR-T cells into GBM. Findings regarding effect on tumor growth and recurrence are less conclusive. One potential limitation is the monovalent approach intrinsic to first-generation CAR T-cell approaches, which can be expanded with cells engineered to target multiple epitopes, but the absolute number of potential targets remains limited.

Oncolytic viruses

Oncolytic virus therapies are designed to infect tumor cells with a virus that affects the innate immune system leading to cytokine release and tumor cell lysis. It promotes generation of an adaptive immune response to new tumor antigens and development of a long-term immunotherapy effect (**Table 3**). Viruses are engineered to replicate and be toxic to tumor cells and/or to deliver an anticancer gene to cells in the tumor microenvironment. Oncolytic viruses are administered intravenously or in situ (peritumorally after resection of the GBM or intratumorally via a stereotactic-guided catheter or via convection-enhanced delivery). No significant improvement in median OS has yet been reported but there have been durable responses in some patients.[67,68] Viral therapies are being explored in combination with check point blockade.

OTHER NOVEL APPROACHES

Treatment of CNS malignancies is different than systemic malignancies due to limited drugs penetrating the brain parenchyma and CSF due to presence of blood-brain barrier (BBB) and blood CSF barrier. One such approach is to use focused ultrasound for BBB disruption. This allows passage of drugs into the cerebral parenchyma. It is currently being investigated in a phase II study for patients with recurrent GBM where an ultrasound device is implanted at the level of an excised bone window after tumor resection. The ultrasound can be transiently activated facilitating BBB disruption.[69,70] Intravenous chemotherapy can then be administered and cross into the brain parenchyma and infiltrating tumor before reconstitution of the BBB (NCT03744026). Other chemotherapeutic agents have undergone preclinical investigation and will soon enter clinical studies.[71,72]

Nanotherapy is another strategy for improving the drug delivery across the BBB. Application of nanomaterials can prolong the circulation time of the drugs and contrasting agents in the brain. Advantages of nanoformulations include drug protection from in vivo and in vitro degradation, increase in the drug solubility, targeted drug delivery by incorporation of ligand molecules, homogenous size distribution, and flexibility in providing controlled drug release behavior.[73,74] Nanotherapeutic approaches provide an attractive option for the treatment of brain-tumors and overcome limitations of current therapeutic approaches.

SUMMARY

Neuro-oncology remains dynamic and exciting. This review has attempted to highlight key studies that have affected clinical management and investigation in the recent past. In addition, the authors have discussed both completed and ongoing clinical trials at all phases of development. Although there remains a need for advances in neuro-oncology, it is hoped that our progressively growing understanding of these diseases will guide us quickly to translation of these findings to clinical improvements for our patients.

CLINICS CARE POINTS

- Discuss update on brain tumor classification.
- Discuss updates in molecular neuro-oncology.
- Discuss update on management of primary brain tumors and future directions.

DISCLOSURE

Jigisha Thakkar and Vikram Prabhu have no disclosures. Katherine Peters: Advisory board: Agios, Bayer Research support: Agios, Novocure. Rimas Lukas: Honoraria for consulting for Abbvie, Eisai. Honoraria for advisory board Monteris. Honoraria for medical editing Medlink Neurology, EBSCO Publishing.

REFERENCES

1. Kam KL, Appin CL, Mao Q, et al. Is next-generation sequencing alone sufficient to reliably diagnose gliomas? J Neuropathol Exp Neurol 2020;79(7):763–6.
2. Louis DN, Wesseling P, Paulus W, et al. cIMPACT-NOW update 1: not otherwise specified (NOS) and not elsewhere classified (NEC). Acta Neuropathol 2018; 135(3):481–4.
3. Louis DN, Giannini C, Capper D, et al. cIMPACT-NOW update 2: diagnostic clarifications for diffuse midline glioma, H3 K27M-mutant and diffuse astrocytoma/anaplastic astrocytoma, IDH-mutant. Acta Neuropathol 2018;135(4):639–42.
4. Brat DJ, Aldape K, Colman H, et al. cIMPACT-NOW update 3: recommended diagnostic criteria for "Diffuse astrocytic glioma, IDH-wildtype, with molecular features of glioblastoma, WHO grade IV". Acta Neuropathol 2018;136(5):805–10.
5. Ellison DW, Hawkins C, Jones DTW, et al. cIMPACT-NOW update 4: diffuse gliomas characterized by MYB, MYBL1, or FGFR1 alterations or BRAF(V600E) mutation. Acta Neuropathol 2019;137(4):683–7.
6. Brat DJ, Aldape K, Colman H, et al. cIMPACT-NOW update 5: recommended grading criteria and terminologies for IDH-mutant astrocytomas. Acta Neuropathol 2020;139(3):603–8.
7. Louis DN, Wesseling P, Aldape K, et al. cIMPACT-NOW update 6: new entity and diagnostic principle recommendations of the cIMPACT-Utrecht meeting on future CNS tumor classification and grading. Brain Pathol 2020;30(4):844–56.
8. Ellison DW, Aldape KD, Capper D, et al. cIMPACT-NOW update 7: advancing the molecular classification of ependymal tumors. Brain Pathol 2020;30(5):863–6.
9. Feldman AZ, Jennings LJ, Wadhwani NR, et al. The essentials of molecular testing in CNS tumors: what to order and how to integrate results. Curr Neurol Neurosci Rep 2020;20(7):23.
10. Horbinski C, Ligon KL, Brastianos P, et al. The medical necessity of advanced molecular testing in the diagnosis and treatment of brain tumor patients. Neuro Oncol 2019;21(12):1498–508.
11. Nabors LB, Portnow J, Ammirati M, et al. National Comprehensive Cancer Network, Central Nervous System Cancers, Version 2.2020. 2020.
12. Schindler G, Capper D, Meyer J, et al. Analysis of BRAF V600E mutation in 1,320 nervous system tumors reveals high mutation frequencies in pleomorphic xanthoastrocytoma, ganglioglioma and extra-cerebellar pilocytic astrocytoma. Acta Neuropathol 2011;121(3):397–405.
13. Vaubel RA, Caron AA, Yamada S, et al. Recurrent copy number alterations in low-grade and anaplastic pleomorphic xanthoastrocytoma with and without BRAF V600E mutation. Brain Pathol 2018;28(2):172–82.
14. Matthias Gromeier MB, Beuabier N, Yan H, et al. Tumor mutational burden predicts response to oncolytic polio/rhinovirus recombinant (PVSRIPO) in malignant glioma patients: assessment of transcriptional and immunological correlates. Neuro Oncol 2019;21(Issue Supplement_6):vi7.
15. Alghamri MS, Thalla R, Avvari RP, et al. Tumor mutational burden predicts survival in patients with low-grade gliomas expressing mutated IDH1. Neurooncol Adv 2020;2(1):vdaa042.
16. van den Bent MJ, Baumert B, Erridge SC, et al. Interim results from the CATNON trial (EORTC study 26053-22054) of treatment with concurrent and adjuvant temozolomide for 1p/19q non-co-deleted anaplastic glioma: a phase 3, randomised, open-label intergroup study. Lancet 2017;390(10103):1645–53.

17. Martin J. Van Den Bent SE, Vogelbaum MA, et al. Second interim and first molecular analysis of the EORTC randomized phase III intergroup CATNON trial on concurrent and adjuvant temozolomide in anaplastic glioma without 1p/19q codeletion. ASCO; May 20, 2019, 2019.

18. Stupp R, Mason WP, van den Bent MJ, et al. Radiotherapy plus concomitant and adjuvant temozolomide for glioblastoma. N Engl J Med 2005;352(10):987–96.

19. Gilbert MR, Wang M, Aldape KD, et al. Dose-dense temozolomide for newly diagnosed glioblastoma: a randomized phase III clinical trial. J Clin Oncol 2013; 31(32):4085–91.

20. Blumenthal DT, Gorlia T, Gilbert MR, et al. Is more better? The impact of extended adjuvant temozolomide in newly diagnosed glioblastoma: a secondary analysis of EORTC and NRG Oncology/RTOG. Neuro Oncol 2017;19(8):1119–26.

21. Herrlinger U, Tzaridis T, Mack F, et al. Lomustine-temozolomide combination therapy versus standard temozolomide therapy in patients with newly diagnosed glioblastoma with methylated MGMT promoter (CeTeG/NOA-09): a randomised, open-label, phase 3 trial. Lancet 2019;393(10172):678–88.

22. Stupp R, Lukas RV, Hegi ME. Improving survival in molecularly selected glioblastoma. Lancet 2019;393(10172):615–7.

23. Stupp R, Taillibert S, Kanner A, et al. Effect of Tumor-Treating Fields Plus Maintenance Temozolomide vs Maintenance Temozolomide Alone on Survival in Patients With Glioblastoma: A Randomized Clinical Trial. JAMA 2017;318(23): 2306–16.

24. Stupp R, Wong ET, Kanner AA, et al. NovoTTF-100A versus physician's choice chemotherapy in recurrent glioblastoma: a randomised phase III trial of a novel treatment modality. Eur J Cancer 2012;48(14):2192–202.

25. Mrugala MM, Ruzevick J, Zlomanczuk P, et al. Tumor Treating Fields in Neuro-Oncological Practice. Curr Oncol Rep 2017;19(8):53.

26. Ingo K, Mellinghoff TFC, Wen PY, et al. A phase I, open label, perioperative study of AG-120 and AG-881 in recurrent IDH1 mutant, low-grade glioma: results from cohort 1. American Society of Clincial Oncology. J Clin Oncol 2019;37(15).

27. Mellinghoff IK, Wen PY, Taylor JW, et al. PL3.1 A phase 1, open-label, perioperative study of ivosidenib (AG-120) and vorasidenib (AG-881) in recurrent, IDH1-mutant, low-grade glioma: results from cohort 1. Neuro Oncol 2019;21(3).

28. Macarena Ines De La Fuente HC, Rosenthal M, Van Tine BA, et al. A phase Ib/II study of olutasidenib in patients with relapsed/refractory IDH1 mutant gliomas: Safety and efficacy as single agent and in combination with azacitidine. J Clin Oncol 2020;38(15).

29. Tawbi HA, Boutros C, Kok D, et al. New era in the management of melanoma brain metastases. Am Soc Clin Oncol Educ Book 2018;38:741–50.

30. Geukes Foppen MH, Boogerd W, Blank CU, et al. Clinical and radiological response of BRAF inhibition and MEK inhibition in patients with brain metastases from BRAF-mutated melanoma. Melanoma Res 2018;28(2):126–33.

31. Drago JZ, Lawrence D, Livingstone E, et al. Clinical experience with combination BRAF/MEK inhibitors for melanoma with brain metastases: a real-life multicenter study. Melanoma Res 2019;29(1):65–9.

32. Shaikh N, Brahmbhatt N, Kruser TJ, et al. Pleomorphic xanthoastrocytoma: a brief review. CNS Oncol 2019;8(3):CNS39.

33. Brown NF, Carter T, Kitchen N, et al. Dabrafenib and trametinib in BRAFV600E mutated glioma. CNS Oncol 2017;6(4):291–6.

34. Schreck KC, Guajardo A, Lin DDM, et al. Concurrent BRAF/MEK Inhibitors in BRAF V600-Mutant High-Grade Primary Brain Tumors. J Natl Compr Canc Netw 2018;16(4):343–7.
35. Kaley T, Touat M, Subbiah V, et al. BRAF Inhibition in BRAF(V600)-Mutant Gliomas: Results From the VE-BASKET Study. J Clin Oncol 2018;36(35):3477–84.
36. Hussain F, Horbinski CM, Chmura SJ, et al. Response to BRAF/MEK Inhibition After Progression With BRAF Inhibition in a Patient With Anaplastic Pleomorphic Xanthoastrocytoma. Neurologist 2018;23(5):163–6.
37. Smith-Cohn M, Davidson C, Colman H, et al. Challenges of targeting BRAF V600E mutations in adult primary brain tumor patients: a report of two cases. CNS Oncol 2019;8(4):CNS48.
38. Karisa C, Schreck MPP, Wemmer J, et al. RAF and MEK inhibitor therapy in adult patients with brain tumors: a case-based overview and practical management of adverse events. Neurooncol Pract 2020;7(4):369–75.
39. Lasorella A, Sanson M, Iavarone A. FGFR-TACC gene fusions in human glioma. Neuro Oncol 2017;19(4):475–83.
40. Singh D, Chan JM, Zoppoli P, et al. Transforming fusions of FGFR and TACC genes in human glioblastoma. Science 2012;337(6099):1231–5.
41. Ziegler DS, Wong M, Mayoh C, et al. Brief Report: Potent clinical and radiological response to larotrectinib in TRK fusion-driven high-grade glioma. Br J Cancer 2018;119(6):693–6.
42. Liu D, Offin M, Harnicar S, et al. Entrectinib: an orally available, selective tyrosine kinase inhibitor for the treatment of NTRK, ROS1, and ALK fusion-positive solid tumors. Ther Clin Risk Manag 2018;14:1247–52.
43. Drilon A, Laetsch TW, Kummar S, et al. Efficacy of Larotrectinib in TRK Fusion-Positive Cancers in Adults and Children. N Engl J Med 2018;378(8):731–9.
44. Brastianos PK, Carter SL, Santagata S, et al. Genomic Characterization of Brain Metastases Reveals Branched Evolution and Potential Therapeutic Targets. Cancer Discov 2015;5(11):1164–77.
45. Warren P, Mason SK, Stupp R, et al. Marie-Laure Casadebaig, Ileana Elias, Benjamin Winograd, Nancy Levin, and Daniela Annenelie Bota. Full enrollment results from an extended phase I, multicenter, open label study of marizomib (MRZ) with temozolomide (TMZ) and radiotherapy (RT) in newly diagnosed glioblastoma (GBM). J Clin Oncol 2019;37(15_suppl):2021.
46. Wilhelm SM, Dumas J, Adnane L, et al. Regorafenib (BAY 73-4506): a new oral multikinase inhibitor of angiogenic, stromal and oncogenic receptor tyrosine kinases with potent preclinical antitumor activity. Int J Cancer 2011;129(1):245–55.
47. Lombardi G, De Salvo GL, Brandes AA, et al. Regorafenib compared with lomustine in patients with relapsed glioblastoma (REGOMA): a multicentre, open-label, randomised, controlled, phase 2 trial. Lancet Oncol 2019;20(1):110–9.
48. Santangelo A, Rossato M, Lombardi G, et al. A Molecular Signature associated with prolonged survival in Glioblastoma patients treated with Regorafenib. Neuro Oncol 2020;noaa156.
49. Weller M, Butowski N, Tran DD, et al. Rindopepimut with temozolomide for patients with newly diagnosed, EGFRvIII-expressing glioblastoma (ACT IV): a randomised, double-blind, international phase 3 trial. Lancet Oncol 2017;18(10):1373–85.
50. Ahluwalia MRD AA, Curry W, Wong E, et al. Phase II trial of a survivin vaccine (SurVaxM) for newly diagnosed glioblastoma. New Orleans: Society for Neuro Oncology; 2018.

51. David A. Reardon SB, Desai AS, et al. INO-5401 and INO-9012 delivered intramuscularly (IM) with electroporation (EP) in combination with cemiplimab (REGN2810) in newly diagnosed glioblastoma (GBM): Interim results. 2020 American Society of Clinical Oncology; 2020.

52. Bloch O, Parsa AT. Heat shock protein peptide complex-96 (HSPPC-96) vaccination for recurrent glioblastoma: a phase II, single arm trial. Neuro Oncol 2014; 16(5):758–9.

53. Bloch O, Shi Q, Keith Anderson S, et al. ATIM-14. ALLIANCE A071101: A PHASE II RANDOMIZED TRIAL COMPARING THE EFFICACY OF HEAT SHOCK PROTEIN PEPTIDE COMPLEX-96 (HSPPC-96) VACCINE GIVEN WITH BEVACIZUMAB VERSUS BEVACIZUMAB ALONE IN THE TREATMENT OF SURGICALLY RESECTABLE RECURRENT GLIOBLASTOMA. Neuro Oncol 2017;19(suppl_6): vi29.

54. Lukas RV, Wainwright DA, Horbinski CM, et al. Immunotherapy Against Gliomas: is the Breakthrough Near? Drugs 2019;79(17):1839–48.

55. Arrieta VA, Iwamoto F, Lukas RV, et al. Can patient selection and neoadjuvant administration resuscitate PD-1 inhibitors for glioblastoma? J Neurosurg 2019; 132(5):1313–74.

56. Touat M, Li YY, Boynton AN, et al. Mechanisms and therapeutic implications of hypermutation in gliomas. Nature 2020;580(7804):517–23.

57. Bouffet E, Larouche V, Campbell BB, et al. Immune Checkpoint Inhibition for Hypermutant Glioblastoma Multiforme Resulting From Germline Biallelic Mismatch Repair Deficiency. J Clin Oncol 2016;34(19):2206–11.

58. Bristol-Myers Squibb Announces Phase 3 CheckMate -498 Study Did Not Meet Primary Endpoint of Overall Survival with Opdivo (nivolumab) Plus Radiation in Patients with Newly Diagnosed MGMT-Unmethylated Glioblastoma Multiforme [press release].

59. Bristol-Myers Squibb Provides Update on Phase 3 Opdivo (nivolumab) CheckMate -548 Trial in Patients with Newly Diagnosed MGMT-Methylated Glioblastoma Multiforme [press release].

60. Reardon DA, Brandes AA, Omuro A, et al. Effect of Nivolumab vs Bevacizumab in Patients With Recurrent Glioblastoma: The CheckMate 143 Phase 3 Randomized Clinical Trial. JAMA Oncol 2020;6(7):1003–10.

61. Ladomersky E, Zhai L, Lenzen A, et al. IDO1 Inhibition Synergizes with Radiation and PD-1 Blockade to Durably Increase Survival Against Advanced Glioblastoma. Clin Cancer Res 2018;24(11):2559–73.

62. Reardon DA, Desjardins A, Rixe O, et al. A phase 1 study of PF-06840003, an oral indoleamine 2,3-dioxygenase 1 (IDO1) inhibitor in patients with recurrent malignant glioma. Invest New Drugs 2020.

63. Migliorini D, Dietrich PY, Stupp R, et al. CAR T-Cell Therapies in Glioblastoma: A First Look. Clin Cancer Res 2018;24(3):535–40.

64. Brown CE, Alizadeh D, Starr R, et al. Regression of Glioblastoma after Chimeric Antigen Receptor T-Cell Therapy. N Engl J Med 2016;375(26):2561–9.

65. O'Rourke DM, Nasrallah MP, Desai A, et al. A single dose of peripherally infused EGFRvIII-directed CAR T cells mediates antigen loss and induces adaptive resistance in patients with recurrent glioblastoma. Sci Transl Med 2017;9(399): eaaa0984.

66. Ahmed N, Brawley V, Hegde M, et al. HER2-Specific Chimeric Antigen Receptor-Modified Virus-Specific T Cells for Progressive Glioblastoma: A Phase 1 Dose-Escalation Trial. JAMA Oncol 2017;3(8):1094–101.

67. Desjardins A, Gromeier M, Herndon JE 2nd, et al. Recurrent Glioblastoma Treated with Recombinant Poliovirus. N Engl J Med 2018;379(2):150–61.
68. Westphal M, Yla-Herttuala S, Martin J, et al. Adenovirus-mediated gene therapy with sitimagene ceradenovec followed by intravenous ganciclovir for patients with operable high-grade glioma (ASPECT): a randomised, open-label, phase 3 trial. Lancet Oncol 2013;14(9):823–33.
69. Idbaih A, Canney M, Belin L, et al. Safety and Feasibility of Repeated and Transient Blood-Brain Barrier Disruption by Pulsed Ultrasound in Patients with Recurrent Glioblastoma. Clin Cancer Res 2019;25(13):3793–801.
70. Carpentier A, Canney M, Vignot A, et al. Clinical trial of blood-brain barrier disruption by pulsed ultrasound. Sci Transl Med 2016;8(343):343re342.
71. Zhang DY, Dmello C, Chen L, et al. Ultrasound-mediated Delivery of Paclitaxel for Glioma: A Comparative Study of Distribution, Toxicity, and Efficacy of Albumin-bound Versus Cremophor Formulations. Clin Cancer Res 2020;26(2):477–86.
72. Beccaria K, Canney M, Bouchoux G, et al. Ultrasound-induced blood-brain barrier disruption for the treatment of gliomas and other primary CNS tumors. Cancer Lett 2020;479:13–22.
73. Agrahari V, Agrahari V, Mitra AK. Next generation drug delivery: circulatory cells-mediated nanotherapeutic approaches. Expert Opin Drug Deliv 2017;14(3):285–9.
74. Meng J, Agrahari V, Youm I. Advances in Targeted Drug Delivery Approaches for the Central Nervous System Tumors: The Inspiration of Nanobiotechnology. J Neuroimmune Pharmacol 2017;12(1):84–98.

Advances in the Surgical Management of Epilepsy

Drug-Resistant Focal Epilepsy in the Adult Patient

Gregory D. Cascino, MD[a],*, Benjamin H. Brinkmann, PhD[b]

KEYWORDS

- Epilepsy • Drug-resistant • Neuroimaging • Surgical treatment

KEY POINTS

- *Pharmacoresistant* seizures may occur in nearly one-third of people with epilepsy, and Intractable epilepsy is associated with an increased mortality.
- Medial temporal lobe epilepsy and lesional epilepsy are the most favorable surgically remediable epileptic syndromes.
- Successful epilepsy surgery may render the patient seizure-free, reduce antiseizure drug(s) adverse effects, improve quality of life, and decrease mortality.
- Surgical management of epilepsy should not be considered a procedure of "last resort."
- Epilepsy surgery despite the results of randomized controlled trials remains an underutilized treatment modality for patients with drug-resistant epilepsy.

INTRODUCTION

Epilepsy is one of the most common chronic neurologic disorders affecting nearly 65 million people in the world.[1] It is estimated that approximately 1.2% of individuals in the United States, or approximately 3.4 million people, have seizure disorders.[1] This includes almost 3 million adults and 470,000 children.[1,2] More than 200,000 individuals in the United States will experience new-onset seizure disorders each year. Nearly 10% of people will have 1 or more seizures during their lifetime.[1–3] The 2012 Institute of Medicine of the National Academy of Sciences report indicated that 1 in 26 Americans will develop a seizure disorder during their lifetime; this is double the risk of those with Parkinson disease, multiple sclerosis, and autism spectrum disorder *combined*.[3] The diagnosis of epilepsy may include patients with 2 or more unprovoked seizures or

[a] Mayo Clinic, 200 First Street Southwest, Rochester, MN 55905, USA; [b] Mayo Clinic, Department of Neurology, 200 First Street Southwest, Rochester, MN 55905, USA
* Corresponding author.
E-mail address: gcascino@mayo.edu

Neurol Clin 39 (2021) 181–196
https://doi.org/10.1016/j.ncl.2020.09.010
0733-8619/21/© 2020 Elsevier Inc. All rights reserved.

neurologic.theclinics.com

those with single seizures with biomarkers that indicate an increased likelihood of seizure recurrence, that is, greater than 60% chance for an additional seizure.[4] Factors that may indicate an increased risk for seizures following a single seizure include the presence of developmental delay or a focal neurologic deficit, autoimmune neurologic disorder, a history of remote symptomatic neurologic disease, and an MRI-identified pathologic substrate or epileptogenic lesion, for example, mesial temporal sclerosis (MTS). The devastating effect of seizure disorders in part relates to the peak onset for the development of new-onset seizure disorders that include the very young (neonates and children) and very old (older than 65 years).[1–4] Approximately one-third of patients with recurrent seizures will have physically, medically, and socially disabling seizure disorders that adversely affect the individual's quality of life, that is, drug-resistant epilepsy (DRE) or *pharmacoresistant* epilepsy.[5] The most common seizure disorder in adults is focal epilepsy associated with focal impaired awareness seizures, also known as complex partial seizures or focal dyscognitive seizures. Such patients are at increased risk for comorbidities and mortality, including cognitive disorders, mood disorders like anxiety and depression, physical trauma related to seizures, and sudden unexpected death in epilepsy (SUDEP).[6–8] Patients with intractable epilepsy may have significant issues obtaining an education, becoming gainfully employed, and living independently. A seizure disorder is considered in remission if the patient is seizure-free for 10 years and has been off antiseizure medication for the past 5 years.[6] Importantly, the psychosocial debilitation associated with epilepsy may be unique compared with other neurologic disorders because of the wide range in age of seizure onset, the variability in response to medical therapy, and the presence of potentially devastating comorbidities.

The most effective medical treatment of epilepsy is the initial antiseizure drug (ASD). The first 2 ASDs are the most likely to be of benefit in rendering the patient seizure-free if the appropriate medication(s) is selected for the seizure type. Most individuals who will be rendered seizure-free and respond to ASD therapy in the initial 2 years of treatment if the patient has *pharmacoresponsive* epilepsy. Perhaps fewer than 10% of individuals with DRE will be rendered seizure-free with additional ASD trials.[6,7] Overreliance on use of antiepileptic drug levels may undermine the success of an ASD. In general, treat the *patient* and not the *drug level*. Patient tolerance and response to ASD medication dosing may be highly variable. Patients who do not respond favorably to 2 antiseizure drugs used appropriately are likely to have DRE and should be investigated for surgery and other alternative forms of treatment. Individuals who fail to respond satisfactorily to 2 or more ASDs would be considered to have DRE.[7] Importantly, medication nonadherence is a significant concern for all individuals with suspected DRE and needs to be carefully assessed in reviewing the efficacy of therapeutic modalities. An estimated one-third of people with epilepsy may have medically refractory seizure disorders and should be considered for alternative forms of treatment such as epilepsy surgery.[6,7]

The goals of treatment for individuals with DRE are to render the patient seizure-free (*No Seizures*), avoid treatment-related adverse effects (*No Side Effects*), and to improve the individual's quality of life allowing the patient to become a participating and productive member of society (*No Lifestyle Limitations*).[9] Often an important rationale for patients considering alternative treatments to ASD therapy is the inability to legally and safely operate a motor vehicle. This may be a significant disability for obtaining an education and being gainfully employed. Potential treatment options for these patients include continued ASD trials, neuromodulation, diet therapy, and surgical management, that is, epilepsy surgery.[8,9] The most effective treatment of DRE is surgical resection of the epileptic brain tissue and the pathologic substrate.

Unfortunately, epilepsy surgery remains a significantly underutilized, but highly effective therapeutic modality.[9] Only a small percentage of patients with focal DRE are referred for surgical treatment. This article discusses the advances in surgical treatment of DRE in adults with focal seizures.

BENEFICIAL EFFECTS OF SURGERY

The rationale for surgical treatment of DRE in patients with focal seizures is to render the individual seizure-free while avoiding neurologic morbidity.[9,10] The putative beneficial effects of surgery may include a reduction in ASD medication and potential adverse effects of medical therapy.[10] Discontinuance of ASD, however, may not be feasible in all patients who have a seizure remission following epilepsy surgery. Successful surgery has been shown to decrease the risk of physical trauma associated with seizures and SUDEP.[11] The overall mortality associated with epilepsy may be reduced following surgical treatment.[11,12] Epilepsy surgery may also improve the symptoms of depression and anxiety that are common comorbidities associated with DRE. A reduction in seizure tendency following surgical treatment in women has also been associated with an apparent increase in fertility and pregnancy.[13] Ultimately, the most common rationale for considering surgical treatment is the improvement in the patient's quality of life allowing them to become more independent and engaged in society.

Goals of Epilepsy Surgery
- Render the patient seizure-free or significantly reduce seizure tendency
- Avoid operative morbidity
- Reduce antiseizure drug(s) adverse effects
- Improve the patient's quality of life
- Decrease risk of seizure-related mortality and SUDEP

DIAGNOSTIC EVALUATION

The care and management of people with focal DRE begins with confirming the classification of the seizure disorder and seizure type(s), determining the presence of an underlying or symptomatic etiology, and evaluating seizure precipitating factors. A comprehensive neurologic history and examination is performed to elucidate the potential underlying etiology, identify the seizure type(s) and precipitating factors, recognize comorbidities and discuss important psychosocial issues including patient education, employment history, and current living situation.[9,14] The presence of a mood disorder such as anxiety and depression should be assessed, as these psychiatric illnesses are overrepresented in people with epilepsy and may significantly impair quality of life. Also, inadequately treated mood disorders may increase seizure tendency. The prior ASD medication and other potential treatment options, for example, diet or neuromodulation, would be reviewed in detail with careful attention to patient compliance and adverse effects of therapy. The presence of dose-related and idiosyncratic side effects associated with ASD need to be recognized. Not uncommonly, patients and their family members may identify certain situations that exacerbate the seizure tendency. These are highly variable but often include ASD noncompliance, sleep deprivation, psychosocial stress, inadequately treated anxiety or depression, or correlation with menstrual cycle. Attempts to manage the precipitating factors that are reversible, for example, irregular ASD intake, may be pivotal to the success of any therapeutic intervention. Patients with cognitive impairment may be at high risk for ASD noncompliance with complicated ASD protocols.

Diagnostic studies obtained initially in the evaluation of suspect DRE include routine electroencephalogram (EEG), neuroimaging procedures, and neuropsychological testing.[8,9,14] Admission to a dedicated epilepsy monitoring unit (EMU) for scalp-recorded long-term video-EEG recordings would be required for evaluation of focal epilepsy to classify seizure type(s) and permit adequate surgical localization. The presence of interictal and ictal epileptiform discharges may assist in localization of the epileptogenic zone, that is, the epileptic brain tissue important for focal seizure activity. The seizure semiologies and behavioral assessment during the seizure activity may be critical in lateralizing and localizing the site of seizure onset. Selected patients with focal epilepsy based on history, seizure type(s), and comorbidities may require additional diagnostic studies including an autoimmune neurology evaluation (serum and cerebrospinal fluid autoantibody determinations) and medical genetics consultation with genetic testing.

Diagnostic Studies for Epilepsy Surgery (Variably performed, indicating these studies may or may not be performed depending on the clinical picture)

- Routine awake-sleep EEG
- MRI head seizure protocol
- Video-EEG monitoring in EMU
- Neuropsychological studies
- 2-Deoxy-2–[18]F-deoxyglucose (FDG)-PET scan*
- Subtraction ictal single-photon emission computed tomography (SPECT) coregistered to MRI*
- Functional MRI (fMRI)*
- Magnetoencephalography*
- Chronic intracranial EEG monitoring*
- Intraoperative electrocorticography*

Electrophysiological Studies

Scalp-recorded EEG studies are performed to record interictal and ictal epileptiform patterns.[15,16] While in the EMU the patients ASD medication may be tapered or withdrawn to increased seizure tendency. Video-EEG monitoring during the individual's habitual clinical seizure type(s) is usually considered pivotal in surgical decision making. Rarely, interictal EEG epileptiform discharges concordant with a structural neuroimaging abnormality may be sufficient for surgical localization. High-density array of EEG electrodes (10–10 electrode placement) may be useful in patients with extratemporal focal seizures; especially involving the mesial frontal lobe such as supplementary motor area seizures. Clinical examination during focal seizures may include language and memory assessments.

Neuroimaging Studies

High-resolution MRI is an essential structural neuroimaging procedure to assess surgical candidacy for patients with DRE and focal seizures.[17] The finding of an MRI-identified pathologic substrate concordant with the site of seizure onset is a major determinant of operative strategy and has significant prognostic importance.[9,17] Specific imaging protocols have been developed to increase the diagnostic yield of these studies. The MRI should include coronal or oblique-coronal T1-weightedd and T2-weighted and fluid-attenuated inversion recovery (FLAIR) sequences (Box 1).[18–21] A 3-T MRI study is routinely performed in patients with seizure disorders.[17] MRI almost invariably reveals an abnormality indicating the focal epileptogenic pathology in patients with low-grade neoplasms like dysembryoplastic neuroepitheliomas tumors (DNET), vascular anomalies including cavernous malformations, large vessel cerebral

Box 1
Standard MRI epilepsy protocol "3D Epilepsy Study" used at Mayo Clinic (3.0-T, 1.5-mm temporal lobe sections)

Imaging sequences:

Scout

Sagittal T1-weighted fluid-attenuated inversion recovery (FLAIR)

Axial 2D T2-weighted fast spin echo with fat saturation

Coronal 2D T2-weighted FLAIR with fat saturation

Sagittal Sampling Perfection with Application optimized Contrasts using different flip angle Evolution (SPACE) double inversion recovery (DIR)

Sagittal magnetization prepared rapid acquisition gradient echo (MPRAGE)

Small Field of View Coronal SPACE T2-weighted FLAIR

Axial diffusion-weighted imaging (DWI)

Axial susceptibility-weighted imaging (SWI)

infarctions, and encephaloceles.[17,22] MRI may reveal hippocampal atrophy and an FLAIR and T2 signal hyperintensity in patients with MTS (**Fig. 1**).[18–21] Quantitative measures of hippocampal volume may be useful in selected patients with bilateral symmetric hippocampal atrophy or subtle unilateral volume loss with MTS.[18–21] Loss of internal structure of the hippocampus may also be seen in these patients. An MRI finding of MTS is predictive of better seizure and memory outcomes following surgery.[17,21] A significant percentage of patients with the common developmental pathologies such as focal cortical dysplasia (FCD) type IIb also may have an imaging alteration.[21] In patients with FCD, MRI findings may be subtle and include mild cortical thickening, a prominent deep sulcus, a cortical signal intensity change, blurring of the gray-white junction, or aberrant cortical architecture, focal atrophy, and hyperintense signal in T2/FLAIR sequences (**Fig. 2**).[21] FCD is characterized by disorganization of the cortical lamination associated with bizarre (dysplastic neurons). The introduction of a 7-T MRI scanner may increase the sensitivity and specificity of selected pathologies. Unfortunately, a significant number of patients referred for epilepsy surgery have MRI-negative focal epilepsy. Additional neuroimaging procedures need to be considered in these individuals and many will require chronic intracranial EEG monitoring for surgical planning (see later in this article).

PET is a functional neuroimaging modality that may localize a focal abnormality for surgical planning in patients with pharmacoresistant epilepsy.[23,24] PET is the most important *interictal* functional neuroimaging procedure in patients with DRE being considered for epilepsy surgery. PET scans use ^{18}F-deoxyglucose (FDG-PET) as a ligand to measure differential glucose consumption as a surrogate for metabolism. A key concept is that FDG-PET measures *interictal* brain metabolism and that the region of seizure onset is *hypometabolic*. FDG-PET has been found to be most useful in temporal lobe epilepsy. In patients with medial temporal lobe epilepsy, temporal hypometabolism may accurately lateralize to the temporal lobe of seizure origin and is associated with favorable surgical outcomes, even when MRI is negative.[23] FDG-PET is less sensitive in patients with extratemporal epilepsy.

SPECT measures cerebral blood flow via the injection of a radiotracer such as technetium-99m-hexamethylpropylene amine oxime (99mTc-HMPAO) with rapid uptake within the brain (30–60 seconds from injection) but a long half-life.[25,26] SPECT

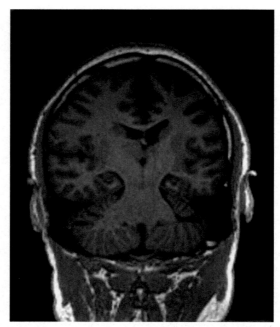

Fig. 1. Patient with left medial temporal lobe epilepsy. MRI head seizure protocol T1-weighted image in the oblique-coronal plane shows volume loss involving the left hippocampal formation and left mesial temporal lobe compatible with MTS. Encephalomalacia within the posterior superior left frontal lobe presumably related to remote meningioma resection. Patient is seizure-free after a left selective amygdalohippocampectomy. Note the left temporal lobe is on the right side of the figure.

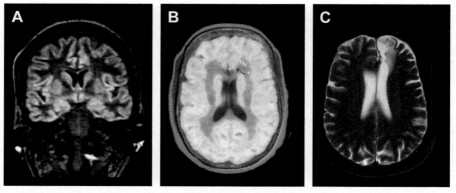

Fig. 2. Patient presenting with focal seizures related to FCD, with scalp EEG maximal over the midline frontal area at onset. (*A*) Double inversion recovery MRI head reveals thickened cortex with blurring of the gray-white matter border over the anterior cingulate (*red arrow*). (*B*) FDG-PET shows bilateral hypometabolism in the anterior cingulate (*red arrow*), and SEEG monitoring shows seizures arising from the left anterior cingulate. (*C*) Focal resection of the FCD lesion including the locations of the seizure onset electrodes rendered the patient seizure free as of 25 months follow-up.

identifies the location of *ictal* activity, which is characterized by *increased* cerebral perfusion. Subtraction ictal SPECT coregistered to MRI (SISCOM) is a modification of the ictal SPECT technique that superimposes ictal and interictal SPECT images and brain MRI. Statistical parametric mapping is a more recent innovation that permits comparison of focal or regional areas of hyperperfusion to a control group that increases the diagnostic yield of the technique in patients with DRE being considered for focal cortical resection.[26]

fMRI is a noninvasive imaging study that may localize selected neurologic clinical functions, for example, language.[27] fMRI detects relative changes in focal blood oxygen levels that occur over time while the patient is given a protocolled computerized task testing specific brain functions and which is alternated with rest or control tasks. Language function can be lateralized and localized to guide surgical resection. This imaging technique may obviate the need for an invasive procedure such as intracarotid amobarbital study.

Neuropsychological Studies

Neuropsychological studies are performed to evaluate the presence of verbal or nonverbal learning and memory deficits in patients with DRE being considered for surgical treatment.[28] These studies may be of highest diagnostic yield in individuals with focal seizures of temporal lobe origin. This is most commonly a standard protocol permitting comparison of results before and after surgery. The preoperative memory assessment may allow appropriate counseling of patients regarding memory outcome following surgery. Neuropsychological studies are often performed to provide a baseline determination of cognitive performance before surgery that can be compared with a postoperative examination.

SURGICAL MANAGEMENT OF FOCAL EPILEPSY

Several surgical strategies may be considered in the management of DRE in the adult patient.[10,29,30] Surgically remediable epileptic syndromes have been identified in patients with focal seizures that are medically, physically, and socially disabling. The patient candidacy and presurgical evaluation depends on the operative intervention. The timing of a consideration of surgical treatment begins with the diagnosis of DRE in individuals with focal seizures. The patients should undergo an appropriate diagnostic evaluation to determine seizure classification, underlying etiology, comorbid conditions, and effective treatment options. Unfortunately, the duration between the diagnosis of DRE and the neurosurgical procedure for epilepsy is often 20 years or longer.[31] This delay may adversely affect the patient's psychosocial development and opportunities to become a participating member of society.

Surgically Remediable Epileptic Syndromes
- Medial temporal lobe epilepsy
- Lesional epilepsy
- MRI-negative focal epilepsy

Medial Temporal Lobe Epilepsy

The most common surgical strategy for DRE is a focal cortical resection of the site of seizure onset and initial seizure propagation. In adult patients with focal seizures this most commonly involves the anteromedial temporal lobe including the amygdala and hippocampus.[9,10,16] The most common pathology is MTS with focal hippocampal neuronal loss.[9,10] The extent of surgical resection is determined by the preoperative investigation including the ictal EEG recordings and the neuroimaging techniques. Selected institutions performed a "standard anterior temporal lobectomy" with the preoperative evaluation determining the operative margins of the focal cortical resection. The resection includes anterior temporal lobe neocortex and an amygdalohippocampectomy.[30,31] Preoperative interictal-ictal EEG recordings and MRI head studies are used for seizure lateralization and localization. The posterior extent of the anterior temporal resection is determined by potential adverse effects on language and vision. Other surgical epilepsy centers perform a "tailored" cortical resection that may use intraoperative electrocorticography and functional mapping of language cortex to guide the excision. Additional operative management of medial temporal lobe epilepsy includes selective amygdalohippocampectomy that limits the excision of the temporal lobe neocortex. There are conflicting results regarding the effectiveness of the specific operative strategies to render individuals with mesial temporal lobe epilepsy seizure-free. Importantly, most individuals experience a significant reduction in seizure tendency with either operative approach. More recently, MRI-guided laser interstitial thermal therapy (LITT) has been introduced in the management of medial temporal lobe epilepsy related to MTS (**Fig. 3**).[32] LITT may be a minimally invasive surgical procedure that is effective in these patients and compares favorably with anterior temporal lobectomy regarding neurocognitive outcome.[32,33]

Surgical management of medial temporal lobe epilepsy has been shown to be safe and effective in randomized clinical trials.[34–36] Surgery was superior in efficacy to "best medical therapy" in a pivotal study involving 80 patients with temporal lobe epilepsy.[34] At 1 year, the cumulative proportion of patients who were seizure-free (focal impaired awareness seizures) was significantly greater in the surgery group than the medical group (58% vs 8%).[34] Quality-of-life ratings were also higher in the surgical-treated group.

The consensus of randomized clinical trials and observational series with large patient cohorts is that approximately 75% of patients with medial temporal lobe epilepsy are seizure-free during long-term follow-up after surgical intervention if the MRI head

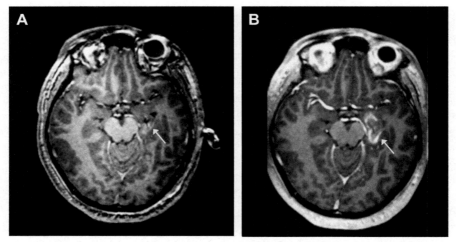

Fig. 3. LITT provides focal ablative therapy without damaging surrounding tissue. (*A*) Intraoperative MRI confirms placement of the water-cooled fiber optic applicator in the hippocampus (*arrow*), and laser energy is used to heat the tissue to ablative levels. (*B*) Gadolinium contrast forms a ring around the damaged tissue following ablation.

shows changes consistent with MTS (focal hippocampal formation atrophy with or without FLAIR-identified mesial temporal signal hyperintensity).[31] The best predictors of a favorable operative outcome include MRI-identified MTS, concordant scalp-recorded EEG and MRI findings, PET-identified hypometabolism concordant with the temporal lobe of seizure origin, and shorter seizure disorder duration.[16] Approximately 90% of patients with unilateral MRI-identified MTS concordant with the interictal epileptiform discharges will be seizure-free or experience auras only or seizures with ASD discontinuance following epilepsy surgery.[16] Poor predictors of operative outcome include normal MRI head study, bilateral MRI-identified MTS, bitemporal epileptiform discharges, normal PET study, and the presence of clinical semiology that suggests seizures emanating from outside the medial temporal lobe region. In a series of 87 patients with a normal MRI undergoing anterior temporal lobectomy, 55% had an excellent operative outcome (seizure-free or auras only).[37] The surgical outcome of patients with a localized temporal lobe PET abnormality and a normal MRI may be equivalent to individuals with MRI-identified unilateral hippocampal sclerosis. Seventy-six percent of patients in one series with temporal lobe PET hypometabolism and a normal MRI were seizure-free following surgery.[23]

Lesional Epilepsy

Patients with DRE due to focal foreign-tissue lesions, that is, lesional epilepsy, may be candidates for surgical treatment of epilepsy.[38–42] A comprehensive evaluation is required to determine the epileptogenicity of the structural-anatomical pathology. The pivotal diagnostic modality in these individuals is almost invariably an MRI head study with and without contrast. The surgical strategy in these patients most commonly involves excision of the pathologic substrate and resection of the epileptogenic tissue. Most individuals with lesional epilepsy become seizure-free or experience a marked reduction in seizure tendency.[38–42] Common pathologic entities responsible for DRE associated with lesional pathology include tumors, cavernous malformations, and FCD.[38–42]

Lesional Epilepsy
- Low-grade neoplasms like DNET and gangliogliomas
- Cavernous hemangiomas
- FCD
- Temporal lobe encephaloceles

The incidence of seizures among patients with primary brain tumors is related to tumor type and grade and cortical localization. Low-grade, slowly growing tumors are most commonly associated with a chronic seizure disorder (**Fig. 4**). Gangliogliomas and DNET together account for approximately three-quarters of all tumors found in adults undergoing epilepsy surgery.[38–41] Some studies have suggested that DNETs are associated with higher seizure relapse rates compared with other epileptogenic tumors. Most patients with DRE related to these low-grade neoplasms are rendered seizure-free with complete lesion resection and excision of the epileptic brain tissue.[38]

Cavernous malformations and arteriovenous malformations are the most common vascular lesions found in patients with focal epilepsy (**Fig. 5**).[42,43] Seizures are a common presenting feature of cavernous malformation. Resection typically leads to complete seizure control or significant improvement. In a case series of 168 patients with symptomatic epilepsy attributed to cavernous malformations, more than two-thirds of patients were seizure free at 3 years after surgery.[43] Predictors for a favorable seizure outcome included medial temporal location, size less than 1.5 cm, and the absence of tonic-clonic seizures.[42]

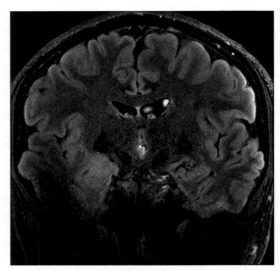

Fig. 4. Patient with right medial temporal lobe epilepsy. Seven-Tesla MRI head T2-weighted image in the oblique-coronal plane shows right medial temporal lobe lesion that is, consistent with a low-grade glial neoplasm. Note the right temporal lobe is on the left side of the figure.

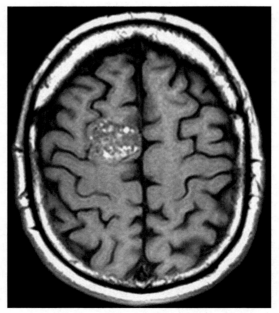

Fig. 5. Patient with right supplementary motor area seizures. MRI head T1-weighted image in the axial plane shows a right mesial frontal cavernous malformation. Note the right frontal lobe is on the left side of the figure.

FCDs are an important etiology for drug-resistant focal epilepsy.[44,45] Patients with MRI-negative focal epilepsy may have evidence of FCD at the time of surgery. Epilepsy surgery is less effective in patients with FCD than in patients with other lesional pathology (eg, tumors or cavernous malformations). Challenging issues in these patients include the difficulty identifying areas of FCD using MRI, the presence of extratemporal neocortical lesions, and multilobar pathology. One center reported that 57% of 166 patients with FCD followed for 2 years or longer after surgery were seizure free.[45] Success rates may be higher in patients with a specific form of focal cortical dysplasia type II in which dysplastic features are maximal at the bottom of the sulcus (referred to as a transmantle sign on MRI). FDG-PET/MRI may improve the surgical outcome in patients with FCD type II associated with balloon cells (Taylor-type focal cortical dysplasia). In a study that included 23 patients who underwent epilepsy surgery, and who had pathologically verified FCD type II, MRI was negative in 13 patients and showed subtle alterations in 10 patients. FDG-PET/MRI revealed a hypometabolic zone in 22 of 23 patients. Twenty of the 23 patients (87%) became seizure free following surgery.[24]

Temporal lobe encephaloceles are a more recently recognized etiology of DRE.[46,47] The encephaloceles may be idiopathic or related to congenital defects, prior head trauma, or surgery. Not all encephaloceles are epileptogenic; therefore, a preoperative evaluation would need to performed and correlate with the structural neuroimaging findings. Surgical strategy may include an encephalocele repair with or without a focal cortical resection.

MRI-Negative Focal Epilepsy

The surgical management of MRI-negative focal seizures of neocortical origin (ie, extrahippocampal) can be challenging because of difficulty defining the boundaries of the epileptogenic zone that must be resected for seizure freedom.[48] There are also increased concerns regarding clinically functional cortex, which may increase the risk of perioperative neurologic deficits. The clinical manifestations of neocortical seizures depend on the localization of seizure onset and initial seizure propagation. Seizures arising from functional cortex can be localized based on neurologic symptoms that occur at seizure onset or during the postictal state. Compared with medial temporal lobe epilepsy, neocortical seizures of temporal lobe origin may have a unique aura and ictal semiology with an increased tendency for tonic-clonic seizures. Frontal lobe seizures tend to be shorter and more frequent than temporal lobe seizures, with ictal manifestations varying from staring to hypermotor behavior. Frontal lobe seizures may be confined to sleep. Parietal and occipital seizures typically have complex sensory symptoms, such as visual hallucinations of objects or scenes. Despite these general principles, extrahippocampal focal seizures often have varied clinical semiology and can be difficult to localize with scalp-recorded ictal EEG studies. In addition, ictal behaviors may relate to seizure propagation and provide few clues regarding the site of actual seizure onset. Another challenge to clinical localization in neocortical epilepsy is that seizures may be tonic-clonic without a clinically recognized focal seizure, or the focal seizure may be very brief or subtle, such as a brief stare with arrest of activity or hypermotor activity. To adequately localize seizures and tailor resections to spare eloquent cortex, the surgical evaluation in patients with neocortical epilepsy often includes functional or metabolic imaging and long-term intracranial EEG monitoring.[49,50]

MRI-negative focal epilepsy
- High-resolution MRI head seizure protocol study is negative for a pathologic substrate
- Patients may have focal seizures of temporal lobe or extratemporal origin

- Chronic intracranial EEG monitoring with stereoelectroencephalography (SEEG) or subdural grid-strip recordings are almost invariably used for surgical localization and functional mapping
- Surgical outcomes in these patients are less favorable than in individuals with an epileptogenic lesion or MTS
- Surgical pathology may reveal FCD

SEEG is an older intracranial EEG technique for seizure localization that has reemerged as a pivotal tool in evaluating patients with DRE being considered for surgical treatment (**Fig. 6**).[49–52] This method for intracranial monitoring does not require a craniotomy and may be a "minimally" invasive diagnostic technique. The overall morbidity and patient tolerance of SEEG compares favorably to subdural grid recordings.[51] SEEG may be preferred in patients with diagnostic uncertainty regarding the lateralization or localization of seizure onset and in seizures suspected to emanate from sequestered cortex, for example, insula.

Unfortunately, despite the use of functional neuroimaging and chronic intracranial EEG monitoring, the surgical outcome is less favorable in patients with MRI-negative compared with medial temporal lobe epilepsy and lesional epilepsy. Perhaps 30% to 40% of patients with MRI-negative focal epilepsy of extratemporal origin are rendered seizure-free following focal cortical resection.[48]

EPILEPSY SURGERY IN CONTEMPORARY PRACTICE

Epilepsy surgery is significantly underutilized despite randomized clinical trials demonstrating the superiority of surgery compared with "best" medical therapy.[34–36]

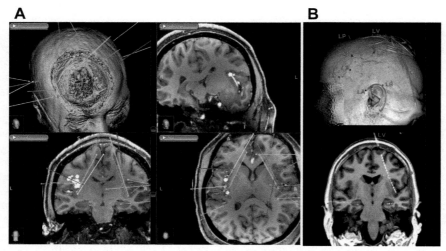

Fig. 6. Stereotactic implantation of electrodes enables invasive EEG monitoring with reduced invasiveness compared with grid and strip electrodes introduced via craniotomy. (*A*) Anatomic structures and functional features (magnetoencephalography dipoles, white spheres) are targeted with linear trajectories in a stereotactic planning system. Gadolinium (MRI) or iodine (CT) contrast-enhanced images (not shown) are used to visualize and avoid vessels when placing trajectories. (*B*) Following electrode implantation, CT images are acquired showing the locations of electrode contacts. The CT images are coregistered to preoperative MRI. Three-dimensional renderings (*top*) illustrate electrode entry points, and oblique slices (*bottom*) show the contact positions in relation to anatomic structures.

A population-based study using the US Nationwide Inpatient Sample found that there were 6653 resective surgeries from 1990 to 2008, and there was no growth trend over this time period.[53] There are several potential reasons for the lack of referral of patients to comprehensive epilepsy centers that have been identified including concerns regarding operative morbidity and the attitude of the neurologists that surgical treatment is a procedure of "last resort."[54–57] Most perioperative complications are relatively "minor" or transient; significant treatment-related adverse effects are relatively uncommon.[57] The use of multiple ASDs in combination with neuromodulation, for example, vagus nerve stimulation, may be preferred to epilepsy surgery in clinical practice. Unfortunately, in patients with DRE medical therapy and neuromodulation are usually *palliative* and not *curative* treatments. An unnecessary delay in referring patients for epilepsy surgery with surgically remediable epileptic syndromes may have devastating effects on the individuals' psychosocial development and quality of life. There are strong compelling reasons to consider early and effective treatment of pharmacoresistant seizure disorders, as DRE can be a progressive and fatal illness.[58,59]

The patient population being referred for epilepsy surgery has changed in the past few years at major epilepsy centers.[60,61] People with medial temporal lobe epilepsy associated with MTS are less commonly being considered for surgical treatment.[60,61] There are a greater number of patients with MRI-negative focal epilepsy and multilobar seizures being considered. This would explain the increase interest in chronic intracranial EEG monitoring using SEEG.[49–51] Finally, an important challenge that remains is the patient disparities that remain regarding access to surgical epilepsy centers. There are racial disparities that have been identified that indicate that people of color are less likely to undergo epilepsy surgery.[62] Treatment gaps have been identified, which suggest that selected patient populations have barriers to access for surgical evaluations and treatment.[53]

RESOURCES

National Association of Epilepsy Centers: www.naec-epilepsy.org.
  American Academy of Neurology: www.aan.com.
  American Epilepsy Society: www.aesnet.org.
  Epilepsy Foundation: www.epilepsy.com.

CLINICS CARE POINTS

- Patients with drug-resistant focal epilepsy should be evaluated for surgical treatment. For many patients surgical resection of a discrete seizure focus represents the best chance for seizure freedom.

REFERENCES

1. Zack MM, Kobau R. National and state estimates of the numbers of adults and children with active epilepsy — United States, 2015. MMWR Morb Mortal Wkly Rep 2017;66:821–5.
2. Russ SA, Larson K, Halfon N. A national profile of childhood epilepsy and seizure disorder. Pediatrics 2012;129:256–64.
3. Hesdorffer DC, Beck V, Begley CE, et al. Research implications of the Institute of Medicine report, epilepsy across the spectrum: promoting health and understanding. Epilepsia 2013;54:207–16.
4. Falco-Walter JJ, Scheffer IE, Fisher RS. The new definition and classification of seizures and epilepsy. Epilepsy Res 2018;139:73–9.

5. Kwan P, Arzimanoglou A, Berg AT, et al. Definition of drug resistant epilepsy: consensus proposal by the Ad Hoc task force of the ILAE Commission on therapeutic strategies. Epilepsia 2010;51:1069–77.

6. Fisher RS, Acevedo C, Arzimanoglou A, et al. ILAE official report: a practical clinical definition of epilepsy. Epilepsia 2014;55:475–82.

7. Kwan P, Arzimanoglou A, Berg AT, et al. Definition of drug resistant epilepsy: consensus proposal by the ad hoc task force of the ILAE commission on therapeutic strategies. Epilepsia 2010;51:1069–77.

8. Jette N, Engel J Jr. Refractory epilepsy is a life-threatening disease: lest we forget. Neurology 2016;86:1932–3.

9. Jobst BC, Cascino GD. Resective epilepsy surgery for drug-resistant focal epilepsy: a review. JAMA 2015;313:285–93.

10. Engel J Jr, Wiebe S, French J, et al. Practice parameter: temporal lobe and localized neocortical resections for epilepsy: report of the Quality Standards Subcommittee of the American Academy of Neurology, in association with the American Epilepsy Society and the American Association of Neurological Surgeons. Neurology 2003;60:538–47.

11. Sperling MR, Harris A, Nei M, et al. Mortality after epilepsy surgery. Epilepsia 2005;46:49–53.

12. Sperling MR, Barshow S, Nei M, et al. A reappraisal of mortality after epilepsy surgery. Neurology 2016;86:1938–44.

13. Fabris RR, Cascino TG, Mandrekar J, et al. Drug-resistant focal epilepsy in women of childbearing age: reproduction and the effect of epilepsy surgery. Epilepsy Behav 2016;60:17–20.

14. Junna MR, Buechler R, Cohen-Gadol AA, et al. Prognostic importance of risk factors for temporal lobe epilepsy in patients undergoing surgical treatment. Mayo Clin Proc 2013;88:332–6.

15. Cascino GD, Trenerry MR, So E, et al. Routine EEG and temporal lobe epilepsy: relation to long-term EEG monitoring, quantitative MRI, and operative outcome. Epilepsia 1996;37:651–6.

16. Radhakrishnan K, So EL, Silbert PL, et al. Predictors of outcome of anterior temporal lobectomy for intractable epilepsy: a multivariate study. Neurology 1998;51:465–71.

17. Jones AL, Cascino GD. Evidence on use of neuroimaging for surgical treatment of temporal lobe epilepsy: a systematic review. JAMA Neurol 2016;73:464–70.

18. Trenerry MR, Jack CR Jr, Ivnik RJ, et al. MRI hippocampal volumes and memory function before and after temporal lobectomy. Neurology 1993;43:1800–5.

19. Jack CR Jr, Rydberg CH, Krecke KN, et al. Mesial temporal sclerosis: diagnosis with fluid-attenuated inversion-recovery versus spin-echo MR imaging. Radiology 1996;199:367–73.

20. Kuzniecky RI, Bilir E, Gilliam F, et al. Multimodality MRI in mesial temporal sclerosis: relative sensitivity and specificity. Neurology 1997;49:774–8.

21. Cendes F, Theodore WH, Brinkmann BH, et al. Neuroimaging of epilepsy. Handb Clin Neurol 2016;136:985–1014.

22. Cascino GD, Jack CR Jr, Parisi JE, et al. Magnetic resonance imaging-based volume studies in temporal lobe epilepsy: pathological correlations. Ann Neurol 1991;30:31–6.

23. LoPinto-Khoury C, Sperling MR, Skidmore C, et al. Surgical outcome in PET-positive, MRI-negative patients with temporal lobe epilepsy. Epilepsia 2012;53:342–8.

24. Chassoux F, Rodrigo S, Semah F, et al. FDG-PET improves surgical outcome in negative MRI Taylor-type focal cortical dysplasias. Neurology 2010;75:2168–75.
25. O'Brien TJ, So EL, Mullan BP, et al. Subtraction ictal SPECT co-registered to MRI improves clinical usefulness of SPECT in localizing the surgical seizure focus. Neurology 1998;50:445–54.
26. Sulc V, Stykel S, Hanson DP, et al. Statistical SPECT processing in MRI-negative epilepsy surgery. Neurology 2014;82:932–9.
27. Szaflarski JP, Gloss D, Binder JR, et al. Practice guideline summary: use of fMRI in the presurgical evaluation of patients with epilepsy: Report of the Guideline Development, Dissemination, and Implementation Subcommittee of the American Academy of Neurology. Neurology 2017;88:395–402.
28. Stroup E, Langfitt J, Berg M, et al. Predicting verbal memory decline following anterior temporal lobectomy (ATL). Neurology 2003;60:1266–73.
29. Engel J Jr, Wiebe S, French J, et al. Practice parameter: temporal lobe and localized neocortical resections for epilepsy. Epilepsia 2003;44:741–51.
30. Jeha LE, Najm IM, Bingaman WE, et al. Predictors of outcome after temporal lobectomy for the treatment of intractable epilepsy. Neurology 2006;66:1938–40.
31. Cohen-Gadol AA, Wilhelmi BG, Collignon F, et al. Long-term outcome of epilepsy surgery among 399 patients with nonlesional seizure foci including mesial temporal lobe sclerosis. J Neurosurg 2006;104:513–24.
32. Brown MG, Drees C, Nagae LM, et al. Curative and palliative MRI-guided laser ablation for drug-resistant epilepsy. J Neurol Neurosurg Psychiatry 2018;89:425–33.
33. Shimamoto S, Wu C, Sperling MR. Laser interstitial thermal therapy in drug-resistant epilepsy. Curr Opin Neurol 2019;32:237–45.
34. Wiebe S, Blume WT, Girvin JP, et al. A randomized, controlled trial of surgery for temporal-lobe epilepsy. N Engl J Med 2001;345:311–8.
35. Engel J Jr, McDermott MP, Wiebe S, et al. Early surgical therapy for drug-resistant temporal lobe epilepsy: a randomized trial. JAMA 2012;307:922–30.
36. Spencer SS, Berg AT, Vickrey BG, et al. Predicting long-term seizure outcome after resective epilepsy surgery: the multicenter study. Neurology 2005;65:912–8.
37. Burkholder DB, Sulc V, Hoffman EM, et al. Interictal scalp electroencephalography and intraoperative electrocorticography in magnetic resonance imaging-negative temporal lobe epilepsy surgery. JAMA Neurol 2014;71:702–9.
38. Tassi L, Meroni A, Deleo F, et al. Temporal lobe epilepsy: neuropathological and clinical correlations in 243 surgically treated patients. Epileptic Disord 2009;11:281–92.
39. Bonney PA, Boettcher LB, Conner AK, et al. Review of seizure outcomes after surgical resection of dysembryoplastic neuroepithelial tumors. J Neurooncol 2016;126:1–10.
40. Giulioni M, Marucci G, Pelliccia V, et al. Epilepsy surgery of "low grade epilepsy associated neuroepithelial tumors": a retrospective nationwide Italian study. Epilepsia 2017;58:1832–41.
41. Nolan MA, Sakuta R, Chuang N, et al. Dysembryoplastic neuroepithelial tumors in childhood: long-term outcome and prognostic features. Neurology 2004;62:2270–6.
42. Kwon CS, Sheth SA, Walcott BP, et al. Long-term seizure outcomes following resection of supratentorial cavernous malformations. Clin Neurol Neurosurg 2013;115:2377–81.

43. Baumann CR, Acciarri N, Bertalanffy H, et al. Seizure outcome after resection of supratentorial cavernous malformations: a study of 168 patients. Epilepsia 2007; 48:559–63.

44. Blümcke I, Thom M, Aronica E, et al. The clinicopathologic spectrum of focal cortical dysplasias: a consensus classification proposed by an ad hoc Task Force of the ILAE Diagnostic Methods Commission. Epilepsia 2011;52:158–74.

45. Kim DW, Lee SK, Chu K, et al. Predictors of surgical outcome and pathologic considerations in focal cortical dysplasia. Neurology 2009;72:211–6.

46. Giulioni M, Licchetta L, Bisulli F, et al. Tailored surgery for drug-resistant epilepsy due to temporal pole encephalocele and microdysgenesis. Seizure 2014;23: 164–6.

47. Urbach H, Jamneala G, Mader I, et al. Temporal lobe epilepsy due to meningoencephaloceles into the greater sphenoid wing: a consequence of idiopathic intracranial hypertension? Neuroradiology 2018;60:51–60.

48. Noe K, Sulc V, Wong-Kisiel L, et al. Long-term outcomes after nonlesional extratemporal lobe epilepsy surgery. JAMA Neurol 2013;70:1003–8.

49. Gonzalez-Martinez J, Mullin J, Bulacio J, et al. Stereoelectroencephalography in children and adolescents with difficult-to-localize refractory focal epilepsy. Neurosurgery 2014;75:258–68.

50. Serletis D, Bulacio J, Bingaman W, et al. The stereotactic approach for mapping epileptic networks: a prospective study of 200 patients. J Neurosurg 2014;121: 1239–46.

51. Tandon N, Tong BA, Friedman ER, et al. Analysis of morbidity and outcomes associated with use of subdural grids vs stereoelectroencephalography in patients with intractable epilepsy. JAMA Neurol 2019;76:672–81.

52. Englot DJ, Ouyang D, Garcia PA, et al. Epilepsy surgery trends in the United States, 1990-2008. Neurology 2012;78:1200–6.

53. Jette N, Sander JW, Keezer MR. Surgical treatment for epilepsy: the potential gap between evidence and practice. Lancet Neurol 2016;15:982–94.

54. Engel J Jr. Why is there still doubt to cut it out? Epilepsy Curr 2013;13:198–204.

55. Roberts JI, Hrazdil C, Wiebe S, et al. Neurologists' knowledge of and attitudes toward epilepsy surgery: a national survey. Neurology 2015;84:159–66.

56. Berg AT, Langfitt JT, Cascino GD. The changing landscape of epilepsy surgery: no longer the "last resort". Neurology 2018;91:55–6.

57. Hader WJ, Tellez-Zenteno J, Metcalfe A, et al. Complications of epilepsy surgery: a systematic review of focal surgical resections and invasive EEG monitoring. Epilepsia 2013;54:840–7.

58. Gomez-Alonso J, Cascino G. Temporal lobe epilepsy is a progressive neurologic disorder: time means neurons! Neurology 2010;74:347.

59. Engel J Jr. Evolution of concepts in epilepsy surgery. Epileptic Disord 2019;21: 391–409.

60. Jehi L, Friedman D, Carlson C, et al. The evolution of epilepsy surgery between 1991 and 2011 in nine major epilepsy centers across the United States, Germany, and Australia. Epilepsia 2015;56:1526–33.

61. Van Gompel JJ, Ottman R, Worrell GA, et al. Use of anterior temporal lobectomy for epilepsy in a community-based population. Arch Neurol 2012;69:1476–81.

62. Burneo JG, Black L, Knowlton RC, et al. Racial disparities in the use of surgical treatment for intractable temporal lobe epilepsy. Neurology 2005;64:50–4.

Treatment of Viral Encephalitis

Allen J. Aksamit Jr, MD

KEYWORDS

- Herpes simplex encephalitis (HSE) • Anti-NMDA receptor (NMDA-R) encephalitis
- Varicella zoster virus (VZV) encephalitis • West Nile virus (WNV) encephalitis
- Eastern equine encephalitis virus (EEE)
- Progressive multifocal leukoencephalopathy (PML)

KEY POINTS

- Herpes simplex encephalitis has standardized therapy that should be started empirically if the diagnosis is considered. Rare cases can have an autoimmune NMDA receptor encephalitis following infection with herpes simplex that can be treated.
- Arthropod-borne encephalitides, such as West Nile virus encephalitis and Eastern equine encephalitis, have limited studies suggesting positive outcome with immunoglobulin treatment. Treatment of these disorders remains supportive.
- Progressive multifocal leukoencephalopathy has no proven treatment, but new attempts using immune stimulation therapy have shown limited promise.

INTRODUCTION

The timing for the submission of this article coincides with a unique time in history, when we are challenged by the pandemic of Coronavirus Disease 2019 (COVID-19). There is great uncertainty about how best to treat the COVID-19 illness, which parallels the challenges of treating viral infections in general. There are few options for treatment of viral encephalitis. Besides herpes simplex encephalitis (HSE), and its rare complication of N-methyl-D-aspartate (NMDA)-receptor encephalitis afterward due to autoimmune mechanisms that can be successfully treated, there are few well-established treatments for viral encephalitis. This discussion seeks to summarize current knowledge of treatment in selected topics of viral encephalitis. It will not cover human immunodeficiency virus (HIV) encephalitis, as its treatment parallels the treatment for HIV disease and is deserving of a discussion by itself. The treatment is nuanced and somewhat controversial, as antiretroviral therapy variably penetrates the central nervous system, although penetration may not dictate success of therapy. Most of the encephalitis-causing viruses are not mentioned in this discussion because they

Department of Neurology, Mayo Clinic, 200 First Street Southwest, Rochester, MN 55905, USA
E-mail address: aksamit@mayo.edu

Neurol Clin 39 (2021) 197–207
https://doi.org/10.1016/j.ncl.2020.09.011
0733-8619/21/© 2020 Elsevier Inc. All rights reserved.

have no specific treatment other than supportive care. Exciting new therapy that may (or may not) succeed in treating progressive multifocal leukoencephalopathy (PML) has emerged and is discussed.

By definition, encephalitis is an inflammation of the parenchyma of the brain. Viral encephalitis implies that a virus directly invades and replicates in cells within the brain. The term "encephalitis" also indicates a clinical syndrome arising from infection and inflammation in the parenchyma, rather than in the leptomeninges. When both the leptomeninges and brain parenchyma are involved, the term "meningoencephalitis" is preferred. In para-infectious encephalitis, a systemic viral infection is associated with a febrile encephalopathy, sometimes with inflammatory spinal fluid but without direct evidence of brain invasion by the virus. When a pathologically purulent infection is produced, the preferred term is cerebritis, which is more connected to bacterial infections.

Viral encephalitis has an estimated incidence of 7 per 100,000 per year.[1] In general, a specific cause is identified in less than 50% of patients in the United States.[2] Many viruses (**Boxes 1** and **2**[3,4]) have been implicated as the cause. Spinal fluid testing by serologic identification or nucleic acid identification (by polymerase chain reaction [PCR]) is generally required to identify the specific etiologic virus.[1,5] The epidemiology of each virus responsible for central nervous system infection is distinct in terms of the patients who are at highest risk, geographic distribution, and seasonal occurrence, which is especially important for the arboviruses and enteroviruses. The details of epidemiology and incidence are beyond the scope of this discussion, which is focused here on the treatment. There are several excellent consensus documents from around the world that summarize much of the data about etiology and diagnostic testing.[6–9]

A common treatment associated with encephalitis is the treatment of seizures. In the context of encephalitis, seizures are common and frequently refractory to antiepileptic drugs. However, the seizures themselves can increase morbidity and mortality,

---

Box 1
Common causes of encephalitis in the United States

A. Nonseasonal
   Herpes simplex virus type 1 (herpes simplex encephalitis)
   Herpes simplex virus type 2 (neonatal encephalitis or adult meningoencephalitis)

B. Seasonal: summer and fall—arboviruses (arthropod-borne)
   West Nile virus
   St. Louis encephalitis virus
   Eastern equine encephalitis virus
   Western equine encephalitis virus
   La Crosse/California encephalitis virus

C. Seasonal: non–arthropod-borne
   Summer and fall: enteroviruses (including coxsackie viruses, echoviruses, polioviruses, and enterovirus 71)
   Winter: influenza virus

D. Immunosuppressed patients
   Human immunodeficiency virus (chronic HIV encephalitis)
   Varicella zoster virus (subacute encephalitis)
   John Cunningham (JC) virus (progressive multifocal leukoencephalopathy)
   Cytomegalovirus (ventriculitis or encephalitis)
   Human herpesvirus 6 (subacute encephalitis)
   Epstein-Barr virus (subacute encephalitis)

> **Box 2**
> **Uncommon causes of viral encephalitis in the United States**
>
> Causes originating within the United States
>   Powassan encephalitis virus
>   Jamestown Canyon virus
>   Cache Valley Virus
>   Zika virus[3]
>   Chikungunya virus[4]
>   Variegated squirrel borna virus
>   Lymphotropic choriomeningitis virus
>   Rabies
>   Measles (subacute sclerosing panencephalitis)
>   Mumps
>   Adenovirus
>   Herpes B virus (of monkeys)
>   Rubella (progressive rubella panencephalitis)
>
> Causes originating outside the United States
>   Zika virus[3]
>   Tick-borne encephalitis virus (Russia, Asia)
>   Japanese encephalitis virus (Japan, Southeast Asia, Malaysia)
>   Venezuelan equine encephalitis virus (Central and South America)
>   Dengue virus (Southern Asia, Africa, South America)
>   Rift Valley fever virus (east central Africa)
>   Murray Valley encephalitis virus (Australia)
>   Powassan encephalitis virus (Canada)
>   Nipah virus (Malaysia and Bangladesh)

so vigorous treatment attempts are required. Epilepsy treatment is beyond the scope of this discussion.

HERPETIC VIRAL ENCEPHALITIDES
Herpes Simplex Encephalitis

HSE remains the most common nonepidemic viral encephalitis in the United States. It causes 10% of encephalitis in the United States.[10] Epidemiology estimates 1 case per 250,000 to 500,000 individuals per year. Great strides have been made in the success of diagnosis, with sensitive PCR techniques, and characteristic MRI findings.[11] Herpes simplex type 1 virus (HSV-1) is the usual virus identified, with more than 90% of cases related to HSV-1. It tends to cause clinical signs of focal cortical neurologic deficits including hemiparesis, aphasia, and seizures. HSE commonly involves limbic parts of the brain, which can lead to prominent behavioral changes at the beginning of the illness before the patient's level of consciousness is depressed. Focal or generalized seizures are particularly common when encephalitis affects the cerebral cortex, especially the temporal lobes.

Before acyclovir (and the drug used to treat it previously, vidarabine), 70% of patients died of infection.[12] Even using acyclovir, which is the current therapy, mortality is still 15%, and fewer than 20% of patients are able to return to full-time employment after treatment, often because of cognitive deficits that persist.

Multicenter prospective trial results emphasize that early treatment affects outcome.[13] When HSE is suspected in the acute setting by the presence of focal signs or symptoms, early empirical treatment is recommended even while the diagnostic evaluation is proceeding. The current therapy-of-choice treatment is intravenous acyclovir (10 mg/kg every 8 hours for 14–21 days). The original trial in the 1980s was performed with 14 days of intravenous therapy.[13] However since that time, given the relatively low toxicity of acyclovir, experts have recommended 21 days of therapy for patients with severe neurologic deficits or at risk for immunosuppression or a more severe course. However, given the difficulty of obtaining prospective data in this rare disease, a controlled trial to support a longer duration of therapy or higher doses of acyclovir to improve neurologic outcomes has not been performed.

A trial of prolonged oral valacyclovir after the standard 2 weeks of intravenous acyclovir was performed in a group of patients who had relatively mild disease (ie, they were able to take oral medications and comply with protocol). However, oral valacyclovir did not change the severity of neurologic deficits between placebo and active oral medication at 6 and 12 months of follow-up.[14]

Herpes Simplex Encephalitis and Steroids

It has been long speculated that the severe injury to the brain as a consequence of HSE and the persistent neurologic deficits occur not only because of active infection but also because of a significant immune response to the virus by the host. Pathology with significant necrotizing immune response has been considered important in generating brain injury and persistent neurologic deficits. Because immune factors play a role in injury, corticosteroids with antiviral therapy were proposed to attenuate the immune response and lessen long-term deficits. This was initially tested in a multicenter, multinational German protocol using acyclovir and corticosteroids; 2 doses of dexamethasone, 40 mg, were given every 24 hours for 4 days with acyclovir and compared with acyclovir alone.[15] The trial closed due to insufficient enrollment, and the results have never been published.

More recently, another European multicenter trial of dexamethasone in herpes simplex virus encephalitis was initiated in the United Kingdom: https://clinicaltrials.gov/ct2/show/NCT03084783?term=encephalitis&cond=NCT03084783&rank=1=.[16,17] It is currently enrolling (Dexamethasone in Herpes Simplex Virus Encephalitis (DexEnceph) - http://www.encephalitis.info/). To combine data and improve power of the study, a trial is currently being carried out in France with the same protocol that compares dexamethasone with placebo with both arms initially treating in combination with acyclovir.[17]

N-Methyl-D-Aspartate Receptor Encephalitis After Herpes Simplex Encephalitis

Autoimmune encephalitis has been described and confirmed as a consequence in a minority of patients who have had HSE. Before this was recognized as a definitive entity, a minority of patients were recognized as having a clinical course that seemingly suggested clinical relapse after HSE. However, this apparent relapse with worsening focal clinical disease and worsening MRI abnormalities, is unaccompanied by the usual viral confirmation of herpes simplex virus PCR in the spinal fluid. This was initially described as a "biphasic illness." It typically occurs as a relapse in the first 1 to 7 weeks after the initial diagnosis of HSE. This was initially described in adults[18] and then in children who experienced HSE.[19] Eventually, once the recognition of autoimmune encephalitis-associated NMDA receptor (NMDAR) antibodies was described, testing revealed that patients who had apparent relapse of HSE without detectable virus actually had NMDAR antibodies in the spinal fluid.[20,21] The exact frequency and risk factors that determine clinical worsening and NMDAR antibodies in the spinal fluid have not been described. This rare complication of a rare disorder makes uncertainty the rule about risks and outcomes of this complication.[22]

In the largest study published to date, which enrolled 51 patients with HSE,[22] none of the patients initially had antibodies to neuronal antigens in the spinal fluid. Fourteen

(27%) of patients developed autoimmune encephalitis (date range: 17−63 days after diagnosis), and all had neuronal antibodies (cerebrospinal fluid [CSF] analysis was most sensitive). Nine (64%) had NMDAR antibodies, and 5 [36%] had other neural antibodies at or before onset of relapse symptoms. The other 37 patients did not develop autoimmune encephalitis. Among the patients who did not develop autoimmune encephalitis after herpes simplex, 11 (30%) developed antibodies (n = 3 to NMDAR, n = 8 to unknown antigens), implying that the presence of antibodies does not always predict the occurrence of autoimmune encephalitis as a complication of HSE. However, antibody detection within 3 weeks of HSE was a statistically significant risk factor for autoimmune encephalitis.

Autoimmune-relapse, post-HSE may respond to corticosteroids, intravenous immunoglobulin (IVIg), or plasma exchange, but no randomized trials are available. There is no universal agreement about how to treat this entity. Once clinical deterioration and worsening imaging has been detected, patients typically receive 5 days of intravenous (IV) methylprednisolone, 1 g each day, followed by oral steroids initiated typically at 60 mg of prednisone per day followed by a taper.[22] IVIg may be considered in patients who cannot tolerate steroids. Plasma exchange may be used in patients with treatment-refractory disease or in patients with contraindications to other treatments.

Other Viruses in the Herpes Virus Group

Varicella zoster virus meningoencephalitis

Although rare, varicella zoster virus (VZV) meningoencephalitis can occur as a complication of cutaneous zoster, occasionally without overt cutaneous manifestations. Older individuals and immunosuppressed hosts are most vulnerable to this complication of zoster encephalitis. Typical treatment is a regimen similar to that for HSE with acyclovir, 10 mg/kg, IV, every 8 hours for 14 days. No prospective trials exist to confirm that this is satisfactory, and some investigators suggest a ≥21-day course of acyclovir, particularly in immunosuppressed hosts with more severe disease.[9,23]

Cytomegalovirus meningoencephalitis

Cytomegalovirus (CMV) produces a characteristic ventriculitis or ascending asymmetric polyradiculopathy in immunosuppressed hosts, best described in patients with acquired immunodeficiency syndrome (AIDS). Improvements in antiretroviral therapy in the past 20 years have made this serious neurologic infection uncommon. MRI shows characteristic ependymal ventricular enhancement with gadolinium imaging. CMV PCR in the spinal fluid is usually positive and confirmatory of CSF dissemination of the virus. Typical treatment for cytomegalovirus is ganciclovir, 5 mg/kg IV every 12 hours plus foscarnet 90 mg/kg for 2 weeks.[9,24] Cidofovir, administered at 5 mg/kg IV weekly for 2 weeks, is more controversial because it does not penetrate the blood-brain barrier.

Epstein-Barr virus encephalitis

Diagnosis of this entity is challenging because the spinal fluid of patients with immunosuppressive illness and other causes for encephalitis can yield false-positive PCR results. Epstein-Barr serology in the blood is ubiquitous in the population and is not sensitive or specific for patients with encephalitis. Furthermore, Epstein-Barr virus (EBV) can reactivate systemically at times of other illness, and lymphocytes carrying EBV from the systemic circulation can be recruited to the nervous system as part of the inflammatory response. This may produce a false-positive PCR, when another agent is responsible for the patient's clinical encephalitis. PCR for EBV has, however, been useful in detecting opportunistic, EBV-driven lymphoma in immunosuppressed hosts and in the AIDS population. Currently, no specific treatments are effective for EBV. Patients have variably been treated with corticosteroids, but the potential risks must be weighed against the benefits.[9]

Human herpes virus 6

Variable success has been reported for treatment of human herpes virus 6 (HHV-6) encephalitis in hematopoietic stem cell transplant recipients using ganciclovir, foscarnet, or valganciclovir, alone or in combination.[25] The treatment recommendation for HHV-6 encephalitis is foscarnet (60 mg/kg every 8 hours for both A and B variants). Ganciclovir (5 mg/kg every 12 hours) is an alternative option only for the B variant of HHV-6 encephalitis.[7]

Effective antiviral therapy does not exist for most forms of viral encephalitis, except for HSE.[12] However, because of the usual delay in establishing or excluding the diagnosis of HSE, patients suspected of having encephalitis should start acyclovir therapy (10 mg/kg IV every 8 hours for 2 weeks), while specific serologic and spinal fluid analyses are being performed to make a diagnosis. Supportive measures for patients with encephalitis typically include intensive care unit treatment in the initial phases of the illness, directed at reducing intracranial pressure, and treating seizures that are a common accompaniment.

NON-HERPETIC VIRAL ENCEPHALITIDES
West Nile Virus Encephalitis

The most common epidemic viral encephalitis in the United States is now West Nile virus (WNV). WNV encephalitis was unknown in the United States until 1999. This is a mosquito-borne arbovirus, introduced presumably by infected animals, with birds being the principal intermediate host. Human disease is not transmissible from human to human, except in unusual circumstances like transplanted organs or blood transfusion. It is estimated that only 1% to 2% of patients infected with WNV develop central nervous system disease. Neuro-invasive disease manifestations include meningitis (25%–40%), encephalitis (55%–60%), or acute flaccid paralysis (5%–10%). Meningitis can occur in any age group, unlike encephalitis, which is more common in the elderly or immune suppressed. Acute flaccid myelitis ("poliomyelitis") can occur in any age group.

The diagnosis is usually confirmed by identification of anti-WNV IgM in CSF in the acute setting of encephalitis symptoms often with impaired consciousness. Positive serum serology indicates exposure but not necessarily neuro-invasive disease. West Nile encephalitis cases show a high incidence of polymorphonuclear cell predominance in the CSF.[26]

Currently, there is no successful treatment for WNV encephalitis. However, some agents have been proposed and used, so far without generalized success. Two patients with serologic confirmation of WNV infection, who presented with deteriorating mental status and progression to coma, were treated with standard interferon alpha-2b within 72 hours of presentation.[27] Within 48 hours after initiation of therapy, both patients demonstrated rapid neurologic improvement. It remains unclear if the change in clinical status was due to interferon or to spontaneous improvement. Scattered reports of open-label interferon alpha used in other patients were regarded as unsuccessful.[28,29]

A large, multicenter, phase-2 trial of IVIg enriched with antibodies against WNV was conceived and organized by the Collaborative Antiviral Study Group. The study with 62 patients enrolled was published recently with negative results.[30]

Ribavirin has been tried in a few cases. It was not considered to be beneficial, and concern was raised that it might actually harmful and therefore not recommended by the Infectious Disease Society of America.[9]

Commercial pharmaceutical attempts have created synthetic anti-sense RNA as inhibitors of WNV replication. Those have not yet come to clinical trial.[31]

Eastern Equine Encephalitis Virus

Eastern equine encephalitis (EEE) is established in the United States, but outbreaks have fortunately been rare. The clinical manifestations can be quite severe, and the disease, transmitted by mosquitos, usually presents with fever, mental status changes, and seizures. This disease has a very high mortality (65% in some series). Focal cerebral signs are common, including increased intracranial pressure, and CSF white blood cell counts can exceed 1000 mm^3. It is typically diagnosed by positive EEE serology in the spinal fluid. Positive serum serology suggests recent exposure and is suspicious for the cause of the encephalitis.

There has been a recent outbreak in the United States. As of December 17, 2019, the Centers for Disease Control and Prevention has received reports of 38 confirmed cases of EEE virus disease for this year including 15 deaths.[32] Treatment is supportive. There have been attempts to treat the disease with IVIg, and 2 case reports have suggested some benefit.[33,34] However, there are no prospective trials.

PROGRESSIVE MULTIFOCAL LEUKOENCEPHALOPATHY

PML is a primary demyelinating disease of the central nervous system caused by infection with John Cunningham (JC) virus, which infects oligodendrocytes, killing those cells selectively and leading to focal demyelination, which spreads in a circumferential pattern to adjacent, uninfected cells. This disease does not present as typical encephalitis. It produces a subacute, focal neurologic deficit, more strokelike that progresses over time without fever, usually with normal spinal fluid cell count. It is a disease of immunosuppressed hosts, most commonly seen in association with AIDS or a lympho-reticular malignancy like lymphoma or chronic lymphocytic leukemia. It can occur in any immunosuppressed state with compromise of cell-mediated immunity. Thus, transplant patients and patients with exogenous immunosuppression, such as rheumatological conditions, are vulnerable. In the past 15 years, much attention has been focused on the occurrence of PML in patients with multiple sclerosis (MS) treated with immunosuppressive drugs, most prominently natalizumab. However, many of the MS disease-modifying agents carry a risk of PML.[35]

Treatment for PML has been disappointingly unsuccessful until recently, when there have been small series of open-label treatments of patients with immune-modifying drugs. Past medications included cytosine arabinoside (ARA-C), which was originally tried in the 1970s and 1980s as a PML treatment because of the antiviral effect of the nucleoside analog ARA-C interfering with DNA replication of JC virus. A small open-label series in non-AIDS patients suggested that approximately one-third had a nonfatal outcome, and some even had neurologic improvement.[36] However, a prospective trial in patients with AIDS was considered unsuccessfull.[37] There were delays in initiating ARA-C in the prospective trial that may have influenced the outcome.

The serologic monitoring of patients of JC virus in patients with MS considering treatment with disease-modifying therapy is based on antibodies in the blood, and the decision to select specific therapy for MS is beyond the scope of this discussion. The diagnosis of PML in MS, however, is similar to the diagnosis of PML in patients with other immunosuppressive illness and relies on JC virus PCR detection in the spinal fluid. That assay is only approximately 70% sensitive.

Treatment of patients with MS who developed PML after taking natalizumab requires specific discussion. When natalizumab was initially released, a higher incidence of PML was recognized than had been noted in clinical trials of the drug. The drug was suspended from use and then reintroduced with safety-monitoring requirements.[36] However, management of the PML, once diagnosed in the context of natalizumab-associated therapy or other immune-modifying therapy for MS, should lead to specific treatment. Management of PML has routinely used plasma exchange (PLEX) to hasten clearance of natalizumab from the bloodstream. The patient's immune system is allowed to reconstitute and clear JC virus from the brain. PLEX has no known role in affecting virus clearing from the brain. However, exacerbation of symptoms and inflammation of lesions on MRI with clinical worsening have occurred indicative of immune reconstitution inflammatory syndrome (IRIS). IRIS seems to be more common and more severe in patients with natalizumab-associated PML than in patients with HIV-associated PML. If IRIS occurs, the treatment is to use high-dose IV methylprednisolone typically 1000 mg IV each day for 5 days and then a tapering dose of oral prednisone usually over 3 to 4 weeks, typically starting with 60 mg per day.

There has been some doubt expressed about whether plasmapheresis (PLEX) removes natalizumab from the body more quickly or, indeed, has any effect on the outcome of PML[37] One study looked at outcomes of patients with MS and natalizumab (NTZ)-associated progressive multifocal leukoencephalopathy in 193 international and 34 Italian NTZ-PML cases. PLEX did not improve the survival or clinical outcomes of Italian or international patients with MS and NTZ-PML,[37] This point is still being debated, but most experts would still recommend plasma exchange in the initial phase of treatment. The newer therapies discussed later in this article, which enhance immunity through the PD-1 pathway, should not be applied to patients with MS. These PD-1 inhibitor drugs are known to exacerbate MS.

AIDS-related PML is typically initially treated with optimizing antiretroviral therapy and attempts to clear virus from the brain by enhancing the patient's immune system with combined antiretroviral therapy (cART). Some other immune reconstitution strategies (see later in this article) have been suggested for patients with AIDS whose immune restoration is refractory to antiretroviral therapy.

For transplant recipients, immunosuppressive therapy can be tapered or discontinued temporarily until there is immune reconstitution and clearing of the virus from the brain. The possibility of organ rejection is a risk. In the case of patients on immunosuppressive therapy for autoimmune disease, the therapy can be discontinued for 2 to 3 months, allowing the patient's own immune system to reconstitute and help to clear the virus. These 2 situations require close clinical reexamination and monitoring with MRI scan to watch for neurologic worsening secondary to IRIS. Repeat spinal fluid PCR for JC virus may also help to guide therapy.

Immune-enhancing drugs like the PD-1 inhibitor pembrolizumab have been suggested as a novel therapy to restore immunity and treat PML. Pembrolizumab has shown promise in patients with leukemia, lymphoma-associated PML, or other conditions in which there is no other ability to reverse immune suppression.[38] This drug works through the PD-1 blockade and attempts to "reinvigorate" anti–JC virus immune activity. In a recent study, 8 adults with PML were administered pembrolizumab, 2 mg per kilogram of body weight every 4 to 6 weeks.[38] Five patients had clinical improvement or stabilization of PML accompanied by a reduction in the JC viral load in the CSF by PCR analysis. The other 3 patients had no meaningful change in outcome. At least 2 other cases have shown no clinical benefit when treated in this fashion.[39,40] The factors determining response to pembrolizumab may be due to exhausted T cells.[40,41] It was concluded that more study of immune checkpoint inhibitors in the treatment of PML is warranted.

Allogeneic BK virus-sensitized T cells have also been proposed as a treatment strategy for PML patients with no ability to reverse their immune-suppressed status, given the strong antigenic overlap between JC virus and BK virus.[42] In a small series, 3 PML-immunosuppressed patients, each with a different kind of immunosuppression, were treated with partially expanded ex vivo, HLA-matched, third-party–produced, cryopreserved BK virus–specific T cells. One patient was undergoing a conditioning regimen for cord-blood transplantation. Another had a myeloproliferative neoplasm treated with rituximab, and the third had AIDS. T-cell infusion in 2 of the patients, led to alleviation of the clinical signs and imaging features of PML, and clearing of JC virus from the cerebrospinal fluid. The other patient had a reduction in JC viral load and stabilization of symptoms that persisted until her death 8 months later. Two of the patients had IRIS and required treatment of IRIS as part of their therapy.

SUMMARY

Therapy for viral encephalitis remains largely supportive in many circumstances. Specific inroads have been achieved in selected virus infections. Strategies to develop immune therapy or more specific viral-targeted therapy appear promising. When dealing with encephalitis, questions about penetration of the central nervous system will remain. Perhaps the lessons learned in the treatment of COVID-19 will translate to future trials of viral encephalitis due to other viruses.

DISCLOSURE

The author has nothing to disclose.

REFERENCES

1. Vora NM, Holman RC, Mehal JM, et al. Burden of encephalitis-associated hospitalizations in the United States, 1998-2010. Neurology 2014;82(5):443–51.
2. Singh TD, Fugate JE, Rabinstein AA. The spectrum of acute encephalitis: causes, management, and predictors of outcome. Neurology 2015;84(4):359–66.
3. Carteaux G, Maquart M, Bedet A, et al. Zika virus associated with meningoencephalitis. N Engl J Med 2016;374(16):1595–6.
4. Gerardin P, Couderc T, Bintner M, et al. Chikungunya virus-associated encephalitis: a cohort study on La Reunion Island, 2005-2009. Neurology 2016;86(1): 94–102.
5. Leber AL, Everhart K, Balada-Llasat JM, et al. Multicenter evaluation of BioFire FilmArray meningitis/encephalitis panel for detection of bacteria, viruses, and yeast in cerebrospinal fluid specimens. J Clin Microbiol 2016;54(9):2251–61.
6. Britton PN, Eastwood K, Paterson B, et al. Consensus guidelines for the investigation and management of encephalitis in adults and children in Australia and New Zealand. Intern Med J 2015;45(5):563–76.
7. Steiner I, Budka H, Chaudhuri A, et al. Viral meningoencephalitis: a review of diagnostic methods and guidelines for management. Eur J Neurol 2010;17(8). 999-e57.
8. Venkatesan A, Tunkel AR, Bloch KC, et al. Case definitions, diagnostic algorithms, and priorities in encephalitis: consensus statement of the international encephalitis consortium. Clin Infect Dis 2013;57(8):1114–28.

9. Tunkel AR, Glaser CA, Bloch KC, et al. The management of encephalitis: clinical practice guidelines by the Infectious Diseases Society of America. Clin Infect Dis 2008;47(3):303–27.

10. Whitley RJ, Kimberlin DW. Herpes simplex encephalitis: children and adolescents. Semin Pediatr Infect Dis 2005;16(1):17–23.

11. Chow FC, Glaser CA, Sheriff H, et al. Use of clinical and neuroimaging characteristics to distinguish temporal lobe herpes simplex encephalitis from its mimics. Clin Infect Dis 2015;60(9):1377–83.

12. Skoldenberg B, Forsgren M, Alestig K, et al. Acyclovir versus vidarabine in herpes simplex encephalitis. Randomised multicentre study in consecutive Swedish patients. Lancet 1984;2(8405):707–11.

13. Whitley RJ, Alford CA, Hirsch MS, et al. Vidarabine versus acyclovir therapy in herpes simplex encephalitis. N Engl J Med 1986;314(3):144–9.

14. Gnann JW Jr, Skoldenberg B, Hart J, et al. Herpes simplex encephalitis: lack of clinical benefit of long-term valacyclovir therapy. Clin Infect Dis 2015;61(5): 683–91.

15. Martinez-Torres F, Menon S, Pritsch M, et al. Protocol for German trial of Acyclovir and corticosteroids in Herpes-simplex-virus-encephalitis (GACHE): a multicenter, multinational, randomized, double-blind, placebo-controlled German, Austrian and Dutch trial [ISRCTN45122933]. BMC Neurol 2008;8:40.

16. Solomon T, Hart IJ, Beeching NJ. Viral encephalitis: a clinician's guide. Pract Neurol 2007;7(5):288–305.

17. Stahl JP. Dexamethasone in herpes simplex virus encephalitis open label randomized controlled trial with an observer-blinded evaluation at 6 months. Grenoble, France Liverpool, UK: University Hospital, Grenoble; 2017.

18. Skoldenberg B, Aurelius E, Hjalmarsson A, et al. Incidence and pathogenesis of clinical relapse after herpes simplex encephalitis in adults. J Neurol 2006;253(2): 163–70.

19. De Tiege X, Rozenberg F, Des Portes V, et al. Herpes simplex encephalitis relapses in children: differentiation of two neurologic entities. Neurology 2003; 61(2):241–3.

20. Armangue T, Leypoldt F, Malaga I, et al. Herpes simplex virus encephalitis is a trigger of brain autoimmunity. Ann Neurol 2014;75(2):317–23.

21. Leypoldt F, Titulaer MJ, Aguilar E, et al. Herpes simplex virus-1 encephalitis can trigger anti-NMDA receptor encephalitis: case report. Neurology 2013;81(18): 1637–9.

22. Armangue T, Spatola M, Vlagea A, et al. Frequency, symptoms, risk factors, and outcomes of autoimmune encephalitis after herpes simplex encephalitis: a prospective observational study and retrospective analysis. Lancet Neurol 2018; 17(9):760–72.

23. De Broucker T, Mailles A, Chabrier S, et al. Acute varicella zoster encephalitis without evidence of primary vasculopathy in a case-series of 20 patients. Clin Microbiol Infect 2012;18(8):808–19.

24. Anduze-Faris BM, Fillet AM, Gozlan J, et al. Induction and maintenance therapy of cytomegalovirus central nervous system infection in HIV-infected patients. AIDS 2000;14(5):517–24.

25. Bhanushali MJ, Kranick SM, Freeman AF, et al. Human herpes 6 virus encephalitis complicating allogeneic hematopoietic stem cell transplantation. Neurology 2013;80(16):1494–500.

26. Tyler KL, Pape J, Goody RJ, et al. CSF findings in 250 patients with serologically confirmed West Nile virus meningitis and encephalitis. Neurology 2006;66(3): 361–5.

27. Kalil AC, Devetten MP, Singh S, et al. Use of interferon-alpha in patients with West Nile encephalitis: report of 2 cases. Clin Infect Dis 2005;40(5):764–6.

28. Chan-Tack KM, Forrest G. Failure of interferon alpha-2b in a patient with West Nile virus meningoencephalitis and acute flaccid paralysis. Scand J Infect Dis 2005; 37(11–12):944–6.

29. Penn RG, Guarner J, Sejvar JJ, et al. Persistent neuroinvasive West Nile virus infection in an immunocompromised patient. Clin Infect Dis 2006;42(5):680–3.

30. Gnann JW Jr, Agrawal A, Hart J, et al. Lack of Efficacy of High-Titered Immunoglobulin in Patients with West Nile Virus Central Nervous System Disease. Emerg Infect Dis 2019;25(11):2064–73.

31. Deas TS, Bennett CJ, Jones SA, et al. In vitro resistance selection and in vivo efficacy of morpholino oligomers against West Nile virus. Antimicrob Agents Chemother 2007;51(7):2470–82.

32. Eastern equine encephalitis. Atlanta (GA): Centers for Disease Control; 2019. Available at: https://www.cdc.gov/easternequineencephalitis/index.html. Accessed October 4, 2020.

33. Mukerji SS, Lam AD, Wilson MR. Eastern equine encephalitis treated with intravenous immunoglobulins. Neurohospitalist 2016;6(1):29–31.

34. Wendell LC, Potter NS, Roth JL, et al. Successful management of severe neuroinvasive eastern equine encephalitis. Neurocrit Care 2013;19(1):111–5.

35. Grebenciucova E, Berger JR. Progressive multifocal leukoencephalopathy. Neurol Clin 2018;36(4):739–50.

36. Clifford DB, De Luca A, Simpson DM, et al. Natalizumab-associated progressive multifocal leukoencephalopathy in patients with multiple sclerosis: lessons from 28 cases. Lancet Neurol 2010;9(4):438–46.

37. Landi D, De Rossi N, Zagaglia S, et al. No evidence of beneficial effects of plasmapheresis in natalizumab-associated PML. Neurology 2017;88(12):1144–52.

38. Cortese I, Muranski P, Enose-Akahata Y, et al. Pembrolizumab treatment for progressive multifocal leukoencephalopathy. N Engl J Med 2019;380(17):1597–605.

39. Kupper C, Heinrich J, Kamm K, et al. Pembrolizumab for progressive multifocal leukoencephalopathy due to primary immunodeficiency. Neurol Neuroimmunol Neuroinflamm 2019;6(6):e628.

40. Pawlitzki M, Schneider-Hohendorf T, Rolfes L, et al. Ineffective treatment of PML with pembrolizumab: Exhausted memory T-cell subsets as a clue? Neurol Neuroimmunol Neuroinflamm 2019;6(6):e627.

41. Du Pasquier RA. Pembrolizumab as a treatment for PML? Waiting for Godot. Neurol Neuroimmunol Neuroinflamm 2019;6(6):e629.

42. Muftuoglu M, Olson A, Marin D, et al. Allogeneic BK virus-specific T cells for progressive multifocal leukoencephalopathy. N Engl J Med 2018;379(15):1443–51.

An Update on Botulinum Toxin in Neurology

Shannon Y. Chiu, MD, Matthew R. Burns, MD, PhD, Irene A. Malaty, MD*

KEYWORDS

- Botulinum toxin • Botox • Dystonia • Spasticity • Blepharospasm
- Hemifacial spasm • Migraine • Emerging

KEY POINTS

- Botulinum neurotoxin (BoNT) reduces acetylcholine neurotransmission at the neuromuscular junction, causing temporary muscle relaxation, with additional secondary mechanisms in certain applications.
- BoNT is a key tool in the armamentarium for many conditions with excessive muscle activity or tone (blepharospasm, hemifacial spasm, cervical, truncal and limb dystonia, spasticity) and for conditions in which acetylcholine impacts nonmotor functions such as sialorrhea.
- Evidence supports that guidance techniques such as electromyography (EMG), ultrasound, and electrical stimulation (E-stim) enhance efficacy.
- Ongoing research is exploring novel indications, toxin formulations, and delivery methods.

BACKGROUND

History

First identified as "sausage poisoning," resulting from unsanitary production of smoked blood sausages in nineteenth century Europe and the Americas, botulism is named after the Latin word for sausages.[1] In the early 1800s, the German physician Dr Justinus Kerner published the first description of botulism, accurately describing classic symptoms through a series of experiments both on animals and himself.[2] He not only proposed the mechanism of action and therapeutic applications of the toxin, but also hypothesized its zoonic origin, a bold suggestion in a scientific era before the discovery of microscopic pathogens.[3] It was not until 73 years later that the microbiologist Dr Emile Pierre van Ermengem[4] first identified and isolated "Bacillus botulinus" from raw, salted pork and victims' postmortem tissue. Over time, the toxin was explored as an agent of warfare before shifting to more therapeutic applications.[5] In the field of neurology, efficacy in blepharospasm[6] and cervical dystonia[7] was first

Department of Neurology, Fixel Institute for Neurological Diseases, University of Florida, 3009 SW Williston Road, Gainesville, FL 32608, USA
* Corresponding author.
E-mail address: Irene.malaty@neurology.ufl.edu

Neurol Clin 39 (2021) 209–229
https://doi.org/10.1016/j.ncl.2020.09.014
0733-8619/21/© 2020 Elsevier Inc. All rights reserved.
neurologic.theclinics.com

reported in 1985, followed by double-blind confirmatory studies shortly thereafter.[8,9] Since this early foundational work, the number of indications and applications has continued to grow with present day global sales estimated to be more than $5 to $6 billion in US dollars.[10]

Mechanisms

The original proposed mechanism of BoNT was a simple blockade of acetylcholine release at the neuromuscular junction, occurring through cleavage and inhibition of the proteins involved in presynaptic vesicle fusion at the synapse, weakening muscle contraction.[11] Additional modes of action and modifying factors are implicated by the dissociation between weakness, pain relief, and efficacy in dystonia.[9] BoNT is preferentially taken up by more highly active axons[12,13] and also inhibits afferent gamma motoneurons of intrafusal stretch muscle fibers[14] and spindle afferents that lead to tonic stretch reflex.[15] Finally, BoNT is retrogradely transported in its active state, which may produce central action both at the level of the spinal cord[16] and brain.[17]

Types of Toxins and Nonconvertability

There are 7 serotypes of the rod-shaped, gram-positive anaerobic bacterium *Clostridium botulinum* (A, B, C, D, E, F, and G), each producing a unique neurotoxin also designated A to G, distinguishable by animal antisera.[18] Serotypes A and B are commonly used in practice. More recent sequencing analysis has identified many genes encoding novel BoNTs with varying amino acid sequences; these "subtypes" are organized under the traditional serotypes followed by numbers (eg, BoNT/A1, BoNT/A2).

Each serotype targets different components of the presynaptic vesicle binding protein complex. These mechanistic differences lead to nonlinear dose conversion from one serotype to the next. However, approximate and empiric attempts exist in the literature to guide ranges of "conversion" ratios (eg, compared with onabotulinumtoxin A [OnaA], estimated ratios are 1:1 for incobotulinumtoxin A [IncoA], 1:2.5 to 4 for abobotulinumtoxin A [AboA], and 1:50 to 100 for rimabotulinumtoxin B [RimaB]).[19–21]

Reconstitution

BoNT complex is packaged in standardized vials, and either vacuum dried (OnaA) or freeze-dried (AboA, IncoA), requiring reconstitution with preservative-free normal saline or in ready to use solution (RimaB). Package inserts of each vial provide specific directions,[22–25] but a few points are worth highlighting. When reconstituting, beware that a lack of vacuum may indicate loss of sterility. Desiccated botulinum is difficult to visualize, and saline should be injected and agitated gently to the bottom of the vial. After mixing, avoid inverting the vial when aspirating into an administration syringe, as small volumes of reconstituted botulinum may get stuck along the walls or cap of the vial.

TREATMENT-RELATED ISSUES
Injection Guidance (Ultrasound, Electromyography)

Regardless of indication, efficacy of BoNT treatment is dependent on accurate targeting. This requires assessment of relative contributions of muscles to the abnormal posture or movement, knowledge of surface anatomic landmarks, palpation, and expert guidance. Targeting may be augmented with ultrasound guidance, electromyography (EMG), or electrical stimulation (E-Stim). Studies consistently show that using these techniques improves outcomes, reduces adverse events and decreases pain across many indications.[26] Head to head comparisons of these guidance techniques, however, are lacking.

Deep Brain Stimulation

Deep brain stimulation (DBS) can be a highly effective treatment for various movement disorders, but residual symptoms may require adjunctive BoNT injections. For DBS patient receiving BoNT injections, clinicians should delineate and palpate the full course of the tunneling wires running behind the ears and down the neck to the implantable pulse generator (IPG) to avoid trauma. In addition, an active IPG can produce significant artifact if EMG or E-stim guidance is used, and the patient or injector must be prepared to temporarily turn off the device during injections.

Immunity

All BoNT serotypes can induce both neutralizing and non-neutralizing antibodies, which may decrease efficacy in treatment.[27,28] Antibodies are not routinely checked in clinic, but blood samples can be screened if there is a concern for acquired immunity. Treatment-related factors such as injection frequency, dose, use of "booster injections" within weeks of initial therapy (which is not recommended), prior exposure, site of injection, and amount of denatured toxin in a given sample may affect rates of immunity. Rates of neutralizing antibody responses among patients have been reported to be ~1% to 3% for BoNT/A1, and 10% to 44% for BoNT/B1.[27–29] However, the precise relationship between neutralizing antibodies and resistance to BoNT is unclear, as a positive titer does not directly indicate non-responsiveness or treatment failure.[30] More research is needed to investigate the association of antibody formation with clinical response.

Expectation Management

It is essential to counsel the patient regarding extent of anticipated benefit, limitations, potential side effects, and expected time to onset and duration of benefit. Effective therapy requires repeated treatments, and dose and injection patterns typically require optimization over multiple injection cycles.

BOTULINUM TOXIN FOR HEAD/NECK INDICATIONS
Migraine

Chronic migraine is the most common primary daily headache seen by headache specialists in the United States and Europe, affecting up to 5% of the general population.[31] OnaA is currently the only toxin approved by the Food and Drug Administration (FDA) for chronic migraine ≥15 days per month with headache lasting 4 hours a day or longer. Efficacy was demonstrated in 2 placebo-controlled trials (PREEMPT1 and 2).[32,33] There are limited studies for efficacy in other serotypes.[34,35]

Current doses and injection sites of OnaA are based on PREEMPT. Typically, dilution is 100 U/1-2 mL, yielding either 10 U/0.1 mL or 5 U/0.1 mL. Higher concentration may reduce diffusion. In each of 31 fixed sites (**Table 1**), 5 U of OnaA are injected. Typically, a total of 155 U is injected; but an additional 40 U can be injected into temporalis (2 sites), occipitalis (2 sites), or trapezius (4 sites).[36] Most common adverse effects included neck pain (4.3%), injection site pain (2.1%), eyelid ptosis (1.9%), and muscular weakness (1.6%).[32]

Possible mechanisms of action in migraine may include axonal transport to trigeminal and dorsal root ganglia, modulation of calcitonin gene–related peptide, substance P and other neurotransmitters, modulation of surface expression of nociceptive receptors and cytokines.[37]

Table 1 Injection paradigm of onabotulinumtoxin A in chronic migraine[22]	
Muscles (Divided Bilaterally Except Procerus)	Total Units (Total no. of Sites)
Frontalis	20 (4)
Corrugators	10 (2)
Procerus	5 (1)
Occipitalis	30 (6)
Temporalis	40 (8)
Trapezii	30 (6)
Cervical paraspinals	20 (4)

Data from Allergan I. Package Insert, BOTOX (Botulinum toxin Type A Purified Neurotoxin Complex). Irvine Allergan Inc. 2019.

Blepharospasm

Blepharospasm is a focal dystonia characterized by involuntary bilateral synchronous tonic or intermittent contraction of orbicularis oculi muscles producing increased blinking or eye closure.[38,39] Blepharospasm can interfere with vision and be exacerbated by bright light. There are primary and secondary forms, all of which can significantly impair quality of life.[40,41] Medical therapies are usually insufficient.[42]

BoNT is first-line therapy for blepharospasm, with more than 90% of patients improving with injections.[40] OnaA and IncoA are FDA-approved with level A evidence.[6,8,43] Several head to head comparisons show increased rate of side effects with AboA[44] resulting in level B evidence for that toxin. A lack of studies for RimaB in blepharospasm relegates this toxin to level U evidence.[43]

Muscles commonly injected are orbicularis oculi, corrugator, and procerus (**Fig. 1**). For patient comfort, injections are usually done with thin 30-gauge needles. EMG guidance is not typically needed. Starting doses per package inserts for OnaA and IncoA are 1.25 to 2.5 U per site for both, with 0.05 to 0.1 mL volume per site. Commonly, starting dose may range from 10 to 15 U per eye and be titrated as needed over time. Most injectors wait 3 months between sessions.

The most common side effect is ptosis, possibly from diffusion to the levator palpebrae muscle. This can be mitigated by avoiding injection near the midline of upper lid and directing the needle away from the midline. Injections should be very superficial with the needle oriented in a trajectory parallel to the eye. Other adverse effects include bruising, tearing, dry eyes, or diplopia. Systemic side effects are rare and longitudinal studies have shown continued efficacy and tolerability.[45]

Apraxia of Eyelid Opening

Apraxia of eyelid opening may be considered a subtype of blepharospasm, a focal eye dystonia, or rarely as its own entity in isolation.[46] Patients describe the inability to voluntarily open their eyes.

BoNT in apraxia of eyelid opening is currently off-label. Small case series have shown that injection into pretarsal fibers of orbicularis oculi with OnaA and AboA can improve eye opening in some patients[46,47] (see **Fig. 1**). Although most experts believe a trial of BoNT is warranted, more controlled studies are needed.

Hemifacial Spasm

Hemifacial spasm (HFS) is a nondystonic, peripheral disorder of the seventh cranial nerve (CN) characterized by intermittent brief tonic or clonic contraction of the

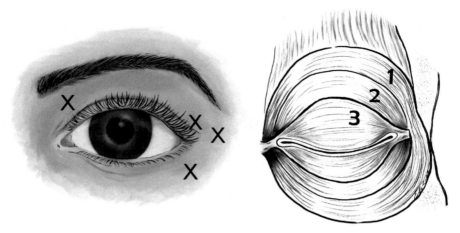

Fig. 1. Orbicularis oculi components. (*A*) Orbicularis oculi: one pattern of potential injection sites. (*B*) The orbicularis oculi muscle is divided into orbital (1) and palpebral (2–3) aspects. The palpebral aspect is further divided into preseptal (2) and pretarsal (3) regions. For both blepharospasm and apraxia of eyelid opening, injections of pretarsal region may be more effective. (*Data from* Jankovic J. Pretarsal injection of botulinum toxin for blepharospasm and apraxia of eyelid opening [13]. *J Neurol Neurosurg Psychiatry*. 1996; and Çakmur R, Ozturk V, Uzunel F, Donmez B, Idiman F. Comparison of preseptal and pretarsal injections of botulinum toxin in the treatment of blepharospasm and hemifacial spasm. *J Neurol*. 2002.)

muscles of facial expression. Fewer than 2% of cases are bilateral.[40] HFS typically starts in one orbicularis oculi muscle and subsequently spreads to the mid and lower face. Medications provide limited benefit.[40] For severe cases in which neurovascular compression of CN VII is identified in neuroimaging, surgical decompression may be considered with ~2% rate of recurrance.[48]

BoNT is effective and well tolerated in HFS but with high risk of facial weakness. There are 2 placebo-controlled studies supporting OnaA,[49,50] and 1 comparison study between OnaA and AboA, which showed equivalent efficacy and side effect profiles.[51] RimaB demonstrated somewhat shorter duration of effect and reports of burning pain with injections.[52] Thus, evidence supports level B recommendation for OnaA; level C for AboA.[43] There are insufficient data for other serotypes.[43]

Table 2 shows typical muscles injected in HFS. The starting dose for HFS is 2.5-5 U/site for OnaA and IncoA; 15 to 20U for AboA. Common adverse effects are facial weakness, followed by facial bruising, ptosis, and diplopia.[40,43]

Orofacial/Oromandibular Dystonia

Orofacial/oromandibular dystonia (OMD) is a focal dystonia involving the jaw, muscles of mastication, mouth/lips, and tongue. It can be primary or secondary to other conditions.[40] OMD is frequently associated with dystonia of the eyes (blepharospasm), tongue (lingual dystonia), neck (cervical dystonia), and larynx (spasmodic dysphonia). Involvement of upper face and lower face/jaw/tongue was previously referred to as Meige syndrome, but it is now more often recognized as cranialfacial dystonia.[53] Typically, OMD is bilateral and classified by primary direction of movement. Common manifestations affect jaw opening, jaw closing, lateral jaw deviation, jaw protrusion or retraction, and tongue protrusion. Medications are often

Table 2
Frequently injected muscles in hemifacial spasm

Characteristic Abnormal Facial Contraction	Muscles to Consider	Comments
Eye spasm(s)	Orbicularis oculi Corrugator Procerus	Injection of pretarsal portion of orbicularis oculi may be more effective
Nasal flare/"snarl"	Levator labii superioris alaeque nasi	Weakness can impact lifting of the lip
Lower face spasm	Zygomaticus major and minor Risorius Orbicularis oris Depressor anguli oris Mentalis	Beware of facial asymmetry (eg, may need contralateral partial injection); beware of weakness of lip closure when injecting orbicularis oris
Neck spasm	Platysma	

insufficient, and alternative therapies for OMD include oral devices and DBS of the globus pallidus interna.[54]

Although BoNT is considered first-line therapy for OMD, evidence for its use is largely based on case reports, small series, and observational studies.[55] Studies with OnaA[8] and AboA[56] consistently report efficacy but with 30% to 45% complication rates including dysarthria and dysphagia. Interestingly, jaw-closing dystonia is typically more responsive to BoNT than jaw-opening dystonia; and complications appear more frequently following injections for jaw opening.[55] Overall, current evidence supports level C recommendation for OnaA and AboA in treatment of OMD; both IncoA and RimaB have level U recommendation due to insufficient data.[43]

Muscle selection is based on clinical features (**Fig. 2**). Common muscles injected in OMD, typically with EMG or ultrasound guidance, are shown in **Table 3**.[53] Total starting doses are typically 50 to 60 U for OnaA, and 100 to 150 U for AboA.[57]

SIALORRHEA

Sialorrhea or drooling can be seen in various neurologic disorders including motor neuron disease, developmental and neurodegenerative disorders. It is particularly prevalent in patients with Parkinson disease (PD) due to reduced automatic swallowing and/or increased speed of saliva excretion.[58] Medications are often limited by side effects, thus BoNT provides an alternative therapy that avoids systemic side effects.

Only RimaB is FDA-approved for treatment of chronic sialorrhea. However, double-blind placebo-controlled trials have demonstrated efficacy of both BoNT-A and BoNT-B formulations,[59,60] and most patients respond to BoNT regardless of type with some variability in time to onset.[61] **Table 4** shows typical targets and BoNT doses. Both blind injection using anatomic landmarks and ultrasound-guided techniques have shown good efficacy and few adverse effects.[62]

CERVICAL DYSTONIA

Cervical dystonia is the most common focal dystonia. It produces abnormal postures of the head, neck and shoulder, and is frequently associated with pain and/or tremor.[64]

Cervical dystonia is further classified based on abnormal posturing, namely horizontal head turning or rotation (torticollis); head tilt or lateral flexion (laterocollis); forward

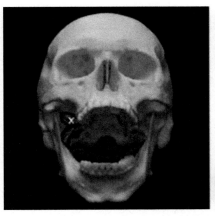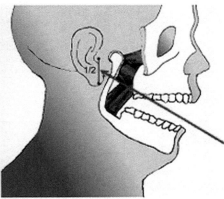

Fig. 2. Intraoral approach to the lateral pterygoid muscle. (*Left*) The injection entry point into the lateral pterygoid muscle, (*Right*) The direction of the injection toward the middle point of a virtual line connecting the ipsilateral ear's tragus and lobe. (Left image from Moscovich M, Chen ZP, Rodriguez R. Successful treatment of open jaw and jaw deviation dystonia with botulinum toxin using a simple intraoral approach. *J Clin Neurosci.* 2015; with permission.)

flexion of head/neck (anterocollis); head/neck extension (retrocollis); lateral displacement from midline (lateral shift); displacement anteriorly ("goose neck") or posteriorly ("double chin") (sagittal displacement); and shoulder elevation or forward rotation.[30] Abnormal postures can be isolated to one plane, or more commonly, have complex combinations. The most common subtype is torticollis (48%), followed by laterocollis (39%); anterocollis and retrocollis are less common (~5%).[65]

BoNT is currently the first-line therapy for cervical dystonia, as medications are often limited by side effects. All 4 currently available US BoNT formulations are FDA-approved for treatment of cervical dystonia, with level A recommendations.[43]

Muscle selection for BoNT injections is dictated by the particular posture and contributing muscles. Patients must be carefully examined in different positions, for example, while sitting comfortably with preferred head positioning, voluntarily moving head along the 3 axes, applying sensory tricks, standing, and walking. Neck palpation helps to detect muscle hypertrophy, elicit pain, and evaluate passive range of

Table 3
Common muscles injected in orofacial/oromandibular dystonia (OMD)

OMD Abnormal Position	Suggested Primary Muscles to Consider	Pearls
Jaw opening	Bilateral lateral pterygoid Bilateral digastric	May approach externally or intraorally Dysphagia risk
Jaw closing	Bilateral masseter Bilateral temporalis	May cause dry mouth (parotid) Avoid temporal artery
Jaw deviation	Contralateral lateral pterygoid	
Tongue protrusion	Bilateral Genioglossus	May inject undersurface of tongue or take submandibular approach Dysarthria risk

Table 4
Typical targets and BoNT doses in sialorrhea[24,63]

Typical Target	BoNT Preparation and Dose Ranges (per Side)		
	OnabotulinumtoxinA (BOTOX), U	IncobotulinumtoxinA (Xeomin), U	RimabotulinumtoxinB (Myobloc), U
Parotid glands	5–75	10–145	1000
Submandibular glands	5–30	70–80	250

Data from Refs.[24,63]

motion.[66] It is important to recognize compensatory muscles, which are secondarily recruited to counter the abnormal posture; compensatory muscles should not be injected as reducing their power may compromise the balance further.[66] **Table 5** shows typical muscles injected in cervical dystonia, with general dose ranges offered for consideration based on our experience and literature review. Adjusting up or down from these ranges may be necessary based on individual patient factors such as muscle size, overall target dose and number of muscles over which to distribute, as well as response over time.

For head tremor associated with cervical dystonia, bilateral injections are often performed in muscles that act synchronously to produce tremor, such as bilateral sternocleidomastoid and splenius capitis muscles in side-to-side head tremor.

Challenges in treatment of cervical dystonia include potential involvement of deeper, poorly accessible muscles.[30,70] Evidence supports using EMG guidance[71] and general consensus is to use the lowest effective dose at the longest tolerated dosing interval. **Table 6** shows product labeling guidelines for maximum recommended doses, though increasing evidence supports flexible treatments above traditionally accepted maximum dosing based on patients' needs.[72,73]

Although 70% to 90% of patients with cervical dystonia benefit from at least one BoNT session,[65] up to 20% of patients discontinue long-term BoNT.[74] Treatment failure may be due to initial or acquired nonresponse, or intolerable adverse effects. Most common adverse effects include dysphagia and neck weakness.[74] Some tips include avoiding (1) injections into lower portion of sternocleidomastoid muscles, and (2) injecting too deeply. Additional risk factors for treatment failure and/or side effects include incorrect diagnosis, wrong muscles injected, inadequate dosing, and unrealistic patient expectations.[75]

LIMB DYSTONIA

Treatment of limb dystonia varies widely based on the specific involuntary movement or position, with a general approach analogous to limb spasticity (see later in this article). This methodology has been well-described.[76]

Initially given level A evidence-based recommendations as a drug class by the American Academy of Neurology (AAN) in 2008, individual BoNT products were subsequently evaluated separately.[77] There is currently level B evidence for AboA and OnaA, but insufficient data for IncoA and RimaB in limb dystonia.[43]

TRUNCAL DYSTONIA

Truncal dystonia is characterized by involuntary contractions of the paraspinal, chest, and/or abdominal muscles. Although primary truncal dystonia is rare and difficult to

Table 5
Botulinum neurotoxin (BoNT) in cervical dystonia[22-25,66-69]

Positional Deviation	Muscles to Consider	Suggested Dose Per Muscle (Units)		
		OnabotulinumtoxinA (BOTOX) or IncobotulinumtoxinA (Xeomin)	AbobotulinumtoxinA (Dysport)	RimabotulinumtoxinB (Myobloc)
Anterocollis	Bilateral sternocleidomastoid (SCM)	(20–80)	(50–300)	(1000–2500)
	Bilateral scalene	(10–50)	(50–200)	(500–1000)
Retrocollis	Bilateral splenius capitis	(20–100)	(75–400)	(1000–5000)
	Bilateral semispinalis capitis	(15–50)	(50–200)	(1000–2500)
	Upper trapezius	(20–70)	(50–250)	(1000–2500)
	Cervical paraspinal muscles	(10–20)	(25–75)	(500–1000)
	Bilateral longissimus capitis	(20–50)	(50–125)	(1000–2500)
Torticollis (turn)	Contralateral SCM	(20–80)	(50–300)	(1000–2500)
	Ipsilateral splenius capitis	(20–100)	(75–400)	(1000–5000)
	Ipsilateral semispinalis capitis	(15–50)	(50–200)	(1000–2500)
	Ipsilateral obliquus capitis inferioris	(20–30)	(50–100)	(1000–1500)
Laterocollis (tilt)	Ipsilateral scalene	(10–50)	(50–200)	(500–1000)
	Ipsilateral SCM	(20–80)	(50–300)	(1000–2500)
	Ipsilateral levator scapulae	(20–70)	(50–200)	(1000–2500)
Shoulder elevation	Ipsilateral trapezius	(20–70)	(50–250)	(1000–2500)
	Ipsilateral levator scapulae	(20–70)	(50–200)	(1000–2500)

Data from Refs.[22-25,66-69]

Table 6
US Food and Drug Administration labeling of botulinum neurotoxin (BoNT) formulations in cervical dystonia[22–25]

BoNT Formulation	Starting Dose	Approved Maximum per Therapy Session	Treatment Interval
OnabotulinumtoxinA (BOTOX)	"Tailored to individual patient"	400 U	3 mo
AbobotulinumtoxinA (Dysport)	500 U (then titrate in 250 U steps based on patient response)	1000 U	12 wk
IncobotulinumtoxinA (Xeomin)	120 U	400 U	≥12 wk
RimabotulinumtoxinB (Myobloc)	2500–5000 U	10,000	12–16 wk

Data from Refs.[22–25]

treat, it is also found in tardive dystonia, segmental and generalized dystonia syndromes, and secondary to other neurodegenerative diseases. Large studies are lacking; and the size, depth, and number of involved muscles make dosing a challenge while increasing the risk of potential side effects.[78] Truncal flexion is the most common clinical syndrome,[79] and although used off-label, case reports support the use of BoNT.[80,81] Such reports describe 25 to 50 U OnaA injected into the paravertebral muscles of the lumbar regions in 4 to 6 sites. Recommended doses for paraspinal muscles are 60 to 100 U per side for OnaA or 240 to 400 U for AboA, and for abdominal muscles between 40 to 80 U OnaA, or 160 to 320 U AboA.[78]

LIMB SPASTICITY

Spasticity results from intermittent or sustained involuntary muscle activation due to upper motor neuron (UMN) lesions,[82] and is often associated with hyperreflexia. Common etiologies include cerebral palsy, stroke, and traumatic brain injury. BoNT is effective for both children and adults with upper extremity spasticity.[39] Primary treatment goals are increasing range of motion and ease of daily hygiene, while decreasing pain, risk of fixed joints, and skin infections. Level A evidence exists for efficacy of AboA, IncoA, and OnaA.[77]

Patients should be counseled that BoNT may improve flexibility but not muscle weakness that is, typically associated with UMN lesion(s). Furthermore, spasticity itself may provide some functionality that may be lost by BoNT-induced limb weakness. Hence, it is critical to thoroughly assess the activities of daily living most important to the patient.

Upper extremity spasticity frequently causes a particular pattern of stiffness or fixed posture, with shoulder adduction and flexion of the elbow, wrist and fingers, often with a clenched fist[83] (**Fig. 3**, **Table 7**). A starting aggregate dose of 200 to 300 U and a total maximum dose of 300 to 400 U is common,[84] although European guidelines suggest doses up to 600 U of OnaA.[85] Escalating IncoA from 400 U to 800 U in patients with spasticity enabled treatment in more affected muscles, was associated with increased treatment efficacy, and maintained safety and tolerability.[86] Although optimal dosing per muscle is not fully known, excellent recommendations have been published based on a structured multistep consensus process of expert panelists.[84] Assistive guidance techniques were considered essential for all common postures.

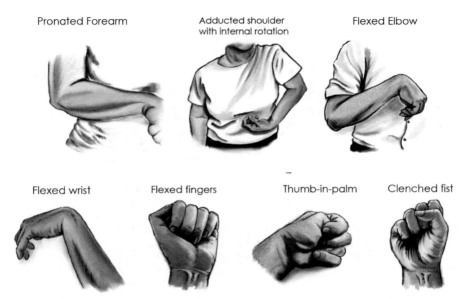

Fig. 3. Common postures of upper limb spasticity. The most common aggregate postures include (1) adducted shoulder, flexed elbow, pronated forearm, flexed wrist and clenched fist; (2) flexed elbow, pronated forearm, flexed wrist and clenched fist; and (3) flexed wrist and clenched fist. (*Data from* Simpson DM, Patel AT, Alfaro A, et al. OnabotulinumtoxinA Injection for Poststroke Upper-Limb Spasticity: Guidance for Early Injectors From a Delphi Panel Process. *PM R.* 2017.)

Table 7	
Upper extremity muscle targets	
Positional Deviation	**Muscles to Consider**
Adducted shoulder	Pectoralis Latissimus dorsi
Flexed elbow	Bicep Brachialis Brachioradialis
Pronated forearm	Pronator teres Pronator quadratus
Flexed wrist	Flexor carpi radialis Flexor carpi ulnaris
Fisted hand: Metacarpophalangeal joint flexion Proximal interphalangeal joint flexion Distal interphalangeal joint flexion	Lumbricals Flexor digitorum superficialis Flexor digitorum profundus
Thumb: Flexion Opposition Adduction	Flexor pollicis brevis and longus Opponens pollicis Adductor pollicis

Similar levels of evidence exist for OnaA and AboA in lower limb spasticity. Based on AAN practice guidelines, there is insufficient evidence for IncoA or RimaB, although additional formulations may be tried if the patient fails first-line toxins. Similar to upper limb spasticity, patterns of abnormal muscle contraction guide injection patterns (**Fig. 4, Table 8**).

BOTULINUM NEUROTOXIN FOR OTHER INDICATIONS
Tics

Tics are brief, repetitive, nonrhythmic motor movements (motor tics) or vocalizations (vocal tics), which can be further categorized as simple or complex. Tics can occur in isolation or as part of Tourette syndrome (TS), and classically manifest before age 18. Current therapeutic options (eg, behavioral therapies; medications) are unable to completely control tics in the majority of patients. Focal or segmental tics may be amenable to BoNT.[88] The mechanism of action is unclear, but some hypothesize that the benefits relate to relaxation of affected muscle and reduction of premonitory sensation.[89]

Injection sites depend on the specific tic and body part(s) involved, focusing on the most bothersome tics. For instance, intense blinking tics may be targeted with an injection pattern similar to that of idiopathic blepharospasm. Rapid, intense and often painful neck tics may be targeted with injection of ipsilateral splenius capitis in a primary rapid sideways jerk. Additional muscles are incorporated based on the tic characteristics. Reduction of tic number and intensity and relief of pain are the typical therapeutic targets. Doses are typically lower than in dystonic or spastic conditions.[88]

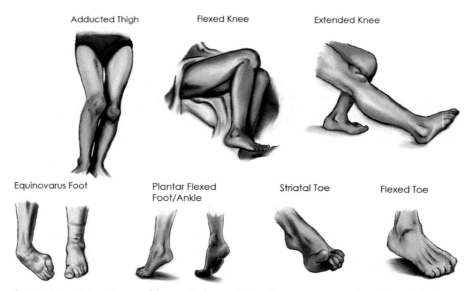

Fig. 4. Common patterns of lower limb spasticity. Common aggregate patterns of lower-limb spasticity include (1) equinovarus foot and flexed toes, (2) extended knee and plantar-flexed foot/ankle, and (3) plantar flexed foot/ankle and flexed toes.[87] Common aggregate starting doses are 300 to 400 U and total maximum dose 500 to 600 U, although may be tailored to patient's needs. (*Data from* Esquenazi A, Alfaro A, Ayyoub Z, et al. Ona-botulinumtoxinA for Lower Limb Spasticity: Guidance From a Delphi Panel Approach. *PM R.* 2017.)

Table 8
Lower extremity muscle targets

Positional Deviation	Muscles to Consider
Flexed hip	Iliopsoas
Adducted thighs	Adductor complex (magnus, longus, brevis)
Flexed knee	Hamstring complex
Extended knee (less common)	Quadricep complex (rectus femoris, vastus medialis, lateralis and intermedius)
Plantar flexion	Gastrocnemius Soleus
Foot inversion	Tibialis posterior
Toe flexion/curling	Flexor digitorum brevis Flexor digitorum longus
Great toe extension	Extensor hallucis longus

BoNT has also been used for phonic tics including coprolalia in small case series.[90] Technique is similar to that used in vocal tremor or spasmodic dysphonia. Most had improvement in phonic tics but 80% developed hypophonia. Interestingly, most still reported improvement in social life. Patients with loud embarrassing coprolalia may prefer hypophonia to the persistent disabling tics.

Despite case reports and uncontrolled studies demonstrating tic improvement with BoNT,[91,92] current evidence supporting BoNT in TS is considered weak. Thus, guidelines suggest that BoNT treatment may be considered in select cases such as simple motor tics or bothersome vocal tics in older adolescents and adults, when potential benefits outweigh risks.[93]

Emerging Applications and Formulations

Novel indications for BoNT continue to emerge. In movement disorders, off-label use has been reported in dystonia (eg, bruxism), tremor (eg, palatal myoclonus, essential tremor [ET], parkinsonian tremor, task-specific tremor, orthostatic tremor), and restless legs syndrome. We will review some of these novel indications. Similarly, there is growing research on alternative BoNT serotypes, formulations, delivery methods, and novel injection techniques.

Novel indications in movement disorders

Tremor Tremor is commonly seen in PD, ET, dystonia, and multiple sclerosis. Medications are often insufficient for severe high amplitude tremors. While DBS and focused ultrasound ablation are surgical options for medically refractory tremor, some limited evidence supports BoNT,[94] though the mechanism is poorly understood.[88]

BoNT has been best studied in ET and parkinsonian limb tremor.[95–97] Muscle selection can be challenging and variable, relying on clinical and electrophysiologic evaluations of patients' tremor to localize active muscles (ie, agonist and antagonist muscles such as flexors/extensors). Injecting finger/wrist extensors sparingly is important to avoid wrist drop. Based on AAN guidelines from 2008, there is insufficient evidence to recommend any particular muscle targeting technique for BoNT limb injection; in fact, evidence for use of BoNT in tremor (particularly ET) is rated as level C by AAN.[98] Most common side effects are forearm and finger weakness.

There is limited literature on use of BoNT in other tremor types, although active trials are ongoing (clinicaltrials.gov).[88]

Novel formulations

DaxibotulinumtoxinA (DAXI) is one of the latest investigational BoNT (RT002) formulations in clinical development for treatment of cervical dystonia, glabellar lines, and plantar fasciitis.[99] It is a purified 150 kDA BoNT type A (RTT150), without accessory proteins and formulated with a proprietary stabilizing excipient peptide (RTP004) in a lyophilized powder. Preliminary data have been promising in showing less diffusion and significantly greater duration of effect compared with OnaA, with tolerability at doses up to 450U.[99,100] There is an active multicenter clinical trial of 2 doses of DAXI for adults with primary cervical dystonia (ASPEN-1, NCT03608397; ASPEN-OLS, NCT03617367). DAXI is also being studied as treatment of upper limb spasticity (JUNIPER, NCT03821402), plantar fasciitis (NCT03825315), topical gel for axillary hyperhidrosis, and canthal lines (NCT03911102).

PrabotulinumtoxinA is also a new BoNT-A preparation, originally developed in South Korea. It is FDA-approved for treatment of glabellar lines.[101] Currently, there are no approved neurologic indications, and it is unclear if scope of application will expand further.

Novel Delivery Methods

BoNT injections can be painful, particularly with injections into palm, foot, and axilla; and risk of bruising in eye/face regions may be undesirable. Thus development of needle-free administration is of great interest. However, biological barriers related to large size of the protein and accurate targeting of muscles remain challenging.[102]

Transdermal drug delivery is currently one of the main needle-free methods in development, aimed at relatively superficial delivery and likely most amenable to indications of facial lines and hyperhidrosis.[103,104] Liquid formulations are also being developed in the treatment of glabellar lines, though neurologic applications are less clear.[105]

Novel Techniques for Muscle Selection and Injection

Precise muscle localization is critical for successful outcomes for BoNT injections. Ongoing trials are exploring ultrasound versus clinical localization in cervical dystonia (Clinical trial NCT03946046), kinematic versus clinical assessments for CD (NCT02662530), and comparing electrical stimulation versus ultrasound in upper extremity dystonia and spasticity (NCT02334683). Augmentation of BoNT benefit with repetitive transcranial magnetic stimulation (rTMS) is also under investigation (NCT02542839).

SUMMARY

BoNT has evolved into an essential therapeutic agent with diverse applications in the field of neurology and beyond. In addition to the growing clinical indications, there are continued efforts to refine the applications, targeting, dosing, and serotypes. New formulations are being explored, and future studies may help expand our understanding of best practices and full scope of benefit.

CLINICS CARE POINTS

- Utilizing guidance techniques for muscle targeting, such as EMG, ultrasound, or electrical stimulation, has been shown to improve outcomes and reduce adverse events across many indications.
- The precise relationship between neutralizing antibodies and resistance to BoNT is unclear, as a positive titer does not directly indicate non-responsiveness or treatment failure.

- In treating abnormal involuntary movements of the head and neck, it is important to recognize compensatory muscles, which are secondarily recruited to counter the abnormal posture; compensatory muscles should not be injected as reducing their power may compromise the balance further.
- Patients should be counseled that BoNT may improve flexibility, range of motion, and abnormal postures but not muscle weakness that is associated with UMN lesions. Furthermore, spasticity itself may provide some functionality, such as leg stiffness that supports weight-baring. Hence, it is critical to thoroughly assess goals of treatment and to customize the treatment plan.

DISCLOSURE

There are no disclosures relevant to this article. Unrelated to this article, in the past year Dr I.A. Malaty has participated in research funded by the Parkinson Foundation of United States, Tourette Association, Dystonia Coalition, AbbVie, Biogen, Boston Scientific, Eli Lilly, Impax, Neuroderm, Prilenia, Revance, and Teva but has no owner interest in any pharmaceutical company. She has received travel compensation or honoraria from the Parkinson Foundation, Tourette Association of America, International Association of Parkinsonism and Related Disorders, Medscape, and Cleveland Clinic, and royalties from Robert Rose publishers. Dr M.R. Burns receives funding from the Parkinson's Foundation, University Of Florida Moonshot Grant, University Of Florida Opportunity Grant, and the Harry T. Mangurian Jr. Foundation. Dr S.Y. Chiu receives funding from the Smallwood Foundation, and the Harry T. Mangurian Jr. Foundation; and has received travel compensation from Movement Disorders Society, International Association of Parkinsonism and Related Disorders, and Cleveland Clinic.

REFERENCE

1. Torrens JK. *Clostridium botulinum* was named because of association with "sausage poisoning. BMJ 1998. https://doi.org/10.1136/bmj.316.7125.151c.
2. Erbguth FJ, Naumann M. Historical aspects of botulinum toxin: Justinus Kerner (1786-1862) and the "sausage poison. Neurology 1999. https://doi.org/10.1212/wnl.53.8.1850.
3. Erbguth FJ. Historical note on the therapeutic use of botulinum toxin in neurological disorders. J Neurol Neurosurg Psychiatry 1996. https://doi.org/10.1136/jnnp.60.2.151.
4. Van Ermengem E. A new anaerobic bacillus and its relation to botulism. Rev Infect Dis 1979. https://doi.org/10.1093/clinids/1.4.701.
5. Schantz EJ, Johnson EA. Botulinum toxin: the story of its development for the treatment of human disease. Perspect Biol Med 1997. https://doi.org/10.1353/pbm.1997.0032.
6. Fahn S, List T, Moskowitz C, et al. Double-blind controlled study of botulinum toxin for blepharospasm. Neurology 1985;35(Suppl):271-2.
7. Tsui JK, Eisen A, Mak E, et al. A pilot study on the use of botulinum toxin in spasmodic torticollis. Can J Neurol Sci 1985. https://doi.org/10.1017/S031716710003540X.
8. Jankovic J, Orman J. Botulinum a toxin for cranial-cervicaldystonia: a double-blind, placebo-controlled study. Neurology 1987. https://doi.org/10.1212/wnl.37.4.616.

9. Tsui JKC, Jon Stoessl A, Eisen A, et al. Double-blind study of botulinum toxin in spasmodic torticollis. Lancet 1986. https://doi.org/10.1016/S0140-6736(86)92070-2.

10. Dressler D. Botulinum toxin drugs: brief history and outlook. J Neural Transm 2016. https://doi.org/10.1007/s00702-015-1478-1.

11. Davletov B, Bajohrs M, Binz T. Beyond BOTOX: Advantages and limitations of individual botulinum neurotoxins. Trends Neurosci 2005. https://doi.org/10.1016/j.tins.2005.06.001.

12. Chen R, Karp BI, Goldstein SR, et al. Effect of muscle activity immediately after botulinum toxin injection for writer's cramp. Mov Disord 1999. https://doi.org/10.1002/1531-8257(199903)14:2<307::AID-MDS1016>3.0.CO;2-3.

13. Eleopra R, Tugnoli V, De Grandis D. The variability in the clinical effect induced by botulinum toxin type A: The role of muscle activity in humans. Mov Disord 1997. https://doi.org/10.1002/mds.870120115.

14. Rosales RL, Arimura K, Takenaga S, et al. Extrafusal and intrafusal muscle effects in experimental botulinum toxin-a injection. Muscle and Nerve; 1996. https://doi.org/10.1002/(SICI)1097-4598(199604)19:4<488::AID-MUS9>3.0.CO;2-8.

15. Trompetto C, Currà A, Buccolieri A, et al. Botulinum toxin changes intrafusal feedback in dystonia: a study with the tonic vibration reflex. Mov Disord 2006. https://doi.org/10.1002/mds.20801.

16. Marchand-Pauvert V, Aymard C, Giboin LS, et al. Beyond muscular effects: depression of spinal recurrent inhibition after botulinum neurotoxin A. J Physiol 2013. https://doi.org/10.1113/jphysiol.2012.239178.

17. Gilio F, Currà A, Lorenzano C, et al. Effects of botulinum toxin type A on intracortical inhibition in patients with dystonia. Ann Neurol 2000. https://doi.org/10.1002/1531-8249(200007)48:1<20::AID-ANA5>3.0.CO;2-U.

18. Smith TJ, Hill KK, Raphael BH. Historical and current perspectives on Clostridium botulinum diversity. Res Microbiol 2015. https://doi.org/10.1016/j.resmic.2014.09.007.

19. Dashtipour K, Chen JJ, Espay AJ, et al. OnabotulinumtoxinA and abobotulinumtoxina dose conversion: a systematic literature review. Mov Disord Clin Pract 2016. https://doi.org/10.1002/mdc3.12235.

20. Scaglione F. Conversion ratio between Botox®, Dysport®, and Xeomin® in clinical practice. Toxins (Basel) 2016. https://doi.org/10.3390/toxins8030065.

21. Bentivoglio AR, Del Grande A, Petracca M, et al. Clinical differences between botulinum neurotoxin type A and B. Toxicon 2015. https://doi.org/10.1016/j.toxicon.2015.08.001.

22. Allergan I. Package insert, BOTOX (botulinum toxin type A purified neurotoxin complex). Madison, NJ: Irvine Allergan Inc; 2019.

23. Merz Pharmaceuticals. Package insert, XEOMIN (incobotulinumtoxintype A). Frankfurt (Germany): Merz Pharmaceuticals GmbH; 2018.

24. Solstice Neurosciences. Package Insert, MYOBLOC (Botulinum toxin type B injectable solution). Louisville (KY): Solstice Neurosciences, LLC; 2019.

25. Ipsen. Package insert, DYSPORT (abobotulinumtoxinA). Basking Ridge (NJ): Ipsen Biopharmaceuticals; 2019.

26. Chan AK, Finlayson H, Mills PB. Does the method of botulinum neurotoxin injection for limb spasticity affect outcomes? A systematic review. Clin Rehabil 2017. https://doi.org/10.1177/0269215516655589.

27. Naumann M, Boo LM, Ackerman AH, et al. Immunogenicity of botulinum toxins. J Neural Transm 2013. https://doi.org/10.1007/s00702-012-0893-9.

28. Naumann M, Dressler D, Hallett M, et al. Evidence-based review and assessment of botulinum neurotoxin for the treatment of secretory disorders. Toxicon 2013. https://doi.org/10.1016/j.toxicon.2012.10.020.

29. Dressler D, Bigalke H. Botulinum toxin type B de novo therapy of cervical dystonia: Frequency of antibody induced therapy failure. J Neurol 2005. https://doi.org/10.1007/s00415-005-0774-3.

30. Bledsoe IO, Comella CL. Botulinum toxin treatment of cervical dystonia. Semin Neurol 2016. https://doi.org/10.1055/s-0035-1571210.

31. Natoli JL, Manack A, Dean B, et al. Global prevalence of chronic migraine: a systematic review. Cephalalgia 2010. https://doi.org/10.1111/j.1468-2982.2009.01941.x.

32. Aurora SK, Dodick DW, Turkel CC, et al. OnabotulinumtoxinA for treatment of chronic migraine: Results from the double-blind, randomized, placebo-controlled phase of the PREEMPT 1 trial. Cephalalgia 2010. https://doi.org/10.1177/0333102410364676.

33. Diener HC, Dodick DW, Aurora SK, et al. OnabotulinumtoxinA for treatment of chronic migraine: results from the double-blind, randomized, placebo-controlled phase of the PREEMPT 2 trial. Cephalalgia 2010. https://doi.org/10.1177/0333102410364677.

34. Ion I, Renard D, Le Floch A, et al. Monocentric prospective study into the sustained effect of Incobotulinumtoxin A (XEOMIN®) botulinum toxin in chronic refractory migraine. Toxins (Basel) 2018. https://doi.org/10.3390/toxins10060221.

35. Herd CP, Tomlinson CL, Rick C, et al. Botulinum toxins for the prevention of migraine in adults. Cochrane Database Syst Rev 2018. https://doi.org/10.1002/14651858.CD011616.pub2.

36. Blumenfeld A, Silberstein SD, Dodick DW, et al. Method of injection of onabotulinumtoxina for chronic migraine: a safe, well-tolerated, and effective treatment paradigm based on the preempt clinical program. Headache 2010. https://doi.org/10.1111/j.1526-4610.2010.01766.x.

37. Do TP, Hvedstrup J, Schytz HW. Botulinum toxin: a review of the mode of action in migraine. Acta Neurol Scand 2018. https://doi.org/10.1111/ane.12906.

38. Hallett M. Blepharospasm: recent advances. Neurology 2002. https://doi.org/10.1212/01.WNL.0000027361.73814.0E.

39. Simpson DM, Hallett M, Ashman EJ, et al. Practice guideline update summary: botulinum neurotoxin for the treatment of blepharospasm, cervical dystonia, adult spasticity, and headache Report of the Guideline Development Subcommittee of the American Academy of Neurology. Neurology 2016. https://doi.org/10.1212/WNL.0000000000002560.

40. Karp BI, Alter K. Botulinum toxin treatment of blepharospasm, orofacial/oromandibular dystonia, and hemifacial spasm. Semin Neurol 2016. https://doi.org/10.1055/s-0036-1571952.

41. Setthawatcharawanich S, Sathirapanya P, Limapichat K, et al. Factors associated with quality of life in hemifacial spasm and blepharospasm during long-term treatment with botulinum toxin. Qual Life Res 2011. https://doi.org/10.1007/s11136-011-9890-y.

42. Peckham EL, Lopez G, Shamim EA, et al. Clinical features of patients with blepharospasm: a report of 240 patients. Eur J Neurol 2011. https://doi.org/10.1111/j.1468-1331.2010.03161.x.

43. Hallett M, Albanese A, Dressler D, et al. Evidence-based review and assessment of botulinum neurotoxin for the treatment of movement disorders. Toxicon 2013. https://doi.org/10.1016/j.toxicon.2012.12.004.

44. Nüßgens Z, Roggenkämper P. Comparison of two botulinum-toxin preparations in the treatment of essential blepharospasm. Graefes Arch Clin Exp Ophthalmol 1997. https://doi.org/10.1007/BF00941758.

45. Streitová H, Bareš M. Long-term therapy of benign essential blepharospasm and facial hemispasm with botulinum toxin A: retrospective assessment of the clinical and quality of life impact in patients treated for more than 15 years. Acta Neurol Belg 2014. https://doi.org/10.1007/s13760-014-0285-z.

46. Krack P, Marion MH. "Apraxia of lid opening," a focal eyelid dystonia: clinical study of 32 patients. Mov Disord 1994. https://doi.org/10.1002/mds.870090605.

47. Jankovic J. Pretarsal injection of botulinum toxin for blepharospasm and apraxia of eyelid opening [13]. J Neurol Neurosurg Psychiatry 1996. https://doi.org/10.1136/jnnp.60.6.704.

48. Miller LE, Miller VM. Safety and effectiveness of microvascular decompression for treatment of hemifacial spasm: a systematic review. Br J Neurosurg 2012. https://doi.org/10.3109/02688697.2011.641613.

49. Yoshimura DM, Aminoff MJ, Tami TASA. Treatment of hemifacial spasm with botulinum toxin. Muscle Nerve 1992;5(9):1045–9.

50. Park YC, Lim JK, Lee DKYS. Botulinum a toxin treatment of hemifacial spasm and blepharospasm. J Korean Med Sci 1993;8(5):334–40.

51. Sampaio C, Ferreira JJ, Simões F, et al. DYSBOT: A single-blind, randomized parallel study to determine whether any differences can be detected in the efficacy and tolerability of two formulations of botulinum toxin type A - Dysport and Botox - Assuming a ratio of 4:1. Mov Disord 1997. https://doi.org/10.1002/mds.870120627.

52. Trosch RM, Adler CH, Pappert EJ. Botulinum toxin type B (Myobloc®) in subjects with hemifacial spasm: Results from an open-label, dose-escalation safety study. Mov Disord 2007. https://doi.org/10.1002/mds.21435.

53. Comella CL. Systematic review of botulinum toxin treatment for oromandibular dystonia. Toxicon 2018. https://doi.org/10.1016/j.toxicon.2018.02.006.

54. Ostrem JL, Marks WJ, Volz MM, et al. Pallidal deep brain stimulation in patients with cranial-cervical dystonia (Meige syndrome). Mov Disord 2007. https://doi.org/10.1002/mds.21580.

55. Tan EK, Jankovic J. Botulinum toxin A in patients with oromandibular dystonia: long-term follow-up. Neurology 1999. https://doi.org/10.1212/wnl.53.9.2102.

56. Scorr LM, Silver MR, Hanfelt J, et al. Pilot single-blind trial of abobotulinumtoxinA in oromandibular dystonia. Neurotherapeutics 2018. https://doi.org/10.1007/s13311-018-0620-9.

57. Cardoso F, Bhidayasiri R, Truong D. Treatment of oromandibular dystonia. In: Truong D, Dressler D, Hallett M, editors. Manual of Botulinum Toxin Therapy. Cambridge Core University Press; 2009. https://doi.org/10.1017/cbo 9780511575761.010.

58. Srivanitchapoom P, Pandey S, Hallett M. Drooling in Parkinson's disease: a review. Parkinsonism Relat Disord 2014. https://doi.org/10.1016/j.parkreldis.2014.08.013.

59. Lagalla G, Millevolte M, Capecci M, et al. Botulinum toxin type A for drooling in Parkinson's disease: a double-blind, randomized, placebo-controlled study. Mov Disord 2006. https://doi.org/10.1002/mds.20793.

60. Ondo WG, Hunter C, Moore W. A double-blind placebo-controlled trial of botulinum toxin B for sialorrhea in Parkinson's disease. Neurology 2004. https://doi.org/10.1212/01.WNL.0000101713.81253.4C.

61. Guidubaldi A, Fasano A, Ialongo T, et al. Botulinum toxin A versus B in sialor-rhea: a prospective, randomized, double-blind, crossover pilot study in patients with amyotrophic lateral sclerosis or Parkinson's disease. Mov Disord 2011. https://doi.org/10.1002/mds.23473.

62. Dogu O, Apaydin D, Sevim S, et al. Ultrasound-guided versus "blind" intrapar-otid injections of botulinum toxin-A for the treatment of sialorrhoea in patients with Parkinson's disease. Clin Neurol Neurosurg 2004. https://doi.org/10.1016/j.clineuro.2003.10.012.

63. Tan EK. Botulinum toxin treatment of sialorrhea: comparing different therapeutic preparations. Eur J Neurol 2006. https://doi.org/10.1111/j.1468-1331.2006.01447.x.

64. van den Dool J, Tijssen MAJ, Koelman JHTM, et al. Determinants of disability in cervical dystonia. Parkinsonism Relat Disord 2016. https://doi.org/10.1016/j.parkreldis.2016.08.014.

65. Jankovic J, Adler CH, Charles D, et al. Primary results from the Cervical Dysto-nia Patient Registry for Observation of OnabotulinumtoxinA Efficacy (CD PROBE). J Neurol Sci 2015. https://doi.org/10.1016/j.jns.2014.12.030.

66. Castagna A, Albanese A. Management of cervical dystonia with botulinum neu-rotoxins and EMG/ultrasound guidance. Neurol Clin Pract 2019;9(1):64–73.

67. Brashear A. Botulinum toxin type A in the treatment of patients with cervical dys-tonia. Biologics 2009. https://doi.org/10.2147/btt.s3113.

68. Walker FO. Botulinum toxin therapy for cervical dystonia. Phys Med Rehabil Clin N Am 2003. https://doi.org/10.1016/S1047-9651(03)00045-7.

69. Trosch RM, Espay AJ, Truong D, et al. Multicenter observational study of abobo-tulinumtoxinA neurotoxin in cervical dystonia: The ANCHOR-CD registry. J Neurol Sci 2017. https://doi.org/10.1016/j.jns.2017.02.042.

70. Bhidayasiri R. Treatment of complex cervical dystonia with botulinum toxin: Involvement of deep-cervical muscles may contribute to suboptimal responses. Parkinsonism Relat Disord 2011. https://doi.org/10.1016/j.parkreldis.2011.06.015.

71. Comella CL, Buchman AS, Tanner CM, et al. Botulinum toxin injection for spas-modic torticollis: increased magnitude of benefit with electromyographic assis-tance. Neurology 1992. https://doi.org/10.1212/wnl.42.4.878.

72. Wissel J. Towards flexible and tailored botulinum neurotoxin dosing regimens for focal dystonia and spasticity – Insights from recent studies. Toxicon 2018. https://doi.org/10.1016/j.toxicon.2018.01.018.

73. Chiu SY, Patel B, Burns MR, et al. High-dose botulinum toxin therapy: safety, benefit, and endurance of efficacy. Tremor Other Hyperkinet Mov (N Y) 2020; 10. https://doi.org/10.7916/tohm.v0.749.

74. Comella CL, Thompson PD. Treatment of cervical dystonia with botulinum toxins. Eur J Neurol 2006. https://doi.org/10.1111/j.1468-1331.2006.01440.x.

75. Evidente VGH, Pappert EJ. Botulinum toxin therapy for cervical dystonia: the science of dosing. Tremor Other Hyperkinet Mov (N Y) 2014. https://doi.org/10.7916/D84X56BF.

76. Karp BI, Alter K. Muscle selection for focal limb dystonia. Toxins (Basel) 2018. https://doi.org/10.3390/toxins10010020.

77. Jankovic J. Botulinum toxin: state of the art. Mov Disord 2017. https://doi.org/10.1002/mds.27072.

78. Benecke R, Dressler D. Botulinum toxin treatment of axial and cervical dystonia. Disabil Rehabil 2007. https://doi.org/10.1080/01421590701568262.

79. Bhatia KP, Quinn NP, Marsden CD. Clinical features and natural history of axial predominant adult onset primary dystonia. J Neurol Neurosurg Psychiatry 1997. https://doi.org/10.1136/jnnp.63.6.788.

80. Ehrlich DJ, Frucht SJ. The phenomenology and treatment of idiopathic adult-onset truncal dystonia: a retrospective review. J Clin Mov Disord 2016. https://doi.org/10.1186/s40734-016-0044-9.

81. Comella CL, Shannon KM, Jaglin J. Extensor truncal dystonia: Successful treatment with botulinum toxin injections. Mov Disord 1998. https://doi.org/10.1002/mds.870130330.

82. Mayer NH, Esquenazi A. Muscle overactivity and movement dysfunction in the upper motoneuron syndrome. Phys Med Rehabil Clin N Am 2003. https://doi.org/10.1016/S1047-9651(03)00093-7.

83. Bhakta BB, Cozens JA, Chamberlain MA, et al. Impact of botulinum toxin type A on disability and carer burden due to arm spasticity after stroke: A randomised double blind placebo controlled trial. J Neurol Neurosurg Psychiatry 2000. https://doi.org/10.1136/jnnp.69.2.217.

84. Simpson DM, Patel AT, Alfaro A, et al. OnabotulinumtoxinA injection for post-stroke upper-limb spasticity: guidance for early injectors from a Delphi Panel Process. PM R 2017. https://doi.org/10.1016/j.pmrj.2016.06.016.

85. Wissel J, Ward AB, Erztgaard P, et al. European consensus table on the use of botulinum toxin type A in adult spasticity. J Rehabil Med 2009;41(1):13–25. https://doi.org/10.2340/16501977-0303.

86. Wissel J, Bensmail D, Ferreira JJ, et al. Safety and efficacy of incobotulinumtoxinA doses up to 800 U in limb spasticity the TOWER study. Neurology 2017. https://doi.org/10.1212/WNL.0000000000003789.

87. Esquenazi A, Alfaro A, Ayyoub Z, et al. OnabotulinumtoxinA for lower limb spasticity: guidance from a Delphi Panel Approach. PM R 2017. https://doi.org/10.1016/j.pmrj.2017.02.014.

88. Lotia M, Jankovic J. Botulinum toxin for the treatment of tremor and tics. Semin Neurol 2016. https://doi.org/10.1055/s-0035-1571217.

89. Patel N, Jankovic J, Hallett M. Sensory aspects of movement disorders. Lancet Neurol 2014. https://doi.org/10.1016/S1474-4422(13)70213-8.

90. Porta M, Maggioni G, Ottaviani F, et al. Treatment of phonic tics in patients with Tourette's syndrome using botulinum toxin type A. Neurol Sci 2004. https://doi.org/10.1007/s10072-003-0201-4.

91. Marras C, Andrews D, Sime E, et al. Botulinum toxin for simple motor tics: a randomized, double-blind, controlled clinical trial. Neurology 2001. https://doi.org/10.1212/WNL.56.5.605.

92. Aguirregomozcorta M, Pagonabarraga J, Diaz-Manera J, et al. Efficacy of botulinum toxin in severe Tourette syndrome with dystonic tics involving the neck. Parkinsonism Relat Disord 2008. https://doi.org/10.1016/j.parkreldis.2007.10.007.

93. Practice guideline: the treatment of tics in people with Tourette syndrome and chronic tic disorders. Minneapolis (MN): American Academy of Neurology; 2019. Available at: https://www.aan.com/Guidelines/Home/GetGuidelineContent/968. Accessed April 2, 2020.

94. Jankovic J. An update on new and unique uses of botulinum toxin in movement disorders. Toxicon 2018. https://doi.org/10.1016/j.toxicon.2017.09.003.

95. Jankovic J, Schwartz K. Botulinum toxin treatment of tremors. Neurology 1991. https://doi.org/10.1212/wnl.41.8.1185.

96. Jankovic J, Schwartz K, Clemence W, et al. A randomized, double-blind, placebo-controlled study to evaluate botulinum toxin type A in essential hand tremor. Mov Disord 1996. https://doi.org/10.1002/mds.870110306.

97. Niemann N, Jankovic J. Botulinum toxin for the treatment of hand tremor. Toxins (Basel) 2018. https://doi.org/10.3390/toxins10070299.

98. Simpson DM, Blitzer A, Brashear A, et al. Assessment: botulinum neurotoxin for the treatment of movement disorders (an evidence-based review): report of the therapeutics and technology assessment subcommittee of the American Academy of Neurology symbol. Neurology 2008. https://doi.org/10.1212/01.wnl.0000311389.26145.95.

99. Jankovic J, Truong D, Patel AT, et al. Injectable daxibotulinumtoxinA in cervical dystonia: a phase 2 dose-escalation multicenter study. Mov Disord Clin Pract 2018. https://doi.org/10.1002/mdc3.12613.

100. Stone HF, Zhu Z, Thach TQD, et al. Characterization of diffusion and duration of action of a new botulinum toxin type A formulation. Toxicon 2011. https://doi.org/10.1016/j.toxicon.2011.05.012.

101. Beer KR, Shamban AT, Avelar RL, et al. Efficacy and safety of prabotulinumtoxinA for the treatment of glabellar lines in adult subjects: results from 2 identical phase III studies. Dermatol Surg 2019. https://doi.org/10.1097/DSS.0000000000001903.

102. Fonfria E, Maignel J, Lezmi S, et al. The expanding therapeutic utility of botulinum neurotoxins. Toxins (Basel) 2018. https://doi.org/10.3390/toxins10050208.

103. Glogau RG. Topically applied botulinum toxin type A for the treatment of primary axillary hyperhidrosis: results of a randomized, blinded, vehicle-controlled study. Dermatol Surg 2007. https://doi.org/10.1111/j.1524-4725.2006.32335.x.

104. Glogau R, Blitzer A, Brandt F, et al. Results of a randomized, double-blind, placebo-controlled study to evaluate the efficacy and safety of a botulinum toxin type A topical gel for the treatment of moderate-to-severe lateral canthal lines. J Drugs Dermatol 2012;11(1):38–45.

105. Ascher B, Kestemont P, Boineau D, et al. Liquid formulation of AbobotulinumtoxinA exhibits a favorable efficacy and safety profile in moderate to severe glabellar lines: a randomized, double-blind, placebo- and active comparator-controlled trial. Aesthet Surg J 2018. https://doi.org/10.1093/asj/sjw272.

Cannabinoids in Neurologic Illnesses

Anup D. Patel, MD

KEYWORDS

- Marijuana • Cannabinoids • CBD • Cannabidiol • Medical marijuana • Cannabis
- Medical cannabis

KEY POINTS

- Evidence for the use of cannabinoids for treating neurologic illness remains scant except in the field of epilepsy and multiple sclerosis.
- In the field of epilepsy, randomized double-blind placebo studies exist demonstrating efficacy and safety for using cannabidiol.
- Good evidence exists for the treatment of pain as it relates to spasticity in multiple sclerosis.
- Synthetic cannabinoid products have been approved by the Food and Drug Administration (FDA) with limited evidence of use for treating neurologic illness.
- A mostly purified plant-based cannabidiol oil has been FDA approved to treat seizures associated with Lennox Gastaut and Dravet syndromes in patients 2 and older.

INTRODUCTION
Brief History and Background

Marijuana has been used to treat medical disease since well before the 1800s.[1] Records exist for the use of marijuana-based products for medical purposes as far back as 2700 BCE.[2] Two species of plants, *Cannabis sativa* and *Cannabis indica*, have been applied to the treatment of neurologic illness for centuries.[3] During the late nineteenth century, Gowers[4] reported on the use of cannabis to treat epilepsy. Cannabis-based and marijuana-based terminology is often used interchangeably. Cannabinoids are the chemical components of marijuana.[5] The 2 major cannabinoids active in the nervous system are the psychoactive D9-tetrahydrocannabinol (D9-THC) and the non-psychoactive cannabidiol (CBD).[6] The psychoactive property of D9-THC is the main reason for use of marijuana for recreational purposes. It is often referred to as THC in studies. Nabiximols are oral mucosal sprays that have a standardized extract of THC, the CBD, and other compounds from the 2 species of the cannabis

Neurology, Nationwide Children's Hospital, The Ohio State University College of Medicine, FOB 41.55, 700 Children's Drive, Columbus, OH 43205, USA
E-mail address: anup.patel@nationwidechildrens.org
Twitter: @pedsepilepsydoc (A.D.P.)

Neurol Clin 39 (2021) 231–241
https://doi.org/10.1016/j.ncl.2020.09.012
0733-8619/21/© 2020 Elsevier Inc. All rights reserved.

plant. However, there are many more cannabinoids within the plant.[7] Most of the cannabinoids are found in the flowering portions of the cannabis plant and little in the stalk; each plant can have varying concentrations of cannabinoids.[5,8] Historically, the Drug Enforcement Agency (DEA) considered all products from the marijuana plant to be considered schedule I, making any product derived from the plant illegal at the federal level.[9]

Mechanism of Action

THC appears to bind within the brain via 2 G-protein–coupled receptors named CB_1 and CB_2, with CB_1 serving as the main site accounting for the psychoactive properties. These 2 receptors were named after studies were performed to demonstrate where in the brain this compound worked. However, these receptors are also found elsewhere within the human body. Many other components of the plant, such as CBD do not bind to these receptors.[8,10]

The mechanism of action is more difficult and complicated as it relates to CBD. Much of the known science is dependent of the concentration of CBD. For example, CBD at lower concentrations blocks the orphan G-protein–coupled receptor GPR55, and the transient receptor potential of Melastatin type 8 (TRPM8) channel.[8,11]

Also, CBD increases the activity of the 5-HT1a receptor, the transient receptor potential of ankyrin type 1 (TRPA1) channel, and the a3 and a1 glycine receptors.[1,8,10] CBD at higher concentrations activation of nuclear peroxisome proliferator-activated receptor-c and the transient receptor potential of vanilloid type 1 (TRPV1) and 2 (TRPV2) channels occurs.[8,10] It is not fully understood which of these known properties is responsible for the potential benefit or therapeutic effect that has been seen for CBD in certain neurologic conditions such as epilepsy. The proposed mechanism of action in epilepsy is related to the following targets: transient receptor potential vanilloid-1 (TRPV1), the orphan G-protein–coupled receptor-55 (GPR55) and the equilibrative nucleoside transporter 1 (ENT-1).[12]

Other Cannabinoids

Based on animal studies, other cannabinoids have potential to treat symptoms of neurologic illness. For example, CBD has preclinical evidence with regard to seizure cessation, which set the foundation for clinical trials.[13] In addition, other cannabinoids such as cannabichromene (CBC) and the propyl homologs of both D9 THC named as D9-tetrahydrocannabivarin (D9-THCV) and CBD named cannabidivarin (CBDV) have shown efficacy in seizure cessation within animal models of epilepsy.

THC named as Δ9-tetrahydrocannabivarin (Δ9-THCV) and CBD named cannabidivarin (CBDV) have shown efficacy in seizure cessation within animal models of epilepsy. In relation to Δ9-THCV, this cannabinoid exhibited a high affinity for cannabinoid receptors (CB_1 and CB_2) and demonstrated efficacy in an animal model of Parkinson disease.[14] However, clinic work using these compounds is mostly lacking and future clinical trials are needed to fully understand if these other cannabinoids may treat neurologic illness and benefit patients.

CONTENT
Drug-to-Drug Interactions

Limited data exist on the potential extent of drug-to-drug interactions between cannabis-based products and common medications. Marijuana is metabolized by the human body in the liver. The P-450 enzyme pathway is involved in metabolizing several exogenous cannabinoids.[15] Tetrahydrocannabinol (THC) is one such cannabinoid due to liver enzyme pathways of CYP2C9 and 3A4, where cannabidiol (CBD) has CYPs 2C19 and 3A4 properties. These preclinical findings are supported by clinical data on THC and CBD metabolism.[15] In contrast, the inhibition or induction of liver containing cytochromes by cannabinoids may potentially affect the metabolism of many drugs that function by using this system. For example, THC is a CYP 1A2 inducer and CBD is a 3A4 inhibitor. Further clinical studies are needed to validate which specific medications that follow these pathways lead to clinical effects in humans. Regarding antiseizure medications, some data have been published. Specifically, a study showed that concomitant administration of a plant-based purified form of CBD significantly changed serum levels of topiramate, rufinamide, clobazam, eslicarbazepine, and zonisamide in adult patients with treatment-resistant (intractable) epilepsy.[16] In other trials using the same formulation of CBD, only increases in a common metabolite of clobazam was noted.[17,18] Elevation in liver transaminases was noted more commonly in patients on concomitant valproic acid despite valproic acid levels not being increased.[17,18]

When given to healthy adults, concomitant administration of fentanyl with CBD did not affect the plasma level of CBD and did not produce cardiovascular complications or respiratory depression and CBD did not increase fentanyl effects.[15] Ketoconazole is a CYP3A4 inhibitor and was found to increase THC and CBD concentrations when studied while rifampin reduced THC and CBD concentration.[15] Rifampin is a well-known CYP3A4 inducer.

Epilepsy

Several studies now exist demonstrating the safety and efficacy of one cannabinoid, CBD, in the field of epilepsy. A Cochrane review detailed 4 controlled studies performed in the 1970s that used various marijuana-based products to treat seizures. Significant flaws existed within these studies making any conclusions on potential therapeutic effect difficult. In these studies, it appeared that doses of 200 to 300 mg of CBD were well tolerated in the few human subjects given this concentration of CBD.[7] Studies evaluating recreational use of marijuana in patients with new-onset seizures had mixed findings showing a potential benefit in men without significant benefit for women.[19,20] Various case reports and series have shown potential benefits of cannabis products for the treatment of seizures.[21,22]

Open-label use of a plant-based and mostly purified form of CBD was studied retrospectively based from an expanded access program available in the United States for compassionate access purposes to patients with treatment-resistant epilepsy.[23] For this open-label trial, patients ages 1 to 30 with treatment-resistant epilepsy were studied. Patients were given oral cannabidiol at 2 to 5 mg/kg per day, up-titrated until intolerance or to a maximum dose of 25 mg/kg per day or 50 mg/kg per day. Some of the study sites had patients with doses of up to 50 mg/kg per day. At all sites, 214 patients were enrolled. The median monthly frequency of motor seizures was 30 at baseline and 15.8 over a 12-week treatment period. The median reduction in monthly motor seizures was 36.5%.[23] Because this was a retrospective open-label study design, no placebo group was present. Adverse events were reported in 79%. Adverse events reported in more than 10% of patients were somnolence (25%), decreased appetite (19%), diarrhea (19%), fatigue (13%), and convulsion (11%). Three percent of patients discontinued treatment because of an adverse event.[23]

These results set the stage for future studies, as several patients had either Lennox Gastaut syndrome (LGS) or Dravet syndrome. The first study was a randomized double-blind placebo-controlled study performed to establish pharmacokinetics and possible dosing of a purified plant-based formulation of CBD, *Epidiolex*, in patients ages 4 to 18 with Dravet syndrome.[18] In this study, patients were randomized 4:1 to CBD (5, 10, or 20 mg/kg per day) or placebo taken twice daily. The trial design consisted of a 4-week baseline, and 3-week treatment portion including titration. Patients who completed the study could continue in an open-label extension. During the study, multiple pharmacokinetic blood samples were taken on the first day of dosing and at end of treatment for measurement of CBD, its metabolites 6-OH-CBD, 7-OH-CBD, and 7-COOH-CBD, and antiepileptic drugs (AEDs; clobazam and metabolite N-desmethylclobazam [N-CLB], valproate, levetiracetam, topiramate, and stiripentol). Several safety assessments included clinical laboratory tests, physical examinations, vital signs, electrocardiograms, adverse events, seizure frequency, and suicidality assessments. Overall, 34 patients were randomized with 32 (94%) who completed treatment. Exposure to CBD and its metabolites was dose-proportional. CBD did not affect concomitant AED levels except an increase in N-CLB. This effect was not present in patients taking stiripentol. The most common adverse effects reported were pyrexia, somnolence, decreased appetite, sedation, vomiting, ataxia, and abnormal behavior. Six patients taking CBD and valproate developed elevated transaminases; none met criteria for drug-induced liver injury. All these patients recovered.[18]

A separate study using a similar study design evaluating the safety and efficacy of this formulation of CBD was performed in patients 2 to 18 with Dravet syndrome.[17] In this double-blind, placebo-controlled study, patients with a clinical confirmed diagnosis of Dravet syndrome and drug-resistant seizures received either the same previously studied cannabidiol oral solution at a dose of 20 mg/kg per day or placebo, in addition to standard antiseizure treatment that was not changed during the study.

The median frequency of convulsive seizures per month decreased from 12.4 to 5.9 with cannabidiol, as compared with a decrease from 14.9 to 14.1 with placebo. This accounted for a 38.9% median convulsive seizure reduction compared with 13.3% for the placebo group. Regarding responder rate for convulsive seizures, reduction in the treatment group (50% reduction in convulsive seizure frequency) was 43% with cannabidiol and 27% with placebo.

The patients' overall condition improved by at least 1 category on the 7-category Caregiver Global Impression of Change (CGIC) scale in 62% of the cannabidiol group as compared with 34% of the placebo group ($P = .02$). The frequency of total seizures of all types was significantly reduced with cannabidiol ($P = .03$). However, no significant reduction in nonconvulsive seizures was noted in this study. The percentage of patients who became seizure-free was 5% with cannabidiol and 0% with placebo. Adverse events that occurred more frequently in the cannabidiol group than in the placebo group included diarrhea, vomiting, fatigue, pyrexia, somnolence, and abnormal results on liver-function tests.[17]

Two similar randomized double-blind placebo-controlled studies evaluating safety and efficacy of this formulation of CBD were performed for patients with LGS. One study evaluated patients ages 2 to 55 with treatment-resistant LGS using a dose of 20 mg/kg per day compared with placebo.[24] The primary endpoint investigated was the efficacy of cannabidiol as add-on therapy for drop seizures with LGS. LGS was defined as a history of slow (<3 Hz) spike-and-wave patterns on electroencephalogram, evidence of more than 1 type of generalized seizure for at least 6 months, at least 2 drop seizures per week during the 4-week baseline period, and had not responded to treatment with at least 2 antiseizure medications. The primary endpoint was percentage change from baseline in monthly frequency of drop seizures during the treatment period. For the study, 171 patients were randomized to receive cannabidiol (n = 86) at a dose of 20 mg/kg per day or placebo (n = 85). The median percentage reduction in monthly drop-seizure frequency from baseline was 43.9% in the treatment group and 21.8% (IQR −45.7–1.7) in the placebo group. Fourteen patients in the cannabidiol group and 1 in the placebo group discontinued study treatment; all randomly assigned patients received at least 1 dose of study treatment and had post-baseline efficacy data. Adverse events occurred in 86% of cannabidiol group and 69% in the placebo group. Most of these adverse effects were reported as mild or moderate. The most common adverse events consisted of diarrhea, somnolence, pyrexia, decreased appetite, and vomiting. Fourteen percent of patients in the cannabidiol group and 1% in the placebo group withdrew from the study because of adverse events.[24]

In another study using a similar study design with 3 arms and the same formulation of CBD: 10 mg/kg per day, 20 mg/kg per day, and placebo, patients 2 to 55 years of age with treatment-resistant LGS were enrolled.[25] Patients with LGS had 2 or more drop seizures per week during a 28-day baseline period and were evaluated over 14 weeks. A total of 225 patients were enrolled into 1 of the 3 groups. The median percent reduction from baseline in drop-seizure frequency during the treatment period was 41.9% in the 20 mg/kg per day group, 37.2% in the 10 mg/kg per day cannabidiol group, and 17.2% in the placebo. The most common adverse events among the patients in the CBD groups were like other studies. Seven patients discontinued the trial medication because of adverse events and were withdrawn from the trial, with 6 of these patients in the 20 mg/kg per day group. Nine percent of patients had elevated liver aminotransferase concentrations in this study.[25]

These Class I studies using this specific formulation of plant-based mostly purified CBD led to the approval of this medication by the Food and Drug Administration (FDA) to treat patients 2 years and older with seizures associated with LGS and Dravet and rescheduled by the DEA allowing all medical providers possessing an active DEA license the ability to prescribe this medication without other regulation or licensure.[26] Long-term data using this formulation have been published demonstrating continued efficacy without significant decrease and a similar adverse effect profile as previously reported.[27–29] Randomized double-blind placebo-controlled studies using other formulations of CBD or different ratios of CBD with THC are not available. Therefore, it is unknown is these products have similar efficacy and safety as demonstrated with the FDA-approved product. A phase II study on a synthetic version of CBD evaluated efficacy in patients with treatment-resistant infantile spasms demonstrating no significant improvement.[30]

Multiple Sclerosis

Studies evaluating various marijuana-based preparations in treating complications related to multiple sclerosis (MS) in adult patients exist. American Academy of Neurology guidelines evaluated these studies to provide recommendations for use in patients with MS.[31,32] This guideline sought to determine the efficacy of marijuana products used to treat patients with MS. For patients with spasticity from MS, oral cannabis extract (OCE) and synthetic preparations are probably effective when evaluating subjective measures with unclear benefit with the evaluation of objective measures; however, smoked preparations were of no benefit.[32]

The investigators determined that OCE is effective and nabiximols and THC are probably effective for reducing patient-centered measures for patients with spasticity from MS. OCE is effective for central pain or painful spasms (including spasticity-related pain, excluding neuropathic pain) with THC and nabiximols listed as probably effective. These oral extracts contain a similar proportion of THC and CBD. When evaluating pain and spasms related to MS, the oral extracts are effective with strong evidence supporting its use.[32] For patients experiencing urinary dysfunction with MS, nabiximols are probably effective for reducing bladder voids/d with THC and OCE determined to be probably ineffective for reducing bladder complaints.

In one study, an orally administered standardized *Cannabis sativa* plant extract was given to patients with a history of MS experiencing poorly controlled spasticity while being evaluated in an inpatient rehabilitation program.[33] Overall, 57 patients were enrolled in a prospective, randomized, double-blind, placebo-controlled crossover study using an OCE capsule standardized to 2.5 mg THC and 0.9 mg CBD. Patients were split into different groups. In one group, patients started with 15 mg and, if well tolerated, increased to a maximum 30 mg THC by 5 mg per day. They were on active medication for 14 days before beginning placebo. A separate group of patients started with placebo for 7 days, then were given the medication for 14 days and switched back to a 3-day placebo period. The measures used to determine potential efficacy included daily self-report of spasm frequency and symptoms, the Ashworth scale, the Rivermead Mobility Index, the 10-m timed walk, the 9-hole peg test, the paced auditory serial addition test, and the digit span test. Fifty patients were included in the analysis. The results demonstrated no statistically significant differences associated with patients given the medication compared with placebo. Thirty-seven patients were reported to have improvements in spasm frequency ($P = .013$) and mobility for patients who received at least 90% of their prescribed dose. Minor adverse events were slightly more frequent and severe for patients who received the medication treatment compared with placebo.[33]

Another class I study was performed to determine whether a cannabis-based medicinal extract (CBME) would benefit a range of symptoms seen in MS.[34] A total of 160 patients with MS experiencing significant problems from at least one of the following: spasticity, spasms, bladder problems, tremor or pain were recruited. The medications used were an oromucosal spray or whole plant CBME containing equal amounts of THC and CBD with divided doses of 2.5 to 120 mg of each daily. The outcome measure used was a Visual Analogue Scale (VAS) score for each patient's most troublesome symptom. Additional measures included VAS scores of other symptoms, and measures of disability, cognition, mood, sleep, and fatigue. No statistical significance was noted for CBME in reducing the primary symptom score. VAS scores related to spasticity were significantly reduced by CBME when compared with placebo ($P = .001$). There were no significant adverse effects reported for cognition or mood. Intoxication from CBME was reported as generally mild.[34]

Another randomized, placebo-controlled trial was performed to evaluate patients with stable MS and muscle spasticity as a symptom. A total of 630 patients were treated with either THC or an OCE combination product with THC/CBD. In this study, the primary outcome measure was change in overall spasticity scores, using the Ashworth scale. No statistically significant difference was noted for the either cannabis-based product on the primary outcome ($P = .40$). However, evidence of a treatment effect on patient-reported spasticity and pain ($P = .003$) was noted for patients receiving the OCE, Delta9-THC, and placebo suggesting a subjective benefit to patient-reported pain as it related to spasticity in the treatment and placebo groups.[35]

A separate study showed a subjective patient-reported response to pain as it relates to spasticity for patients with MS when compared with placebo.[36] In this double-blind, placebo-controlled study, patients received an OCE that was increased weekly from 5 mg to a maximum of 25 mg of THC daily. They were followed for 10 weeks with the primary outcome measure being a category rating scale (CRS) measuring patient-reported change in muscle stiffness from baseline. Further CRSs assessed body pain, spasms, and sleep quality. In addition, 3 other validated MS-specific patient-reported outcome measures evaluating various aspects of spasticity, physical and psychological impact, and walking ability were collected. The relief from muscle stiffness was reported to be approximately 2 times as high with OCE when compared with placebo (P = .004) with similar reports from the other validated MS patient-reported outcome measures. Adverse events in participants treated with OCE were consistent with the known side effects from previous studies and no new safety concerns were raised.[36]

Evaluation of spasticity using an oral mucosal spray with a 50/50 preparation containing THC and CBD compared with placebo was performed.[37] In this study, the primary endpoint was a spasticity 0 to 10 numeric rating scale (NRS). A statistically significant improvement was not seen in patients receiving the medication compared with placebo. However, the investigators reported a per protocol population (79% of subjects) change in NRS score and showed a statistically significant improvement for the medication group when compared with placebo (0.035). In addition, a responder rate that was based on a greater than or equal to 30% improvement from baseline was reported for the medication group when compared with placebo (P = .040). Further, CGIC assessment (P = .013) and timed 10-m walk (P = .042) demonstrated significance in the treatment group when compared with the placebo group. This preparation was well tolerated with most adverse events reported being mild-to-moderate in severity.[37]

Movement Disorders and Tourette Syndrome

Overall, data are either lacking or cannabis-related products have not been found to benefit patients with various movement disorders. A class I randomized placebo-controlled crossover study was performed in 19 patients with Parkinson disease. These patients were randomized to receive OCE followed by placebo or vice versa. The treatment phase lasted for 4 weeks with an intervening 2-week washout phase. The primary outcome measure used was a change in the Unified Parkinson's Disease Rating Scale (UPDRS) dyskinesia score. Several secondary outcome measures were evaluated and included: the Rush scale, the Bain scale, the tablet arm drawing task, and the total UPDRS score following a levodopa challenge, a patient-completed measures of a dyskinesia activities of daily living scale, the PDQ-39, the on-off diaries, and a range of category rating scales. Of the 19 patients, 17 completed the trial. No statistical significance was noted for a treatment effect on levodopa-induced dyskinesia as assessed by the UPDRS, or any of the secondary outcome measures.

Interestingly, survey data suggest patients are receiving cannabis-related products to treat various symptoms of movement disorders despite lack of evidence and source of information is often other families and not medical providers.[38] In other studies, oral cannabinoids have limited data and are of unknown benefit for non–chorea-related symptoms of Huntington disease, Tourette syndrome, and cervical dystonia.[32]

Headache and Migraine

No randomized double-blind placebo-controlled trials have been performed in the use of any marijuana-based product in the treatment of specific headache syndromes or migraine.[39] Retrospective reviews have demonstrated patient reports of improvement with cannabis products.[40] Reports from the late 1800s described the use of marijuana to treat migraine and various other forms of neurologic pain and headache.[41] A meta-analysis evaluating all randomized control trials reported in the literature was performed as it relates to chronic pain and found that pain relief was achieved with some marijuana products with the investigators noting significant central nervous system adverse effects were commonly reported within the specific studies.[42] Patients were given oral or a nasal mucosal spray and compared with a placebo group in adult patients with pain due to various diseases; however, headache was not specifically studied.[42] Therefore, it is unclear whether marijuana-based products can specifically treat patients with headache or migraine.[43]

SUMMARY

Recently, an increased interest in studying cannabis-based products for medical use has occurred.[15] However, studies still lack in the field of neurology with more randomized double-blind placebo studies needing to be performed.[32] For patients with seizures associated with certain epilepsy syndromes and for patients with pain from spasticity from MS, class I evidence exists that has demonstrated both efficacy and tolerability of the products studied.

It is important to note that not all cannabis-based products are equal and offer truth in labeling.[44] Products sold and marketed outside the purview of the FDA are not regulated nor tested reliably.[45] In addition, controversy remains as to the brain inhibition properties of some marijuana compounds[46] and other potential symptom worsening.[6] Drug-to-drug interactions exist for the chemical compounds found in marijuana with more study needed.[15] Information about use of these products is often obtained via other patients, advertisements, or media sources and not by medical providers.[47] Therefore, it is important all neurology providers understand the current level of evidence for using marijuana-based products to treat neurologic illnesses.

CLINICS CARE POINTS

- The medical literature on the use of cannabis in neurological illness is scant.
- Evidence does exist for the use of a plant based mostly purified form of cannabidiol (CBD) to treat seizures in patients with Lennox Gastaut syndrome, Dravet syndrome, and Tuberous Sclerosis Complex.
- Not all CBD products are the same as testing is not always robust or consistent.
- Caution should be had when using medical cannabis for the treatment of neurological illness.

DISCLOSURE

Institutional research funding from Greenwich Biosciences.

REFERENCES

1. Russo E. Cannabis for migraine treatment: the once and future prescription? An historical and scientific review. Pain 1998;76(1–2):3–8.
2. Brill H. Marihuana: the first twelve thousand years. J Psychoactive Drugs 1981; 13(4):397–8.
3. Grundy RI. The therapeutic potential of the cannabinoids in neuroprotection. Expert Opin Investig Drugs 2002;11(10):1365–74.
4. Gowers W. Epilepsy and other chronic convulsive disorders. London: Churchill; 1881.
5. Mechoulam R, Hanus L. A historical overview of chemical research on cannabinoids. Chem Phys Lipids 2000;108(1–2):1–13.
6. Fusar-Poli P, Crippa JA, Bhattacharyya S, et al. Distinct effects of {delta}9-tetrahydrocannabinol and cannabidiol on neural activation during emotional processing. Arch Gen Psychiatry 2009;66(1):95–105.
7. Gloss D, Vickrey B. Cannabinoids for epilepsy. Cochrane Database Syst Rev 2014;(3):CD009270.

8. Pertwee RG. The diverse CB1 and CB2 receptor pharmacology of three plant cannabinoids: delta9-tetrahydrocannabinol, cannabidiol and delta9-tetrahydro-cannabivarin. Br J Pharmacol 2008;153(2):199–215.
9. Joffe A. Legalization of marijuana: potential impact on youth. Pediatrics 2004; 113(6):1825–6.
10. Pertwee RG. Ligands that target cannabinoid receptors in the brain: from THC to anandamide and beyond. Addict Biol 2008;13(2):147–59.
11. Devinsky O, Cilio MR, Cross H, et al. Cannabidiol: pharmacology and potential therapeutic role in epilepsy and other neuropsychiatric disorders. Epilepsia 2014;55(6):791–802.
12. Gray RA, Whalley BJ. The proposed mechanisms of action of CBD in epilepsy. Epileptic Disord 2020;22(S1):10–5.
13. Hill AJ, Williams CM, Whalley BJ, et al. Phytocannabinoids as novel therapeutic agents in CNS disorders. Pharmacol Ther 2012;133(1):79–97.
14. Garcia C, Palomo-Garo C, Garcia-Arencibia M, et al. Symptom-relieving and neuroprotective effects of the phytocannabinoid Delta(9)-THCV in animal models of Parkinson's disease. Br J Pharmacol 2011;163(7):1495–506.
15. Alsherbiny MA, Li CG. Medicinal cannabis-potential drug interactions. Medicines (Basel, Switzerland) 2018;6(1):3.
16. Gaston TE, Bebin EM, Cutter GR, et al. Interactions between cannabidiol and commonly used antiepileptic drugs. Epilepsia 2017;58(9):1586–92.
17. Devinsky O, Cross JH, Laux L, et al. Trial of cannabidiol for drug-resistant seizures in the Dravet syndrome. N Engl J Med 2017;376(21):2011–20.
18. Devinsky O, Patel AD, Thiele EA, et al. Randomized, dose-ranging safety trial of cannabidiol in Dravet syndrome. Neurology 2018;90(14):e1204–11.
19. Brust JC, Ng SK, Hauser AW, et al. Marijuana use and the risk of new onset seizures. Trans Am Clin Climatological Assoc 1992;103:176–81.
20. Ng SK, Brust JC, Hauser WA, et al. Illicit drug use and the risk of new-onset seizures. Am J Epidemiol 1990;132(1):47–57.
21. Ladino LD, Hernandez-Ronquillo L, Tellez-Zenteno JF. Medicinal marijuana for epilepsy: a case series study. Can J Neurol Sci Le J canadien des Sci neurologiques 2014;41(6):753–8.
22. Maa E, Figi P. The case for medical marijuana in epilepsy. Epilepsia 2014;55(6): 783–6.
23. Devinsky O, Marsh E, Friedman D, et al. Cannabidiol in patients with treatment-resistant epilepsy: an open-label interventional trial. Lancet Neurol 2016;15(3):270–8.
24. Thiele EA, Marsh ED, French JA, et al. Cannabidiol in patients with seizures associated with Lennox-Gastaut syndrome (GWPCARE4): a randomised, double-blind, placebo-controlled phase 3 trial. Lancet 2018;391(10125): 1085–96.
25. Devinsky O, Patel AD, Cross JH, et al. Effect of cannabidiol on drop seizures in the Lennox-Gastaut Syndrome. N Engl J Med 2018;378(20):1888–97.
26. Nabbout R, Thiele EA. The role of cannabinoids in epilepsy treatment: a critical review of efficacy results from clinical trials. Epileptic Disord 2020;22(S1):23–8.
27. Szaflarski JP, Bebin EM, Comi AM, et al. Long-term safety and treatment effects of cannabidiol in children and adults with treatment-resistant epilepsies: expanded access program results. Epilepsia 2018;59(8):1540–8.
28. Devinsky O, Nabbout R, Miller I, et al. Long-term cannabidiol treatment in patients with Dravet syndrome: an open-label extension trial. Epilepsia 2019; 60(2):294–302.

29. Laux LC, Bebin EM, Checketts D, et al. Long-term safety and efficacy of canna-bidiol in children and adults with treatment resistant Lennox-Gastaut syndrome or Dravet syndrome: Expanded access program results. Epilepsy Res 2019;154: 13–20.

30. Hussain SA, Dlugos DJ, Cilio MR, et al. Synthetic pharmaceutical grade canna-bidiol for treatment of refractory infantile spasms: a multicenter phase-2 study. Epilepsy Behav 2020;102:106826.

31. Yadav V, Bever C Jr, Bowen J, et al. Summary of evidence-based guideline: com-plementary and alternative medicine in multiple sclerosis: report of the guideline development subcommittee of the American Academy of Neurology. Neurology 2014;82(12):1083–92.

32. Koppel BS, Brust JC, Fife T, et al. Systematic review: efficacy and safety of med-ical marijuana in selected neurologic disorders: report of the Guideline Develop-ment Subcommittee of the American Academy of Neurology. Neurology 2014; 82(17):1556–63.

33. Vaney C, Heinzel-Gutenbrunner M, Jobin P, et al. Efficacy, safety and tolerability of an orally administered cannabis extract in the treatment of spasticity in patients with multiple sclerosis: a randomized, double-blind, placebo-controlled, cross-over study. Mult Scler 2004;10(4):417–24.

34. Wade DT, Makela P, Robson P, et al. Do cannabis-based medicinal extracts have general or specific effects on symptoms in multiple sclerosis? A double-blind, randomized, placebo-controlled study on 160 patients. Mult Scler 2004;10(4): 434–41.

35. Zajicek J, Fox P, Sanders H, et al. Cannabinoids for treatment of spasticity and other symptoms related to multiple sclerosis (CAMS study): multicentre rando-mised placebo-controlled trial. Lancet 2003;362(9395):1517–26.

36. Zajicek JP, Hobart JC, Slade A, et al. Multiple sclerosis and extract of cannabis: results of the MUSEC trial. J Neurol Neurosurg Psychiatry 2012; 83(11):1125–32.

37. Collin C, Ehler E, Waberzinek G, et al. A double-blind, randomized, placebo-controlled, parallel-group study of Sativex, in subjects with symptoms of spas-ticity due to multiple sclerosis. Neurol Res 2010;32(5):451–9.

38. Wilson JL, Gregory A, Wakeman K, et al. Cannabis use in children with pantothe-nate kinase-associated neurodegeneration. J Child Neurol 2020;35(4):259–64.

39. Rajapakse T, Davenport WJ. Phytomedicines in the treatment of migraine. CNS Drugs 2019;33(5):399–415.

40. Rhyne DN, Anderson SL, Gedde M, et al. Effects of medical marijuana on migraine headache frequency in an adult population. Pharmacotherapy 2016; 36(5):505–10.

41. McGeeney BE. Cannabinoids and hallucinogens for headache. Headache 2013; 53(3):447–58.

42. Martin-Sanchez E, Furukawa TA, Taylor J, et al. Systematic review and meta-analysis of cannabis treatment for chronic pain. Pain Med 2009;10(8): 1353–68.

43. Whiting PF, Wolff RF, Deshpande S, et al. Cannabinoids for medical use: a sys-tematic review and meta-analysis. JAMA 2015;313(24):2456–73.

44. Bonn-Miller MO, Loflin MJE, Thomas BF, et al. Labeling accuracy of cannabidiol extracts sold online. JAMA 2017;318(17):1708–9.

45. Freedman DA, Patel AD. Inadequate regulation contributes to mislabeled online cannabidiol products. Pediatr Neurol Briefs 2018;32:3.

46. deShazo RD, Parker SB, Williams D, et al. Marijuana's effects on brain structure and function: what do we know and what should we do? A brief review and commentary. Am J Med 2019;132(3):281–5.
47. Leos-Toro C, Fong GT, Meyer SB, et al. Cannabis labelling and consumer understanding of THC levels and serving sizes. Drug and Alcohol Dependence 2020; 208:107843.

Therapeutic Pitfalls in the Transition of Neurologic Patients from Pediatric to Adult Health Care Providers

Eugene R. Schnitzler, MD[a,b],*, Michael J. Schneck, MD[c,d]

KEYWORDS

- Transitions of care • Pediatric neurology • Adult neurology

KEY POINTS

- Transitions of care from the pediatric to adult setting are fraught with difficulty.
- For patients whose neurologic problems began in childhood, there is often a lack of organized multidisciplinary care with the desired neurologic expertise in the adult setting.
- This monograph highlights those difficulties and reviews disease-specific instances of the problems with transition from pediatric to adult neurologic care.
- The authors suggest that the use of an arbitrary chronologic age cutoff for transition from pediatric to adult expertise in specific disease state may be a disservice in provision of care, and in certain circumstances, the disease-specific expertise of providers may outweigh the benefit of an age-related provider focus.

Transition is synonymous with the process of change, and change has been philosophized as life's only constant. The practice of modern medicine requires the accurate and efficient implementation of frequent transitions of care. These transitions can occur between and across multiple timeframes and locations. The World Health Organization (WHO) has recognized that there are risks inherent in health care transitions and has issued position statements with recommendations on how to facilitate and improve these processes.[1] Similarly, in the United States, The Joint Commission on

[a] Department of Neurology, Division of Pediatric Neurology, Loyola University Chicago, Stritch School of Medicine, Maguire Building Suite 2700, 2160 South First Avenue, Maywood, IL 60153, USA; [b] Department of Pediatrics, Loyola University Chicago, Stritch School of Medicine, Maywood, IL, USA; [c] Department of Neurology, Loyola University Chicago, Stritch School of Medicine, Maywood, IL, USA; [d] Department of Neurosurgery, Loyola University Chicago, Stritch School of Medicine, Maywood, IL, USA
* Corresponding author. Department of Neurology, Division of Chicago Neurology, Loyola University Chicago, Stritch School of Medicine, Maguire Building Suite 2700, 2160 South First Avenue, Maywood, IL 60153.
E-mail address: Eschnitzler@lumc.edu

Neurol Clin 39 (2021) 243–256
https://doi.org/10.1016/j.ncl.2020.09.015
0733-8619/21/© 2020 Elsevier Inc. All rights reserved.

Accreditation of Healthcare Organizations has examined transitions of care and identified several root causes of suboptimal outcomes.[2] Problems include breakdown in communications between providers and between providers and patients, as well as breakdowns in patient education. Failure of physicians and other clinicians to be accountable for the care coordination required for successful transitions is also a major concern.

Specifically, transitions of care equate to a repositioning of patients between and among providers and settings. As such, a transition can occur within a hospital, such as from emergency department (ED) to intensive care unit (ICU), or between settings, such as from a hospital to a primary care provider's (PCP's) office or the patient's home. Accompanying such processes will also be transfers of responsibility for care between physician providers as well as nonphysician health care providers, including nurses, psychologists, physical and occupational therapists, pharmacists, and other health care personnel. Transitions can also be long term, such as from hospital to nursing home or pediatrician to internist. Similarly, short-term care transitions occur daily with changes in nursing shifts and resident on-call schedules.

All transitions have the intrinsic commonality of an exchange of patient data between "senders" and "receivers," that is, the providers on either end of the transfer of care.[3] Recognizing patient vulnerability, the WHO has cited numerous risks inherent in the transition process, including increases in mortality, morbidity, adverse events, and treatment delays. Also noted were increased ED and PCP visits, lost or duplicated test results, and preventable hospital readmissions. The Joint Commission has suggested several strategies to mitigate these risks.[4] These strategies include establishment of national guidelines for care transition with standardization of terminology and systems of information transfer. Additional recommendations include systems for tracking of diagnostic tests, referrals, and appointments and comprehensive discharge planning. In particular, medication reconciliation, that is, review, updating, and revisions of patient medication lists, was deemed to be a crucial component of successful care transition.[5]

The essential mechanism of the transition process is the "handoff."[6] The Joint Commission defines a handoff as "a transfer and acceptance of patient care responsibility achieved through effective communication." Handoffs can be conceptualized as transactions between senders and receivers of essential patient data. As such, they are a crucial component of modern health care delivery, which should be structured and standardized. In the case of inpatient care, resident handoffs should include the patient's diagnosis, vital signs, hospital course, care plan, laboratory tests, medications, and a to-do list with contingency plans. Standardized handoff protocols should be added to the medical record.[7] Mnemonics have been devised that can remind providers of the essential components of the handoff. One such mnemonic is "I-PASS," which stands for "illness severity, patient summary, action list, situation awareness and contingency plans, and synthesis by receiver." The use of this mnemonic resulted in a 23% reduction in medical error rates at a major American university hospital.[8]

Miscommunications during handoffs occur for many reasons, including lack of sufficient provider training, language barriers, poor documentation, unrealistic assumptions, and ongoing distractions. Cornish and associates[9] screened the medication lists of 151 patients at the time of admission to a teaching hospital. They found that more than half of these patients had at least 1 unintended medication discrepancy. Omissions of a regularly used medication were the most frequent error. Although most of these errors were benign, 38.6% were deemed potentially serious. Similarly, Arora and colleagues[10] found a 27% rate of discrepancies between daily medication lists on residents' daily sign-out sheets and patient charts. Most of these (80%) were medication omissions. Moreover, distractions may be a contributing factor in medication errors. Bonafide and associates[11] found a significant association between cell phone call interruptions and nursing medication errors in a pediatric ICU. Thus, although successful handoffs are a crucial part of day-to-day health care, they are vulnerable to multiple sources in inefficiency and miscommunication with the potential for medical errors. Accordingly, it would seem to be a prudent management strategy to minimize the frequency of medical handoffs, as well as the amount of data transferred per handoff. Nevertheless, paradoxically, the decrease in weekly resident duty hours mandated by the ACGME has necessarily resulted in an increase in resident handoffs and a decrease in resident continuity of care.[12]

A permanent and usually irrevocable transition of care occurs when a pediatric patient is transferred to an adult provider. In the case of primary care, such transitions typically happen between the ages of 18 and 22. The American Academy of Pediatrics, American Academy of Family Practice, American College of Physicians, and American Society of Internal Medicine issued a joint position statement on transition of care of adolescents in 2002[13] and again in 2011[14] and 2018.[15] The initial statement emphasizes that several steps are necessary for successful transitions. It is important to identify appropriate adult providers with the required interest and knowledge base. Patient and family readiness for transition must be established. Medical records must be up-to-date and accessible and should contain a transition plan. Maintenance of health insurance coverage during and following transition must be assured. In the follow-up position statements, it was noted that there were continued issues with the implementation of effective transitions. A persistent problem was the lack of adult providers with the willingness and training to take on the care of adolescents with chronic medical problems. The prevalence of this subset of the adolescent population is estimated to be 18.4%, many of whom have neurologic conditions. Additional concerns include the extra professional time involved in developing transition plans and the lack of insurance reimbursement for those nonencounter patient services.[16] In 2016, the American Academy of Neurology issued a consensus statement endorsing the stepwise transition of pediatric neurology patients. It emphasizes 8 common principles for transition of care.[17] These are as follows:

1. Expectation of transition
2. Yearly self-management assessment
3. Annual discussion of medical condition and age-appropriate consensus
4. Evaluation of legal competency
5. Annual review of transition plan of care
6. Child neurology team responsibilities
7. Identification of adult provider
8. Transfer complete

These principles are elaborated in detail in the statement. The concepts of introduction of transition planning by age 13 and annual reassessment of readiness and planning are emphasized. The statement concedes that there is a lack of research on transition and whether it will result in optimal outcomes. Numerous challenges remain to be overcome, in particular, selection of adult providers with the appropriate training and comfort level to manage young adults with developmental disabilities. Alternatively, neurologic care may be transferred to other adult providers, such as PCPs, psychiatrists, and/or disease-focused clinics. Interestingly, the Got Transition guidelines for PCPs recognizes that in the case of family medicine and combined medicine-pediatrics providers, transition of care to an adult model does not require a change in the health care provider.[18] Paradoxically, the same reasoning has not been adapted to the neurology transition models. This is despite the fact that the training and board certi-fication of child neurologists traditionally have included demonstration of expertise in adult neurology.[19]

The consensus statement also acknowledges that "transfer of care is fraught with high rates of anxiety" for both patients and their families. The recommended age for completion of transition is 18 years, which coincides with the age of majority (achieve-ment of adult legal status) in the United States. However, for the many neurologic pa-tients who are developmentally disabled, age 18 brings the added stressors of applying for guardianship, extending high-school programs, and seeking out addi-tional community resources for adaptive employment and housing. Therefore, perhaps it would be prudent to rethink the timing of the proposed transition models and to realize that a "one-size-fits-all" approach is not always feasible. An alternative idea might be to restructure transition plans and tailor them to disease or disorder spe-cific models. Some examples are as follows.

EPILEPSY

According to recent data, PCPs manage a third of the 3.4 million adult American pa-tients with epilepsy. Two-thirds of adults with epilepsy are followed by a neurologist or epileptologist, but over half of those patients still have breakthrough seizures despite medications.[20] Children with epilepsy are typically managed by a pediatric neurolo-gist, some of whom have also subspecialized in epilepsy or neurophysiology. Many childhood-onset epileptic syndromes, such as benign rolandic, benign occipital, and childhood absence epilepsy, will be outgrown in adolescence. However, other conditions, such as infantile spasms, Dravet syndrome, and Lennox-Gastaut syn-drome (LGS), will result in refractory seizures with cognitive impairment and develop-mental delays which will persist into adulthood.

Complex partial seizures can occur as a consequence of mesial temporal sclerosis (MTS). In some cases, MTS is thought to follow childhood febrile status epilepticus.[21] Seizures from MTS that are refractory to medications may be amenable to surgical resection. Juvenile myoclonic epilepsy (JME) presents in adolescence with myoclonic jerks and generalized convulsions. Although most cases of JME are readily controlled with medication, it is usually a condition that will persist well into adulthood.[22]

Logically, the childhood epilepsies that predictably will remit in adolescence will not require transitional care or planning. However, in the case of the refractory epilepsies, such as LGS, it may be prudent to transition care to an "adult" epileptologist or comprehensive epilepsy center sooner rather than later. The complexities of multiple drug regimens with numerous potential drug interactions make this all the more imper-ative. Similarly, the adolescent with new onset primary generalized epilepsy should be promptly referred to an epileptologist who can provide lifelong care and monitor the patient for potential medication side effects, as well as drug teratogenicities. Patients with MTS and other surgically remediable epilepsies should be referred to a compre-hensive epilepsy center for specialized imaging and video-EEG monitoring in anticipa-tion of an operative intervention. Epileptologists can also offer patients with refractory epilepsy nonpharmacologic options, such as vagal nerve stimulation, deep brain stim-ulation, and the ketogenic diet.

HEADACHES

Migraine is not uncommon among children. It is prevalent in 7.7% of adolescents with a significant female predominance.[23] Migraine precursors, such as cyclic vomiting syndrome, benign paroxysmal vertigo, and paroxysmal torticollis, may be early childhood presentations. Common migraine with diffuse or bifrontal localization, nausea, and vomiting is more typical than classical adult hemicrania. Tension headaches are also seen in children and are often an indicator of underlying anxiety or school stress. These headaches typically occur daily in the afternoon or evening hours. Chronic daily headaches typically occur in adolescent women and may have both tension and migrainous features.

Most pediatric and adolescent headaches are managed by PCPs with counseling, diet changes, and lifestyle modification. Refractory chronic migraine in children presents diagnostic and therapeutic challenges and may require pediatric neurologic consultations. Preventative medications, such as topiramate or amitriptyline, may be prescribed, although there are conflicting data on their efficacy in adolescence.[24] Gabapentin and valproic acid are other preventative options. Some triptans have shown efficacy in aborting pediatric migraine, particularly nasal sumatriptan and oral rizatriptan.[25]

Pediatric and adolescent migraines are often outgrown. However, for those adolescents with refractory migraine, prompt referral and transition of care to a headache medicine specialist may offer an earlier opportunity to use newer therapies, including botulinum toxin and monoclonal antibodies against calcitonin gene related peptide.[26] These innovative treatments are not yet Food and Drug Administration (FDA) approved for patients less than age 18, and it is therefore difficult to obtain insurance preauthorization. However, these drugs are more likely to be compassionately approved if prescribed by a headache specialist who has systematically tried all other available options.

ATTENTION-DEFICIT HYPERACTIVITY DISORDER

Attention-deficit/hyperactivity disorder (ADHD) is typically diagnosed in childhood, often coinciding with entry in the school system. In 2016, the Center for Disease Control and Prevention reported that 8.4% of children ages 2 to 17 had a current diagnosis of ADHD and that two-thirds of them were receiving medications.[27] The core symptoms of ADHD are hyperactivity, impulsivity, distractibility, and lack of concentration. *Diagnostic and Statistical Manual of Mental Disorders* (Fifth Edition) (*DSM-5*) recognizes 3 ADHD subtypes: hyperactive-impulsive, inattentive, and combined.[28] Comorbidities of ADHD include oppositional defiant disorder, autism spectrum disorder (ASD), learning disabilities, tic disorders, Tourette syndrome, anxiety, and depression. Medications for pediatric ADHD are primarily prescribed by PCPs. However, pediatric neurologists and child psychiatrists are often consulted, particularly when comorbidities are suspected.

Pharmacologic management of ADHD typically consists of stimulant medications, such as methylphenidate or mixed amphetamine salts.[29] These medications are FDA approved for use in children ages 6 and older. However, they are Schedule II controlled substances, which are highly regulated. Prescriptions must be signed originals or securely e-mailed to pharmacies, and they are limited to a 1-month supply. Stimulant medications are available in intermediate and extended-release formulations. For younger children, there are now liquid preparations, as well as a methylphenidate skin patch. Common side effects include loss of appetite, poor weight gain, and insomnia. These side effects are usually transient and manageable. Mild tachycardia and blood pressure increases are not uncommon. On occasion, tics may develop or exacerbate, and very rarely hallucinations and psychotic reactions have occurred.

Although formerly thought to be a disorder unique to childhood, ADHD persists into adolescence and adulthood.[30] As such, it is really a lifelong disorder. However, transition of adolescent patients with ADHD to adult providers is difficult. Most internists and adult neurologists lack training, expertise, and comfort with ADHD management. Therefore, many pediatric neurologists continue to manage ADHD well into adulthood. This continuity of care can be safely accomplished if the provider is cognizant of adult psychiatric comorbidities, including anxiety, depression, and substance abuse, as well as systemic disorders, such as hypertension and cardiovascular diseases.

AUTISM SPECTRUM DISORDERS

ASD usually present by age 2 and are characterized by delays in speech and language development, cognition, and socialization. Echolalic speech is common as are stereotypic mannerisms, such as hand flapping, rocking, and spinning. Social withdrawal and poor eye contact are also typical.[31] Children with higher functioning ASD are reclassified under *DSM-5* as social communication disorder or semantic pragmatic disorder. They are socially maladroit and tend to self-isolate with a narrow range of interests.

The prevalence of ASD has been continuously increasing over the past 2 decades and as of 2016 is estimated to be 1 in 54.[32] The reasons for this increase are unclear, but may reflect increasing awareness, as well as a broadening of the diagnostic criteria. The causes of ASD are usually undetermined, but genetic factors are undoubtedly implicated. ASD is a recognized comorbidity of numerous genetic disorders, including tuberous sclerosis, and Fragile X, Down, Rett, and Angelman syndromes.

Maladaptive behaviors are commonly seen in ASD and create difficult therapeutic challenges. Anxiety, depression, mood swings, agitation, aggression, and self-injurious behaviors begin in childhood and often exacerbate in adolescence. Applied behavioral analysis (ABA) is a highly specialized form of individualized therapy with demonstrated efficacy in diminishing these behaviors in ASD.[33] However, ABA is necessarily intensive and long term, requiring a recommended 25 to 40 hours per week for at least a year.[34] As such, it is an expensive treatment, and insurance reimbursement is often denied.

As an alternative or adjunct to therapy, pediatric neurologists are often requested to provide pharmacologic management for children with ASD. An estimated 10% to 30% of autistic children have comorbid epilepsy and will require anticonvulsant medications.[35] Some seizure drugs, such as levetiracetam and barbiturates, can exacerbate irritability. However, others, such as carbamazepine, oxcarbazepine, and lamotrigine, have a role as mood stabilizers.[36] The stimulant drugs discussed above may have a beneficial effect for autistic children with comorbid ADHD.[37] The atypical antipsychotics risperidone and aripiprazole have FDA approval for treating irritability and aggressive behaviors.[38] Selective serotonin reuptake inhibitors may have beneficial effects on anxiety and mood as well. Naltrexone has shown some benefit in modulating self-injurious behaviors.[39]

Medication management of children with ASD can be extraordinarily challenging because of polypharmacy with the potential for numerous side effects and drug interactions. Transitioning autistic adolescents to adult providers at age 18 may therefore be particularly difficult because of the many nuances of the patient's treatment plan. Parents of children with developmental disabilities who turn 18 are also confronted with obtaining court-appointed guardianship and finding suitable adult educational and rehabilitation services. Autistic individuals are inherently resistant to change so that these multiple changes may be overwhelming. Moreover, there is a lack of adult neurologists with the necessary training and motivation to take on the multifaceted care of this medically and psychiatrically complex population. In reality, it is not uncommon for transition of care to be indefinitely delayed in adults with autism. Perhaps this is not unreasonable because the ASD can be conceptualized as a developmental delay, which essentially results in a prolonged persistence of childhood.

CEREBROVASCULAR DISEASE

Pediatric stroke is an uncommon but not rare disease. In fact, approximately 15% of all ischemic strokes occur in adolescents and young adults.[40] The causes of stroke in the young are varied.[41] Although classical vascular risk factors often play an etiologic role even in young persons, nonatherosclerotic causes are far more typical in this population. Because of the lesser frequency of stroke in this population and atypical presentations, awareness of stroke onset is low.[42] Furthermore, because stroke is less frequent and the causes are more heterogeneous, there is a lesser degree of robust evidence regarding the acute, and long-term, management of stroke in children and young adults.[43] Stroke mortality among children and young adults is low. In 1 series, most strokes in children and young adults were not severe (median NIHSS 56), and the initial stroke severity was the most important predictor of good outcome.[44]

Long-term, pediatric stroke patients will live longer with their disabilities, and the impact of incident stroke on stroke recurrence, other vascular events, poststroke complications (ie, poststroke seizures), cognitive and psychological issues, quality-of-life issues, and financial burdens are long-term issues that have been inadequately addressed.[40] Pediatric stroke is a nascent subspecialty of pediatric neurology.[45] As such, expertise in acute treatment of pediatric stroke and the long-term implications of these strokes are less studied than in adults. These limitations also affect the transitions when pediatric stroke patients enter adulthood.

For pediatric stroke patients, data about transitions of care are limited. For patients at risk of stroke, data about transitions are most robust for congenital heart disease and sickle cell disease (SCD). A systematic review of care transitions for these heart disease patients noted that many patients, leaving pediatric congenital heart disease clinics, were lost to follow-up or experienced long gaps in care.[46] Patients were more likely to have a successful transition with pediatric referral to an adult congenital heart clinic. Patients were also more likely to successfully transition their care if they had worse overall health status, were not dependent on parents for follow-up care, and had personal recognition of a possible benefit of specialized adult care.

For SCD patients (with or without stroke), transitions to adult care have been studied by several investigators. Patients in 1 series transitioning to adult care were less likely to receive stroke preventive treatments for SCD, such as transfusions or hydroxyurea. In addition, these patients were less likely to receive iron chelation therapies. They also had more SCD-related complications than pediatric patients and had higher health care costs.[47] Debaun and Telfair[48] noted that the high proportion of clinical stroke or silent cerebral infarcts, estimated around 30% of SCD patients, is a factor affecting cognition and subsequent likelihood of follow-up. Additional significant factors included a higher proportion of SCD patients with limited insurance and high rates of comorbid conditions. Andemariam and colleagues[49] also described the difficulty of transitions to adult SCD care. In their study, insurance barriers were a lesser issue than access to care based on location of adult SCD centers. Older age at first modified combined transition clinic visit was a significant risk factor for lack of transition. Similar to patients with congenital heart disease, worse SCD severity was associated with a greater likelihood for successful transition to an adult center. Stollon and colleagues[50] interviewed 13 SCD experts and reported that successful transitions to adult SCD care were mediated by patients' stronger relationships with parents and providers, and higher patient levels of developmental maturity. Significantly, these experts noted that neurocognitive deficits related to strokes were one of the barriers to successful transitions in care. Other negative factors included developmental maturity problems, sociodemographic issues, and negative ED experiences.

HYDROCEPHALUS

Brain tumors, shunted hydrocephalus, and myelomeningocele (MMC) are three of the most common examples of pediatric neurosurgical patients with long-term postoperative sequelae that persist into adulthood.[51,52] In regard to hydrocephalus, the clinical spectrum of hydrocephalus in adults includes those with acquired hydrocephalus owing to other risk factors (ie, trauma or hemorrhage) and idiopathic causes, such as normal pressure hydrocephalus. Hydrocephalus in the pediatric population leading to transitions of care in adulthood includes those with unrecognized congenital problems that were not treated before age 18 and so-called transition hydrocephalus representing those patients treated before age 18.[53,54] The Adult Hydrocephalus Clinical Research Network series reported that 43% of the patients in their series had childhood onset of symptoms.[55] Impairments in all groups were related to the underlying cause of neurologic injury; those with unrecognized congenital hydrocephalus had the least impairment.

The Hydrocephalus Association reported that approximately 5000 to 6000 US adolescents and young adults transition from the pediatric to adult health care systems Long-term outcome of adult patients with shunted pediatric hydrocephalus is poor, however.[55] The poor outcome can be partly related to available technologies at the time of initial shunting. Gmeiner and colleagues[56] reported their series of patients whose initial shunt was placed in the years1982 to 1992. Many of these patients had underlying neurologic comorbidities in addition to hydrocephalus that contributed to poor cognitive status. In this series, verbal intelligence of 31 patients (47.7%) was within the normal range, but 19 patient (29.2%) had severe verbal deficits. Factors in adult patients who had a pediatric shunt that led to worse outcome included shunt infections ($P = .0025$), epilepsy ($P < .0001$), and the number of shunt operations ($P = .0082$). Most patients with average or above average verbal intelligence had deficits in detailed neuropsychological testing. Another study found that patients requiring a shunt revision in childhood, patients with shunt infection, and patients with proximal shunt complications were more likely to have worse outcome and greater need for adult revisions.[53]

Unfortunately, coordination of care for these patients is common in the pediatric world, but multidisciplinary care is less organized in the adult population.[52,56,57] The Hydrocephalus Association consensus statement on transition of care notes that pediatric and adult neurologists and neurosurgeons must develop an organized system for transition of care in this vulnerable population[55]

MYELOMENINGOCELE

MMC is the most common form of spina bifida.[58] Associated hydrocephalus is a common problem among this population. Tethered cords with associated nonambulatory status are another serious problem. With the addition of folic acid into grain products, the United States has had a 31% decrease in the frequency of spina bifida, from 5.04 cases per 10,000 births to 3.49 per 10,000 births.[59] Still, MMC remains a significant pediatric neurology/neurosurgery issue, and with advances in neonatal and pediatric neurosurgery, more of these patients are living to adulthood. As these children transition to adulthood, support services to provide independent functional status are critically lacking in scope and availability. In addition to the hydrocephalus problems discussed above, adult MMC patients have the added ongoing problems of mobility, and other problems associated with spinal dysfunction (ie, mobility and urologic issues). Maintaining independence and functionality in activities of daily living is an important part of transitioning MMC patients to adulthood.[60] Spina bifida care is frequently delivered through multidisciplinary clinics, encompassing disciplines such as neurosurgery physical medicine and other rehabilitation services, orthopedic surgery, urology, and social work. In a pediatric neurosurgery clinic, one-third of these clinics saw both pediatric and adult patients, one-third provided a formal transition program to adult care, and one-third had no organized transition program.[61] Unfortunately the needs of spina bifida/MMC patients are incompletely addressed in terms of transition of the patients in adolescence and adulthood particularly as the needs relate to transition of health insurance coverage, adult provider care, and, of particular note, sexuality and reproductive issues.[62]

BRAIN TUMORS

Central nervous system tumors are the most common form of nonhematologic cancer in children, and these tumors the leading cause of solid tumor pediatric cancer death in the United States.[51,63] The frequency of pediatric brain tumors is increasing, but survival of these patients is also increasing. Pediatric brain tumor types are more diverse in the pediatric population with astrocytoma comprising 53% of pediatric brain tumors; the most common type is pilocytic astrocytoma (17.6% of all tumors). As more patients survive to adulthood, the challenges in the care of these patients include managing the complications that arise as sequelae of treatment, including cognitive dysfunction and other developmental delay and the development of secondary malignancies.

The types of long-term sequelae of pediatric brain tumors will depend on the tumor type, tumor location, and type and location of craniospinal radiation or chemotherapy.[64,65] Long-term problems may include hydrocephalus, necessitating ventriculoperitoneal shunt, speech/language problems, vision or visual-motor impairments, and problems with attention or cognition.[65] Children with midline tumors in particular may also have endocrinopathies, obesity, arrested physical development, hypersomnia, and autonomic dysfunction. Additional complications of radiotherapy include cognitive dysfunction and arrested or delayed mental development. Radiation therapy can also cause accelerated cerebrovascular disease related to radiation-induced vasculopathy as well as radiation-induced secondary brain malignancies.

Long-term surveillance imaging may only be indicated in select patients, but knowledge of the patient's clinical status at the time of transition of care to adult providers is critical, as clinicians should have a lower threshold for neuroimaging with any new or worsening symptoms. Regular imaging of the brain is *not* indicated in the absence of clinical change unless the survivor has an inherited predisposition to cancer or vasculopathy.

The provision of care for patients as they transition to adulthood necessitates a detailed "handoff" to adult providers of the patient's history, treatment course, and current clinical status.[51] Ideally, these patients would transition to an adult multidisciplinary neurooncology program, but this option, regretfully, is often not available. These patients need annual neurologic surveillance and continued treatment of medical and psychiatric comorbidities. As noted, coordinated multidisciplinary care of adult patients with a history of childhood brain tumor survivors, including social services, vocational supports, and cognitive rehabilitation, can contribute to better long-term function.[65] Coordination of care with additional specialists for problems with hearing, vision, endocrine, sleep, and mental health is indicated for these patients with a high risk for ongoing and new medical, neurologic, cognitive, and psychological problems.

NEUROMUSCULAR DISORDERS

Pediatric onset neuromuscular disorders consist of an array of diseases of anterior horn cells, peripheral nerves, the myoneural junction, and muscle. Examples include relatively rare conditions, such as spinal muscular atrophies (SMA), hereditary neuropathies, such as Charcot-Marie-Tooth and Duchenne muscular dystrophy (DMD). Historically, such disorders have been challenging to diagnose and essentially untreatable. However, in recent years, remarkable therapeutic innovations have been developed, including antisense oligonucleotides and gene replacement therapy for SMA and exon skipping therapy for DMD.[66–68] Earlier diagnosis through neonatal screening offers further hope for improved outcomes.

The necessity for multidisciplinary care for neuromuscular disorders has led to the development of a national network of regional clinics under the auspices of the Muscular Dystrophy Association. These clinics provide a broad range of clinical specialties and support services for patients across the lifespan. This disease-based care model could serve as a prototype, which demonstrates smoother and more collaborative transition of care from pediatric to adult providers.

SUMMARY

The concept of transition of care from pediatric to adult providers was introduced more than 2 decades ago and is still an idea in evolution. The goals of transition should be improvement of quality of care, increased patient and family satisfaction, and measurable meaningful outcomes. Currently, outcomes and risk benefit ratios appear to be variable and difficult to quantify. Transition results in a handoff of care, and handoffs have been shown to have intrinsic risks. Inaccurate or incomplete information, lack of patient and/or provider readiness, and failure of providers to accept patient care responsibility continue to be major concerns.

It is not entirely clear why the patient's age should be a major determinant of transition. Physiologic and metabolic pathways are generally fully mature by adolescence, and therefore, pharmacologic management of young adults should be well within the scope and training of both pediatric and adult health care providers. Conversely, it is increasingly clear that brain maturation is a slower process, which can extend behavioral adolescence well into the third decade of life.

A more cogent approach to the transition process would be to consider it from the standpoint of disease states. In the case of neurologic disorders, the conditions discussed herein: epilepsy, migraine, ADHD, autism, pediatric cerebrovascular diseases, hydrocephalus, myelomeningocoele, pediatric brain tumors, and pediatric neuromuscular disorders, begin in childhood and persist into adulthood. The chronicity of these neurologic conditions demands knowledgeable providers who are capable of providing uninterrupted care across the lifespan. As discussed, patients with ADHD and ASD may therefore be better served by pediatric neurologists who are willing to continue their care into adulthood. Conversely, perhaps those children with adolescent-onset epilepsy and chronic migraine should be considered for earlier transition to adult providers. For other disorders, more innovative models with shared patient care responsibilities and cross coverage between pediatric and adult subspecialists may offer the option of a more gradual transition process with less "separation anxiety" for patients, parents, and providers. The new age of telehealth will also usher in new possibilities for patient access and open up a myriad of models for joint patient management, continuity of care, and, it is hoped, increased patient satisfaction.

CLINICS CARE POINTS

- Transitions of health care are a necessary reality of patient management in all modern medical settings.
- Effective transitions require accurate and efficient "handoffs" between responsible senders and receivers of health care information.
- Transition of care from pediatric to adult providers during adolescence is a desirable outcome which has been advocated by numerous medical societies and organizations.
- However, unanticipated pitfalls may preclude effective transitions for patients with chronic neurological disorders with onset in childhood, suggesting the need for alternative care models.

REFERENCES

1. Dawda P, Russell K. Transitions of care: technical series on safer primary care. Geneva (Switzerland): World Health Organization; 2016. License CCBY-NC-SA 3.0 IGO.
2. Labson M. Adapting the joint commission's seven foundations of safe and effective transitions of care to home. Home Healthc Now 2015;33(3):142–6.
3. Joint Commission Resources: Transitions of Care: The Need For a More Effective Approach to Continuing Patient Care (8), (2012).
4. The Joint Commission. Hot Topics in Health Care, Issue #2: Transitions of Care: The need For Collaboration across entire care continuum. February, 2013.
5. The Joint Commission. Quick Safety, Issue 26; Transitions of Care: Managing Medications. August, 2016.
6. The Joint Commission. Sentinel Event Alert. Issue 58, September 12, 2017.
7. Benjamin MF, Hargrave S, Klaus N. Using the targeted solutions tool to improve emergency department handoffs in a community hospital. Jt Comm J Qual Patient Saf 2016;42(3):107–14.
8. Starmer AJ, Spector ND, Srivastava R, et al. Changes in medical errors after implementation of a handoff program. N Engl J Med 2014;371:1803–12.
9. Cornish PL, Knowles SR, Marchesano R, et al. Unintended medication discrepancies at the time of hospital admission. Arch Intern Med 2005;165(4):424–9.
10. Arora VM, Kao J, Lovinger D, et al. Medication discrepancies in resident sign-outs and their potential to harm. J Gen Intern Med 2007;22(12):1751–5.
11. Bonafide CP, Miller JM, Localio AR, et al. Association between mobile telephone interruption and medication administration errors in a pediatric intensive care unit. JAMA Pediatr 2020;174(2):162–9.
12. Tapia NM, Fallon SC, Brandt ML, et al. Assessment and standardization of resident handoff practices: PACJ project. Surg Res 2013;184(1):71–7.
13. American Academy of Pediatrics (AAP), American Academy of Family Physicians (AAFP) and American Society of Internal Medicine (ASIM). A consensus statement on health care transitions for young adults with special health care needs. Pediatrics 2002;110(6, pt.2):1304–6.
14. American Academy of Pediatrics (AAP), American Academy of Family Physicians (AAFP), American College of Physicians (ACP); Transitions Clinical Report Authoring Group. Supporting the health care transition from adolescence to adulthood in the medical home. Pediatrics 2011;128(1):182–200.

15. American Academy of Pediatrics (AAP), American Academy of Family Physicians (AAFP), American College of Physicians (ACP); Transitions Clinical Report Authoring Group. Supporting the health care transition from adolescence to adulthood in the medical home. Pediatrics 2018;142(5):2018–587.

16. Okumura MJ, Kerr EA, Cabana MD, et al. Physician views on barriers to primary care for young adults with childhood onset chronic disease. Pediatrics 2010; 125(4):745–e754.

17. Brown LW, Camfield P, Capers M, et al. The neurologist's role in supporting transition to adult health care. Neurology 2016;87:1–6.

18. White PH, Cooley WC. www.GotTransition.org, Transition Clinical Authoring Group, American Academy of Pediatrics, American Academy of Family Physicians, American College of Physicians, September, 2020.

19. Faulkner LR, Juul D, Aminoff MJ, et al. Trends in American Board of Psychiatry and Neurology specialties and neurologic subspecialties. Neurology 2010; 75(12):1110–7.

20. Tian N, Boring M, Kobau R, et al. Active epilepsy and seizure control in adults-United States, 2013 and 2015. MMWR 2018;67(15):437–42.

21. Shinnar S, Bello JA, Chan S, et al. MRI abnormalities following febrile status epilepticus in children. The FEBSTAT study. Neurology 2012;79(9):871–7.

22. Baykan B, Martinez-Juarez I, Altindag E. Lifetime prognosis of juvenile myoclonic epilepsy. Epilepsy Behav 2013;28:S18–24.

23. Abu-Arafeh I, Razak S, Sivaraman B, et al. Prevalence of headache and migraine in children and adolescents: a systematic review of population-based studies. Dev Med Child Neurol 2010;52(12):1088–97.

24. Powers SW, Coffey CS, Chamberlin LA, et al, CHAMP Investigators. Trial of amitriptyline, topiramate, and placebo for pediatric migraine. N Engl J Med 2017;376:115–24 [Abstract].

25. Eiland LS, Hunt MO. The use of triptans for pediatric migraines. Pediatr Drugs 2010;12(6):379–89.

26. Schreiber AM. Erenumab (Aimovig) for migraine prophylaxis in adults. Am Fam Physician 2019;99(12):781–2.

27. Danielson ML, Bitsko RH, Ghandour RM, et al. Prevalence of parent-reported ADHD diagnosis and associated treatment among U.S. children and adolescents, 2016. J Clin Child Adolesc Psychol 2018;47(2):199–212.

28. Shaffer D, Castellanos FX. ADHD and Disruptive Behavior Disorders. In: Diagnostic and Statistical Manuel of Mental Disorders. 5th edition. Arlington, VA: American Psychiatric Association; 2013.

29. Froehlich TE, Delgado SV, Anixt JS. Expanding medication options for pediatric ADHD. Curr Psychiatry 2013;12(12):20–9.

30. Kolar D, Keller A, Golfinopoulos M, et al. Treatment of adults with attention-deficit/hyperactivity disorder. Neuropsychiatr Dis Treat 2008;4(2):389–403.

31. Lord C, Risi S, Lambrecht L, et al. The autism diagnostic observation schedule –generic: a standard measure of the social and communication deficits associated with the spectrum of autism. J Autism Dev Disord 2000;30:205–23.

32. Maenner MJ, Shaw KA, Baio J, et al. Prevalence of autism spectrum disorder among children aged 8 years-autism and developmental disabilities monitoring network, 11 sites, United States, 2016. MMWR 2020;69(4):1–12.

33. Foxx RM. Applied behavioral analysis treatment of autism: the state of the art. Child Adolesc Psychiatr Clin N Am 2008;17(4):821–34.

34. Fortunato JA, Sigafoos J, Morsillo-Searls LM. A communication plan for autism and its applied behavioral analysis treatment: a framing strategy. Child Youth Care Forum 2007;36:87–97.
35. Gabis L, Pomeroy J, Andriola MR. Autism and epilepsy: cause, consequence, co-morbidity or coincidence. Epilepsy Behav 2005;7:652–6.
36. Canitano R. Mood stabilizers in children and adolescents with autism spectrum disorders. Clin Neuropharmacol 2015;38(5):177–82.
37. Nickels KC, Katusic SK, Colligan RC, et al. Stimulant medication treatment of target behaviors in children with autism: a population-based study. J Dev Behav Pediatr 2008;9(2):75–81.
38. Blankenship K, Erickson CA, Stigler KA, et al. Aripiprazole for irritability associated with autistic disorder in children and adolescents, aged 6-17 years. Ped Health 2010;4(4):375–81.
39. Symons FJ, Thompson A, Rodriguez MC. Self-injurious behavior and the efficacy of naltrexone treatment: a quantitative synthesis. Ment Retard Dev Disabil Res Rev 2004;10(3):193–200.
40. Singhal AB, Biller J, Elkind MS, et al. Recognition and management of stroke in young adults and adolescents. Neurology 2013;81(12):1089–97.
41. Cardenas JF, Jong M, Rho JM. Pediatric stroke. Childs Nerv Syst 2011;27(9): 1375–90.
42. Rivkin MJ, Bernard TJ, Dowling MM, et al. Guidelines for urgent management of stroke in children. Pediatr Neurol 2016;56:8–17.
43. Buckowski A, Rose E. Pediatric stroke: diagnosis and management in the emergency department. Pediatr Emerg Med Pract 2019;16(11):1–20.
44. Bigi S, Fischer U, Wehrli E, et al. Acute ischemic stroke in children versus young adults. Ann Neurol 2011;70(2):245–54.
45. Fullerton HJ, GanesanV, Jordan LC, et al. Building a career as a pediatric stroke neurologist. Stroke 2019;50:e287–9.
46. Heery E, Sheehan AM, Although AE, et al. Experiences and outcomes of transition from pediatric to adult health care services for young people with congenital heart disease: a systematic review. Congenit Heart Dis 2015;10:413–27.
47. Blinder MA, Vekeman F, Sasane M, et al. Age-related treatment patterns in sickle cell disease patients and the associated sickle cell complications and healthcare costs. Pediatr Blood Cancer 2013;60(5):828–35.
48. Debaun MR, Telfair J. Transition and sickle cell disease. Pediatrics 2012;130(5): 926–35.
49. Andemariam B, Owarish-Gross J, Grady J, et al. Identification of risk factors for an unsuccessful transition from pediatric to adult sickle cell disease care. Pediatr Blood Cancer 2014;61(4):697–701.
50. Stollon NB, Pain CW, Lucas MS, et al. Transitioning adolescents and young adults with sickle cell disease from pediatric to adult health care: provider perspectives multicenter study. J Pediatr Hematol Oncol 2015;37(8):577–83.
51. Rothstein DH, Li V. Transitional care in pediatric neurosurgical patients. Semin Pediatr Surg 2015;24(2):79–82.
52. Vinchon M, Baroncini M, Delestret I. Adult outcome of pediatric hydrocephalus. Childs Nerv Syst 2012;28(6):847–54.
53. Reddy GK, Bollam P, Caldito G, et al. Ventriculoperitoneal shunt surgery outcome in adult transition patients with pediatric-onset hydrocephalus. Neurosurgery 2012;70(2):380–8.
54. Williams MA, Nagel SJ, Luciano MG, et al. The clinical spectrum of hydrocephalus in adults: report of the first 517 patients of the adult hydrocephalus clinical

research network registry. J Neurosurg 2019;1–12. https://doi.org/10.3171/2019. 2.JNS183538.

55. Williams MA, van der Willigen T, White PH, et al. Improving health care transition and longitudinal care for adolescents and young adults with hydrocephalus: report from the hydrocephalus association transition summit. J Neurosurg 2018;1–9. https://doi.org/10.3171/2018.6.JNS188.

56. Gmeiner M, Wagner H, Schlögl C, et al. Adult outcome in shunted pediatric hydrocephalus: long-term functional, social, and neurocognitive results. World Neurosurg 2019;132:e314–23.

57. Rekate HL. The pediatric neurosurgical patient: the challenge of growing up Semin Pediatr Rey-Casserly C, Diver T. Late effects of pediatric brain tumors. Curr Opin Pediatr 2019;31(6):789–96.

58. Spoor JKH, Gadjradj PS, Eggink AJ. Contemporary management and outcome of myelomeningocele: the Rotterdam experience. Neurosurg Focus 2019;47(4):E3.

59. Le JT, Mukherjee S. Transition to adult care for patients with spina bifida. Phys Med Rehabil Clin N Am 2015;26(1):29–38.

60. Patel SK, Staarmann B, Heilman A, et al. Growing up with spina bifida: bridging the gaps in the transition of care from childhood to adulthood. Neurosurg Focus 2019;47(4):E16.

61. Alford EN, Hopson BD, Safyanov F, et al. Care management and contemporary challenges in spina bifida: a practice preference survey of the American Society of Pediatric Neurosurgeons. J Neurosurg Pediatr 2019;1–10. https://doi.org/10.3171/2019.5.PEDS18738.

62. Kelly MS, Thibadeau J, Struwe S. Evaluation of spina bifida transitional care practices in the United States. J Pediatr Rehabil Med 2017;10(3–4):275–81.

63. Available at: https://akidsbraintumorcure.org/childhood-brain-tumors/childrens-brain-tumor-facts/. Accessed June 15, 2015.

64. Rey-Casserly C, Diver T. Late effects of pediatric brain tumors. Curr Opin Pediatr 2019;31(6):789–96.

65. Janss AJ, Mazewski C, Patterson B. Guidelines for treatment and monitoring of adult survivors of pediatric brain tumors. Curr Treat Options Oncol 2019;20(1):10.

66. Schorling DC, Pechmann A, Kirschner J. Advances in treatment of spinal muscular atrophy-new phenotypes, new challenges, new implications for care. J Neuromuscul Dis 2020;7(1):1–13.

67. Kole R, Krieg AM. Exon skipping therapy for Duchenne muscular dystrophy. Adv Drug Deliv Rev 2015;87:104–7.

68. Baker M, Griggs R, Byrne B, et al. Maximizing the benefit of life-saving treatments for Pompe disease, spinal muscular atrophy, and Duchenne muscular dystrophy through newborn screening: essential steps. JAMA Neurol 2019. https://doi.org/10.1001/jamaneurol.2019.1206.

Moving?

Make sure your subscription moves with you!

To notify us of your new address, find your **Clinics Account Number** (located on your mailing label above your name), and contact customer service at:

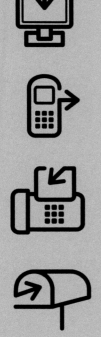

Email: journalscustomerservice-usa@elsevier.com

800-654-2452 (subscribers in the U.S. & Canada)
314-447-8871 (subscribers outside of the U.S. & Canada)

Fax number: 314-447-8029

Elsevier Health Sciences Division
Subscription Customer Service
3251 Riverport Lane
Maryland Heights, MO 63043